REFERENCE EDITION

ESAP™ 2024

Endocrine Society's Endocrine Self-Assessment Program Questions, Answers, and Discussions

Thomas J. Weber, MD, Program Co-Chair
Professor of Medicine
Division of Endocrinology, Metabolism, and Nutrition
Duke University Medical Center

Deepika Reddy, MD, Program Co-Chair
Assistant Professor
Division of Diabetes, Endocrinology, and Metabolism
University of Utah Healthcare

Danit Ariel, MD, MS
Associate Professor
Division of Endocrinology, Gerontology, and Metabolism
Stanford University

Gregory Clines, MD, PhD
Associate Professor of Internal Medicine
Metabolism, Endocrinology, and Diabetes Division
University of Michigan

Nazanene H. Esfandiari, MD
Professor of Medicine
Metabolism, Endocrinology, and Diabetes Division
University of Michigan

Mathis Grossmann, MD, PhD
Professor of Medicine
University of Melbourne
Austin Health

Mark Gurnell, MBBS, MA (Med Ed), PhD
Professor of Clinical Endocrinology & Clinical SubDean
Wellcome Trust-MRC Institute of Metabolic Science & School of Clinical Medicine
University of Cambridge

Erik Imel, MD
Professor of Medicine and Pediatrics
Indiana University School of Medicine

Adriana G. Ioachimescu, MD, PhD
Professor of Medicine
Endocrinology and Molecular Medicine Division
Medical College of Wisconsin

Sarah E. Mayson, MD
Associate Professor of Medicine
Director of the Endocrinology Fellowship Program
Division of Endocrinology, Metabolism, and Diabetes
University of Colorado School of Medicine

Kevin M. Pantalone, DO
Professor of Medicine
Director of Diabetes Initiatives
Department of Endocrinology
Cleveland Clinic

Meera Shah, MB ChB
Assistant Professor of Medicine
Mayo Clinic College of Medicine
Consultant, Division of Endocrinology
Mayo Clinic – Rochester

Anu Sharma, MBBS
Assistant Professor of Medicine
Division of Endocrinology, Diabetes, and Metabolism
University of Florida

Aniket R. Sidhaye, MD
Associate Professor of Clinical Medicine
Program Director, Adult Endocrinology Fellowship
Johns Hopkins University School of Medicine

Vinaya Simha, MBBS, MD
Associate Professor of Medicine
Mayo Clinic College of Medicine
Mayo Clinic – Rochester

Elias Spanakis, MD
Associate Professor of Medicine
University of Maryland School of Medicine

Adina F. Turcu, MD, MS
Associate Professor of Internal Medicine
Metabolism, Endocrinology, and Diabetes Division
University of Michigan

Abbie L. Young, MS, CGC, ELS(D)
Medical Editor

Endocrine Society
2055 L Street NW, Suite 600, Washington, DC 20036
1-888-ENDOCRINE • www.endocrine.org

ENDOCRINE SOCIETY
Hormone Science to Health

ENDOCRINE SOCIETY
Hormone Science to Health

The Endocrine Society is the world's largest, oldest, and most active organization working to advance the clinical practice of endocrinology and hormone research. Founded in 1916, the Society now has more than 18,000 global members across a range of disciplines. The Society has earned an international reputation for excellence in the quality of its peer-reviewed journals, educational resources, meetings, and programs that improve public health through the practice and science of endocrinology.

For between-edition updates, visit us at:
endocrine.org/education-and-training/book-updates

Other publications:
endocrine.org/publications

The statements and opinions expressed in this publication are those of the individual authors and do not necessarily reflect the views of the Endocrine Society. The Endocrine Society is not responsible or liable in any way for the currency of the information, for any errors, omissions, or inaccuracies, or for any consequences arising therefrom. With respect to any drugs mentioned, the reader is advised to refer to the appropriate medical literature and the product information currently provided by the manufacturer to verify appropriate dosage, method and duration of administration, and other relevant information. In all instances, it is the responsibility of the treating physician or other health care professional, relying on independent experience and expertise, as well as knowledge of the patient, to determine the best treatment for the patient.

ISBN: 978-1-936704-38-5

Library of Congress Control Number: 2023952021

On the Cover: 3D rendering of DNA structure, abstract background.

OVERVIEW

The Endocrine Self-Assessment Program (ESAP™) is a self-study curriculum aimed at physicians wanting a self-assessment and a broad review of endocrinology. The ESAP Reference Edition consists of 120 brand-new multiple-choice questions in all areas of endocrinology, diabetes, and metabolism. There is extensive discussion of each correct answer, a comprehensive syllabus, and references. ESAP is updated annually with new questions.

The ESAP reference book is intended primarily for consultation and self-assessment of knowledge relating to endocrinology. As a reference book, educational credits are not available upon completion of the multiple-choice questions included. For information on educational products that include educational credit, please visit endocrine.org/store.

LEARNING OBJECTIVES

ESAP 2024 will allow learners to assess their knowledge of all aspects of endocrinology, diabetes, and metabolism.

Completion of this educational activity enables learners to accomplish key objectives:

- Recognize clinical manifestations of endocrine and metabolic disorders and select among current options for diagnosis, management, and therapy.
- Identify risk factors for endocrine and metabolic disorders and develop strategies for prevention.
- Evaluate endocrine and metabolic manifestations of systemic disorders.
- Use existing resources pertaining to clinical guidelines and treatment recommendations for endocrine and related metabolic disorders to guide diagnosis and treatment.

TARGET AUDIENCE

ESAP is a self-study curriculum aimed at physicians seeking initial certification or recertification in endocrinology, program directors interested in a testing and training instrument, and clinicians simply wanting a self-assessment and broad review of endocrinology.

STATEMENT OF INDEPENDENCE

The Endocrine Society has a policy of ensuring that the content and quality of this educational activity are balanced, independent, objective, and scientifically rigorous. The scientific content of this activity was developed under the supervision of the Endocrine Society's ESAP Faculty Working Group.

DISCLOSURE POLICY

The faculty, committee members, and staff who are in position to control the content of this activity are required to disclose to the Endocrine Society and to learners any relevant financial relationship(s) of the individual or spouse/partner that have occurred within the last 12 months with any commercial interest(s) whose products or services are related to the content. Financial relationships are defined by remuneration in any amount from the commercial interest(s) in the form of grants; research support; consulting fees; salary; ownership interest (eg, stocks, stock options, or ownership interest excluding diversified mutual funds); honoraria or other payments for participation in speakers' bureaus, advisory boards, or boards of directors; or other financial benefits. The intent of this disclosure is not to prevent planners with relevant financial relationships from planning or delivering content, but rather to provide learners with information that allows them to make their own judgments of whether these financial relationships may have influenced the educational activity with regard to exposition or conclusion. The Endocrine Society has reviewed all disclosures and resolved or managed all identified conflicts of interest, as applicable.

The following faculty reported relevant financial relationship(s): **Mathis Grossmann, MD, PhD**, receives funding from Bayer Pharma and Otsuka. He is a speaker for Bayer Pharmaceuticals and Besins Healthcare and is an associate editor for the *European Journal of Endocrinology*. **Mark Gurnell, MBBS, MA (Med Ed), PhD**, serves on the advisory board for AstraZeneca, HRA Pharma, and Recordati. He is on the speakers bureau for AstraZeneca and Novartis. **Adrianna Ioachimescu, MD, PhD**, is a consultant for Chiasma, Crinetics, Camurus, HRA Pharma, Strongbridge, Recordati, and Tiburio Therapeutics. Her institution has also received grants from Chiasma, Strongbridge, and Recordati. **Erik Imel, MD**, is a clinical trial investigator for Amgen, Calciolytix, Spruce, Neurocrine, Sanofi, and Ultragenyx. He serves on advisory boards for Kyowa Hakko Kirin and Ultragenyx. He is a consultant for Alexion, and serves on data and safety monitoring boards for Inozyme and Agios. **Kevin M. Pantalone, DO**, receives research support from Bayer, Merck, Novo Nordisk, and Twinhealth. He is a speaker for AstraZeneca, Corcept Therapeutics, Merck, and Novo Nordisk and is a consultant for AstraZeneca, Bayer, Corcept Therapeutics, Diasome, Eli Lilly, Merck, Novo Nordisk, and Sanofi. He is a principal investigator for Eli Lilly, Novo Nordisk, and Twinhealth. **Meera Shah, MB ChB**, is a research collaborator for Pendulum Therapeutics, Inc. Compensation for her time is paid to her institution, Mayo Clinic. **Vinaya Simha, MD**, serves on an advisory board for Pfizer. **Elias Spanakis, MD**, has received unrestricted research support from Dexcom (to Baltimore VA Medical Center and to the University of Maryland) for conducting clinical trials. **Adina Turcu, MD, MS**, receives grant funds from the National Institutes of Health. She is an advisor for CinCor. She is an investigator in a sponsor-initiated clinical trial for Novartis and is a consultant for Crinetics, Poxel, Chiasma, and PhaseBio. **Thomas J. Weber, MD**, serves as a primary investigator and consultant for Ultragenyx. He is on the FDA Endocrine and Metabolic Drug Advisory Committee.

The following faculty reported no relevant financial relationships: **Danit Ariel, MD, MS; Gregory A. Clines, MD, PhD; Nazanene H. Esfandiari, MD; Sarah E. Mayson, MD; Deepika Reddy, MD; Anu Sharma, MD; Aniket Sidhaye, MD**

The medical editor for this program, **Abbie L. Young, MS, CGC, ELS(D)**, reported no relevant financial relationships.

The Endocrine Society staff associated with the development of content for this activity reported no relevant financial relationships.

DISCLAIMERS

The information presented in this activity represents the opinion of the faculty and is not necessarily the official position of the Endocrine Society.

USE OF PROFESSIONAL JUDGMENT:

The educational content in this self-assessment test relates to basic principles of diagnosis and therapy and does not substitute for individual patient assessment based on the health care provider's examination of the patient and consideration of laboratory data and other factors unique to the patient. Standards in medicine change as new data become available.

DRUGS AND DOSAGES:

When prescribing medications, the physician is advised to check the product information sheet accompanying each drug to verify conditions of use and to identify any changes in drug dosage schedule or contraindications.

POLICY ON UNLABELED/OFF-LABEL USE

The Endocrine Society has determined that disclosure of unlabeled/off-label or investigational use of commercial product(s) is informative for audiences and therefore requires this information to be disclosed to the learners at the beginning of the presentation. Uses of specific therapeutic agents, devices, and other products discussed in this educational activity may not be the same as those indicated in product labeling approved by the Food and Drug Administration (FDA). The Endocrine Society requires that any discussions of such "off-label" use be based on scientific research that conforms to generally accepted standards of experimental design, data collection, and data analysis. Before recommending or prescribing any therapeutic agent or device, learners should review the complete prescribing information, including indications, contraindications, warnings, precautions, and adverse events.

ACKNOWLEDGMENT OF COMMERCIAL SUPPORT

This activity is not supported by educational grant(s) or other funds from any commercial supporter.

PUBLICATION DATE: February 2024

Laboratory Reference Ranges

Reference ranges vary among laboratories. The listed reference ranges should be used when interpreting laboratory values presented in ESAP™. Conventional units are listed first with SI units in parentheses.

Lipid Values

High-density lipoprotein (HDL) cholesterol
- Optimal---------------------------- >60 mg/dL (SI: >1.55 mmol/L)
- Normal --------------------- 40-60 mg/dL (SI: 1.04-1.55 mmol/L)
- Low-------------------------------- <40 mg/dL (SI: <1.04 mmol/L)

Low-density lipoprotein (LDL) cholesterol
- Optimal-- <100 mg/dL (SI: <2.59 mmol/L) (for primary prevention); <70 mg/dL (SI: <1.81 mmol/L) (for secondary prevention)
- Low---------------------- 100-129 mg/dL (SI: 2.59-3.34 mmol/L)
- Borderline-high --------- 130-159 mg/dL (SI: 3.37-4.12 mmol/L)
- High --------------------- 160-189 mg/dL (SI: 4.14-4.90 mmol/L)
- Very high ------------------------ ≥190 mg/dL (SI: ≥4.92 mmol/L)

Non-HDL cholesterol
- Optimal-------------------------- <130 mg/dL (SI: <3.37 mmol/L)
- Borderline-high --------- 130-159 mg/dL (SI: 3.37-4.12 mmol/L)
- High ----------------------------- ≥240 mg/dL (SI: ≥6.22 mmol/L)

Total cholesterol
- Optimal-------------------------- <200 mg/dL (SI: <5.18 mmol/L)
- Borderline-high --------- 200-239 mg/dL (SI: 5.18-6.19 mmol/L)
- High ----------------------------- ≥240 mg/dL (SI: ≥6.22 mmol/L)

Triglycerides
- Optimal-------------------------- <150 mg/dL (SI: <1.70 mmol/L)
- Borderline-high --------- 150-199 mg/dL (SI: 1.70-2.25 mmol/L)
- High --------------------- 200-499 mg/dL (SI: 2.26-5.64 mmol/L)
- Very high ------------------------ ≥500 mg/dL (SI: ≥5.65 mmol/L)

Lipoprotein (a) --------------------------≤30 mg/dL (SI: ≤1.07 μmol/L)

Apolipoprotein B -------------------- 50-110 mg/dL (SI: 0.5-1.1 g/L)

Hematologic Values

Erythrocyte sedimentation rate ------------------------- 0-20 mm/h

Haptoglobin -------------------- 30-200 mg/dL (SI: 300-2000 mg/L)

Hematocrit------------------------- 41%-51% (SI: 0.41-0.51) (male); 35%-45% (SI: 0.35-0.45) (female)

Hemoglobin A_{1c}----------------------- 4.0%-5.6% (20-38 mmol/mol)

Hemoglobin --------------- 13.8-17.2 g/dL (SI: 138-172 g/L) (male); 12.1-15.1 g/dL (SI: 121-151 g/L) (female)

International normalized ratio --------------------------------0.8-1.2

Mean corpuscular volume (MCV)---------80-100 μm^3 (SI: 80-100 fL)

Platelet count----------------150-450 × $10^3/\mu L$ (SI: 150-450 × $10^9/L$)

Protein (total) ----------------------------6.3-7.9 g/dL (SI: 63-79 g/L)

Reticulocyte count--- 0.5%-1.5% of red blood cells (SI: 0.005-0.015)

White blood cell count-------- 4500-11,000/μL (SI: 4.5-11.0 × $10^9/L$)

Thyroid Values

Thyroglobulin --------- 3-42 ng/mL (SI: 3-42 μg/L) (after surgery and radioactive iodine treatment: <1.0 ng/mL [SI: <1.0 μg/L])

Thyroglobulin antibodies -----------------≤4.0 IU/mL (SI: ≤4.0 kIU/L)

Thyrotropin (TSH) -------------------------------------0.5-5.0 mIU/L

Thyrotropin-receptor antibodies (TRAb) ----------------- ≤1.75 IU/L

Thyroid-stimulating immunoglobulin-------- ≤120% of basal activity

Thyroperoxidase (TPO) antibodies --------<2.0 IU/mL (SI: <2.0 kIU/L)

Thyroxine (T_4) (free) ----------0.8-1.8 ng/dL (SI: 10.30-23.17 pmol/L)

Thyroxine (T_4) (total)------- 5.5-12.5 μg/dL (SI: 94.02-213.68 nmol/L)

Free thyroxine (T_4) index -------------------------------------- 4-12

Triiodothyronine (T_3) (free)------2.3-4.2 pg/mL (SI: 3.53-6.45 pmol/L)

Triiodothyronine (T_3) (total)----- 70-200 ng/dL (SI: 1.08-3.08 nmol/L)

Triiodothyronine (T_3), reverse ---- 10-24 ng/dL (SI: 0.15-0.37 nmol/L)

Triiodothyronine uptake, resin -----------------------------25%-38%

Radioactive iodine uptake-- 3%-16% (6 hours); 15%-30% (24 hours)

Endocrine Values

Serum

Aldosterone-------------------- 4-21 ng/dL (SI: 111.0-582.5 pmol/L)

Alkaline phosphatase ------------- 50-120 U/L (SI: 0.84-2.00 μkat/L)

Alkaline phosphatase (bone-specific)---------≤20 μg/L (adult male); ≤14 μg/L (premenopausal female); ≤22 μg/L (postmenopausal female)

Androstenedione - 65-210 ng/dL (SI: 2.27-7.33 nmol/L) (adult male); 30-200 ng/dL (SI: 1.05-6.98 nmol/L) (adult female)

Antimullerian hormone ------- 0.7-19.0 ng/mL (SI: 5.0-135.7 pmol/L) (male, >12 years); 0.9-9.5 ng/mL (SI: 6.4-67.9 pmol/L) (female, 13-45 years); <1.0 ng/mL (SI: <7.1 pmol/L) (female, >45 years)

Calcitonin ----------------<16 pg/mL (SI: <4.67 pmol/L) (basal, male); <8 pg/mL (SI: <2.34 pmol/L) (basal, female); ≤130 pg/mL (SI: ≤37.96 pmol/L) (peak calcium infusion, male); ≤90 pg/mL (SI: ≤26.28 pmol/L) (peak calcium infusion, female)

Carcinoembryonic antigen ----------------<2.5 ng/mL (SI: <2.5 μg/L)

Chromogranin A --------------------------- <93 ng/mL (SI: <93 μg/L)

Corticosterone---53-1560 ng/dL (SI: 1.53-45.08 nmol/L) (>18 years)

Corticotropin (ACTH) ------------- 10-60 pg/mL (SI: 2.2-13.2 pmol/L)

Cortisol (8 AM) ----------------- 5-25 μg/dL (SI: 137.9-689.7 nmol/L)

Cortisol (4 PM)-------------------2-14 μg/dL (SI: 55.2-386.2 nmol/L)

C-peptide -----------------------0.5-2.0 ng/mL (SI: 0.17-0.66 nmol/L)

C-reactive protein -------------0.8-3.1 mg/L (SI: 7.62-29.52 nmol/L)

Cross-linked N-telopeptide of type 1 collagen ---------------------- 5.4-24.2 nmol BCE/mmol creat (male); 6.2-19.0 nmol BCE/mmol creat (female)

Dehydroepiandrosterone sulfate (DHEA-S)

Patient Age	Female	Male
18-29 years	44-332 μg/dL (SI: 1.19-9.00 μmol/L)	89-457 μg/dL (SI: 2.41-12.38 μmol/L)
30-39 years	31-228 μg/dL (SI: 0.84-6.78 μmol/L)	65-334 μg/dL (SI: 1.76-9.05 μmol/L)
40-49 years	18-244 μg/dL (SI: 0.49-6.61 μmol/L)	48-244 μg/dL (SI: 1.30-6.61 μmol/L)
50-59 years	15-200 μg/dL (SI: 0.41-5.42 μmol/L)	35-179 μg/dL (SI: 0.95-4.85 μmol/L)
≥60 years	15-157 μg/dL (SI: 0.41-4.25 μmol/L)	25-131 μg/dL (SI: 0.68-3.55 μmol/L)

Deoxycorticosterone ------ <10 ng/dL (SI: <0.30 nmol/L) (>18 years)

1,25-Dihydroxyvitamin D_3----- 16-65 pg/mL (SI: 41.6-169.0 pmol/L)

Estradiol -------------- 10-40 pg/mL (SI: 36.7-146.8 pmol/L) (male);
10-180 pg/mL (SI: 36.7-660.8 pmol/L) (follicular, female);
100-300 pg/mL (SI: 367.1-1101.3 pmol/L) (midcycle, female);
40-200 pg/mL (SI: 146.8-734.2 pmol/L) (luteal, female);
<20 pg/mL (SI: <73.4 pmol/L) (postmenopausal, female)

Estrone --------------- 10-60 pg/mL (SI: 37.0-221.9 pmol/L) (male);
17-200 pg/mL (SI: 62.9-739.6 pmol/L) (premenopausal female);
7-40 pg/mL (SI: 25.9-147.9 pmol/L) (postmenopausal female)

α-Fetoprotein -------------------------------- <6 ng/mL (SI: <6 μg/L)

Follicle-stimulating hormone (FSH) --------------------------------
1.0-13.0 mIU/mL (SI: 1.0-13.0 IU/L) (male);
<3.0 mIU/mL (SI: <3.0 IU/L) (prepuberty, female);
2.0-12.0 mIU/mL (SI: 2.0-12.0 IU/L) (follicular, female);
4.0-36.0 mIU/mL (SI: 4.0-36.0 IU/L) (midcycle, female);
1.0-9.0 mIU/mL (SI: 1.0-9.0 IU/L) (luteal, female);
>30.0 mIU/mL (SI: >30.0 IU/L) (postmenopausal, female)

Free fatty acids ---------------- 10.6-18.0 mg/dL (SI: 0.4-0.7 nmol/L)

Gastrin --------------------------------- <100 pg/mL (SI: <100 ng/L)

Growth hormone (GH) -- 0.01-0.97 ng/mL (SI: 0.01-0.97 μg/L) (male);
0.01-3.61 ng/mL (SI: 0.01-3.61 μg/L) (female)

Homocysteine -------------------------- ≤1.76 mg/L (SI: ≤13 μmol/L)

β-Human chorionic gonadotropin (β-hCG) --------------------------
<3.0 mIU/mL (SI: <3.0 IU/L) (nonpregnant female);
>25 mIU/mL (SI: >25 IU/L) indicates a positive pregnancy test

β-Hydroxybutyrate ------------------ <3.0 mg/dL (SI: <288.2 μmol/L)

17-Hydroxypregnenolone ------ 29-189 ng/dL (SI: 0.87-5.69 nmol/L)

17α-Hydroxyprogesterone <220 ng/dL (SI: <6.67 nmol/L) (adult male);
<80 ng/dL (SI: <2.42 nmol/L) (follicular, female);
<285 ng/dL (SI: <8.64 nmol/L) (luteal, female);
<51 ng/dL (SI: <1.55 nmol/L) (postmenopausal, female)

25-Hydroxyvitamin D ---- <20 ng/mL (SI: <49.9 nmol/L) (deficiency);
21-29 ng/mL (SI: 52.4-72.4 nmol/L) (insufficiency);
30-80 ng/mL (SI: 74.9-199.7 nmol/L) (optimal levels);
>80 ng/mL (SI: >199.7 nmol/L) (toxicity possible)

Inhibin B --------------------------- 15-300 pg/mL (SI: 15-300 ng/L)

Insulinlike growth factor 1 (IGF-1)

Patient Age	Female	Male
18 years	162-541 ng/mL (SI: 21.2-70.9 nmol/L)	170-640 ng/mL (SI: 22.3-83.8 nmol/L)
19 years	138-442 ng/mL (SI: 18.1-57.9 nmol/L)	147-527 ng/mL (SI: 19.3-69.0 nmol/L)
20 years	122-384 ng/mL (SI: 16.0-50.3 nmol/L)	132-457 ng/mL (SI: 17.3-59.9 nmol/L)
21-25 years	116-341 ng/mL (SI: 15.2-44.7 nmol/L)	116-341 ng/mL (SI: 15.2-44.7 nmol/L)
26-30 years	117-321 ng/mL (SI: 15.3-42.1 nmol/L)	117-321 ng/mL (SI: 15.3-42.1 nmol/L)
31-35 years	113-297 ng/mL (SI: 14.8-38.9 nmol/L)	113-297 ng/mL (SI: 14.8-38.9 nmol/L)
36-40 years	106-277 ng/mL (SI: 13.9-36.3 nmol/L)	106-277 ng/mL (SI: 13.9-36.3 nmol/L)
41-45 years	98-261 ng/mL (SI: 12.8-34.2 nmol/L)	98-261 ng/mL (SI: 12.8-34.2 nmol/L)
46-50 years	91-246 ng/mL (SI: 11.9-32.2 nmol/L)	91-246 ng/mL (SI: 11.9-32.2 nmol/L)
51-55 years	84-233 ng/mL (SI: 11.0-30.5 nmol/L)	84-233 ng/mL (SI: 11.0-30.5 nmol/L)
56-60 years	78-220 ng/mL (SI: 10.2-28.8 nmol/L)	78-220 ng/mL (SI: 10.2-28.8 nmol/L)
61-65 years	72-207 ng/mL (SI: 9.4-27.1 nmol/L)	72-207 ng/mL (SI: 9.4-27.1 nmol/L)
66-70 years	67-195 ng/mL (SI: 8.8-25.5 nmol/L)	67-195 ng/mL (SI: 8.8-25.5 nmol/L)
71-75 years	62-184 ng/mL (SI: 8.1-24.1 nmol/L)	62-184 ng/mL (SI: 8.1-24.1 nmol/L)
76-80 years	57-172 ng/mL (SI: 7.5-22.5 nmol/L)	57-172 ng/mL (SI: 7.5-22.5 nmol/L)
>80 years	53-162 ng/mL (SI: 6.9-21.2 nmol/L)	53-162 ng/mL (SI: 6.9-21.2 nmol/L)

Insulinlike growth factor binding protein 3 ------------- 2.5-4.8 mg/L

Insulin ------------------------ 1.4-14.0 μIU/mL (SI: 9.7-97.2 pmol/L)

Islet-cell antibody assay ------- 0 Juvenile Diabetes Foundation units

Luteinizing hormone (LH) --- 1.0-9.0 mIU/mL (SI: 1.0-9.0 IU/L) (male);
<1.0 mIU/mL (SI: <1.0 IU/L) (prepuberty, female);
1.0-18.0 mIU/mL (SI: 1.0-18.0 IU/L) (follicular, female);
20.0-80.0 mIU/mL (SI: 20.0-80.0 IU/L) (midcycle, female);
0.5-18.0 mIU/mL (SI: 0.5-18.0 IU/L) (luteal, female);
>30.0 mIU/mL (SI: >30.0 IU/L) (postmenopausal, female)

Metanephrines (plasma fractionated)
Metanephrine ---------------------- <99 pg/mL (SI: <0.50 nmol/L)
Normetanephrine ---------------- <165 pg/mL (SI: <0.90 nmol/L)

75-g oral glucose tolerance test blood glucose values --------------
60-100 mg/dL (SI: 3.3-5.6 mmol/L) (fasting);
<200 mg/dL (SI: <11.1 mmol/L) (1 hour);
<140 mg/dL (SI: <7.8 mmol/L) (2 hour); between 140-200 mg/dL (SI: 7.8-11.1 mmol/L) is considered impaired glucose tolerance or

prediabetes; greater than 200 mg/dL (SI: >11.1 mmol/L) is a sign of diabetes mellitus

50-g oral glucose tolerance test for gestational diabetes ---------- <140 mg/dL (SI: <7.8 mmol/L) (1 hour)

100-g oral glucose tolerance test for gestational diabetes ---------- <95 mg/dL (SI: <5.3 mmol/L) (fasting); <180 mg/dL (SI: <10.0 mmol/L) (1 hour); <155 mg/dL (SI: <8.6 mmol/L) (2 hour); <140 mg/dL (SI: <7.8 mmol/L) (3 hour)

Osteocalcin ---------------------- 9.0-42.0 ng/mL (SI: 9.0-42.0 μg/L)

Parathyroid hormone, intact (PTH) ---- 10-65 pg/mL (SI: 10-65 ng/L)

Parathyroid hormone–related protein (PTHrP) ----------- <2.0 pmol/L

Progesterone -------------------- ≤1.2 ng/mL (SI: ≤3.8 nmol/L) (male); ≤1.0 ng/mL (SI: ≤3.2 nmol/L) (follicular, female); 2.0-20.0 ng/mL (SI: 6.4-63.6 nmol/L) (luteal, female); ≤1.1 ng/mL (SI: ≤3.5 nmol/L) (postmenopausal, female); >10.0 ng/mL (SI: >31.8 nmol/L) (evidence of ovulatory adequacy)

Proinsulin ------------------- 26.5-176.4 pg/mL (SI: 3.0-20.0 pmol/L)

Prolactin ----------------- 4-23 ng/mL (SI: 0.17-1.00 nmol/L) (male); 4-30 ng/mL (SI: 0.17-1.30 nmol/L) (nonlactating female); 10-200 ng/mL (SI: 0.43-8.70 nmol/L) (lactating female)

Prostate-specific antigen (PSA) ------------------------------------ <2.0 ng/mL (SI: <2.0 μg/L) (≤40 years); <2.8 ng/mL (SI: <2.8 μg/L) (≤50 years); <3.8 ng/mL (SI: <3.8 μg/L) (≤60 years); <5.3 ng/mL (SI: <5.3 μg/L) (≤70 years); <7.0 ng/mL (SI: <7.0 μg/L) (≤79 years); <7.2 ng/mL (SI: <7.2 μg/L) (≥80 years)

Renin activity, plasma, sodium replete, ambulatory ---------------- 0.6-4.3 ng/mL per h

Renin, direct concentration ---------- 4-44 pg/mL (SI: 0.1-1.0 pmol/L)

Sex hormone–binding globulin (SHBG) -------------- 1.1-6.7 μg/mL (SI: 10-60 nmol/L) (male); 2.2-14.6 μg/mL (SI: 20-130 nmol/L) (female)

α-Subunit of pituitary glycoprotein hormones ---------------------- <1.2 ng/mL (SI: <1.2 μg/L)

Testosterone (bioavailable) ----- 0.8-4.0 ng/dL (SI: 0.03-0.14 nmol/L) (20-50 years, female on oral estrogen); 0.8-10.0 ng/dL (SI: 0.03-0.35 nmol/L) (20-50 years, female not on oral estrogen); 83.0-257.0 ng/dL (SI: 2.88-8.92 nmol/L) (male 20-29 years); 72.0-235.0 ng/dL (SI: 2.50-8.15 nmol/L) (male 30-39 years); 61.0-213.0 ng/dL (SI: 2.12-7.39 nmol/L) (male 40-49 years); 50.0-190.0 ng/dL (SI: 1.74-6.59 nmol/L) (male 50-59 years); 40.0-168.0 ng/dL (SI: 1.39-5.83 nmol/L) (male 60-69 years)

Testosterone (free) ----- 9.0-30.0 ng/dL (SI: 0.31-1.04 nmol/L) (male); 0.3-1.9 ng/dL (SI: 0.01-0.07 nmol/L) (female)

Testosterone (total) ---- 300-900 ng/dL (SI: 10.4-31.2 nmol/L) (male); 8-60 ng/dL (SI: 0.3-2.1 nmol/L) (female)

Vitamin B_{12} ------------------- 180-914 pg/mL (SI: 133-674 pmol/L)

Chemistry Values

Alanine aminotransferase ---------- 10-40 U/L (SI: 0.17-0.67 μkat/L)

Albumin --------------------------------- 3.5-5.0 g/dL (SI: 35-50 g/L)

Amylase -------------------------- 26-102 U/L (SI: 0.43-1.70 μkat/L)

Anion gap ---------------------------- 3-11 mEq/L (SI: 3-11 mmol/L)

Aspartate aminotransferase ------- 20-48 U/L (SI: 0.33-0.80 μkat/L)

Bicarbonate ----------------------- 21-28 mEq/L (SI: 21-28 mmol/L)

Bilirubin (total) ------------------ 0.3-1.2 mg/dL (SI: 5.1-20.5 μmol/L)

Blood gases

Po_2, arterial blood ----------- 80-100 mm Hg (SI: 10.6-13.3 kPa)

Pco_2, arterial blood --------------- 35-45 mm Hg (SI: 4.7-6.0 kPa)

Blood pH -- 7.35-7.45

Calcium ------------------------ 8.2-10.2 mg/dL (SI: 2.1-2.6 mmol/L)

Calcium (ionized) ------------- 4.60-5.08 mg/dL (SI: 1.2-1.3 mmol/L)

Carbon dioxide -------------------- 22-28 mEq/L (SI: 22-28 mmol/L)

CD_4 cell count --------------------- 500-1400/μL (SI: 0.5-1.4 × 10^9/L)

Chloride ------------------------- 96-106 mEq/L (SI: 96-106 mmol/L)

Creatine kinase -------------------- 50-200 U/L (SI: 0.84-3.34 μkat/L)

Creatinine ------------ 0.7-1.3 mg/dL (SI: 61.9-114.9 μmol/L) (male); 0.6-1.1 mg/dL (SI: 53.0-97.2 μmol/L) (female)

Ferritin ----------------------- 15-200 ng/mL (SI: 33.7-449.4 pmol/L)

Folate ------------------------------------ ≥4.0 ng/mL (SI: ≥4.0 μg/L)

Glucose --------------------------- 70-99 mg/dL (SI: 3.9-5.5 mmol/L)

γ-Glutamyltransferase -------------- 2-30 U/L (SI: 0.03-0.50 μkat/L)

Iron ---------------------- 50-150 μg/dL (SI: 9.0-26.8 μmol/L) (male); 35-145 μg/dL (SI: 6.3-26.0 μmol/L) (female)

Lactate dehydrogenase ----------- 100-200 U/L (SI: 1.7-3.3 μkat/L)

Lactic acid --------------------- 5.4-20.7 mg/dL (SI: 0.6-2.3 mmol/L)

Lipase ---------------------------- 10-73 U/L (SI: 0.17-1.22 μkat/L)

Magnesium ---------------------- 1.5-2.3 mg/dL (SI: 0.6-0.9 mmol/L)

Osmolality -------------- 275-295 mOsm/kg (SI: 275-295 mmol/kg)

Phosphate ----------------------- 2.3-4.7 mg/dL (SI: 0.7-1.5 mmol/L)

Potassium ----------------------- 3.5-5.0 mEq/L (SI: 3.5-5.0 mmol/L)

Prothrombin time --------------------------------------- 8.3-10.8 s

Serum urea nitrogen --------------- 8-23 mg/dL (SI: 2.9-8.2 mmol/L)

Sodium ---------------------- 136-142 mEq/L (SI: 136-142 mmol/L)

Transferrin saturation ------------------------------------ 14%-50%

Troponin I --------------------------------- <0.6 ng/mL (SI: <0.6 μg/L)

Tryptase ----------------------------- <11.5 ng/mL (SI: <11.5 μg/L)

Uric acid -------------------- 3.5-7.0 mg/dL (SI: 208.2-416.4 μmol/L)

Urine

Albumin ------------ 30-300 μg/mg creat (SI: 3.4-33.9 μg/mol creat)

Albumin-to-creatinine ratio ------------------------- <30 mg/g creat

Aldosterone ---------------------- 3-20 μg/24 h (SI: 8.3-55.4 nmol/d) (should be <12 μg/24 h [SI: <33.2 nmol/d] with oral sodium loading—confirmed with 24-hour urinary sodium >200 mEq)

Calcium ---------------------- 100-300 mg/24 h (SI: 2.5-7.5 mmol/d)

Catecholamine fractionation

Normotensive normal ranges:

Dopamine ------------------- <400 μg/24 h (SI: <2610 nmol/d)

Epinephrine -------------------- <21 μg/24 h (SI: <115 nmol/d)

Norepinephrine ----------------- <80 µg/24 h (SI: <473 nmol/d)

Citrate -------------------- 320-1240 mg/24 h (SI: 16.7-64.5 mmol/d)

Cortisol --------------------------- 4-50 µg/24 h (SI: 11-138 nmol/d)

Cortisol following dexamethasone-suppression test (low-dose: 2 day, 2 mg daily) ----------------- <10 µg/24 h (SI: <27.6 nmol/d)

Creatinine ---------------------- 1.0-2.0 g/24 h (SI: 8.8-17.7 mmol/d)

Glomerular filtration rate (estimated) ------- >60 mL/min per 1.73 m^2

5-Hydroxyindole acetic acid ----- 2-9 mg/24 h (SI: 10.5-47.1 µmol/d)

Iodine (random) -- >100 µg/L

17-Ketosteroids ---- 6.0-21.0 mg/24 h (SI: 20.8-72.9 µmol/d) (male); 4.0-17.0 mg/24 h (SI: 13.9-59.0 µmol/d) (female)

Metanephrine fractionation

Normotensive normal ranges:

Metanephrine -------- <261 µg/24 h (SI: <1323 nmol/d) (male); <180 µg/24 h (SI: <913 nmol/d) (female)

Normetanephrine --------------------- age and sex dependent

Total metanephrine ------------------- age and sex dependent

Osmolality ------------ 150-1150 mOsm/kg (SI: 150-1150 mmol/kg)

Oxalate ----------------------------- <40 mg/24 h (SI: <456 mmol/d)

Phosphate -------------------- 0.9-1.3 g/24 h (SI: 29.1-42.0 mmol/d)

Potassium --------------------- 17-77 mEq/24 h (SI: 17-77 mmol/d)

Sodium ---------------------- 40-217 mEq/24 h (SI: 40-217 mmol/d)

Uric acid ---------------------------- <800 mg/24 h (SI: <4.7 mmol/d)

Saliva

Cortisol (salivary), midnight ------------ <0.13 µg/dL (SI: <3.6 nmol/L)

Semen

Semen analysis --------------- >20 million sperm/mL; >50% motility

Abbreviations

ACTH -- corticotropin

ACE inhibitor --------------- angiotensin-converting enzyme inhibitor

ALT --------------------------------------- alanine aminotransferase

AST ------------------------------------ aspartate aminotransferase

BMI --- body mass index

CDC -------------------- Centers for Disease Control and Prevention

CNS --- central nervous system

CT --- computed tomography

DHEA -------------------------------------- dehydroepiandrosterone

DHEA-S ---------------------------- dehydroepiandrosterone sulfate

DNA -- deoxyribonucleic acid

DPP-4 inhibitor ---------------------- dipeptidyl-peptidase 4 inhibitor

DXA ------------------------------ dual-energy x-ray absorptiometry

FDA ---------------------------------- Food and Drug Administration

FGF-23 --------------------------------- fibroblast growth factor 23

FNA --- fine-needle aspiration

FSH ------------------------------------ follicle-stimulating hormone

GH --- growth hormone

GHRH ------------------------- growth hormone–releasing hormone

GLP-1 receptor agonist ----- glucagonlike peptide 1 receptor agonist

GnRH ----------------------------- gonadotropin-releasing hormone

hCG --------------------------------- human chorionic gonadotropin

HDL -- high-density lipoprotein

HIV ---------------------------------- human immunodeficiency virus

HMG-CoA reductase inhibitor ---------- 3-hydroxy-3-methylglutaryl coenzyme A reductase inhibitor

IGF-1 ------------------------------------ insulinlike growth factor 1

LDL -- low-density lipoprotein

LH --- luteinizing hormone

MCV -------------------------------------- mean corpuscular volume

MIBG ------------------------------------ *meta*-iodobenzylguanidine

MRI ---------------------------------- magnetic resonance imaging

NPH insulin -------------------- neutral protamine Hagedorn insulin

PCSK9 inhibitor ---- proprotein convertase subtilisin/kexin 9 inhibitor

PET --------------------------------- positron emission tomography

PSA --------------------------------------- prostate-specific antigen

PTH --- parathyroid hormone

PTHrP ------------------------ parathyroid hormone–related protein

SGLT-2 inhibitor ----------- sodium-glucose cotransporter 2 inhibitor

SHBG ------------------------------- sex hormone–binding globulin

T_3 --- triiodothyronine

T_4 --- thyroxine

TPO antibodies ------------------------- thyroperoxidase antibodies

TRH --------------------------------- thyrotropin-releasing hormone

TRAb -------------------------------------- TSH-receptor antibodies

TSH -- thyrotropin

VLDL ---------------------------------- very low-density lipoprotein

QUESTIONS

ENDOCRINE SELF-ASSESSMENT PROGRAM 2024

Part I

1 A 50-year-old man presents for follow-up of a left thyroid nodule. The nodule was detected as an incidental finding on neck CT performed after a motor vehicle crash 10 years ago. Initially, the left thyroid nodule measured 2.4 cm, but 5 years later it had increased to a maximum diameter of 4 cm, and 2 years later to 5.2 cm. The patient underwent ultrasound-guided FNA at initial diagnosis and again 5 years later, both with benign results. Over the past year, he has noticed increased anterior neck pressure, such that he is no longer comfortable wearing neck ties and has a choking sensation on occasion. He has decided to undergo a left thyroid lobectomy to alleviate these symptoms.

On physical examination, his blood pressure is 120/78 mm Hg, and pulse rate is 63 beats/min. His height is 72 in (182.9 cm), and weight is 217 lb (98.4 kg) (BMI = 29.4 kg/m^2). There is a firm nodule in the mid to inferior aspect of the left thyroid lobe extending to level of the clavicle. The right thyroid lobe is normal in size and without nodules. The rest of the examination findings are normal.

Laboratory test results:
TSH = 1.2 mIU/L (0.5-5.0 mIU/L)
TPO antibodies, negative

Which of the following most strongly predicts this patient's likelihood of remaining euthyroid after surgery?

A. Isthmus-sparing operation
B. Male sex
C. Preoperative serum TSH concentration
D. Technical expertise of the surgeon
E. TPO antibody status

2 A 75-year-old man with a 30-year history of type 2 diabetes mellitus presents for a follow-up appointment. His medical history is notable for stage G3b chronic kidney disease, coronary artery disease, atrial fibrillation, hypertension, dyslipidemia, diabetic neuropathy, and mild diabetic retinopathy. His medication regimen consists of insulin glargine, 80 units subcutaneous daily; metformin, 500 mg twice daily; empagliflozin, 25 mg daily; glipizide, 10 mg daily; and semaglutide, 1 mg subcutaneously once weekly (which was initiated at his last visit). He checks his blood glucose levels mainly in the morning, and he states that the values are usually in the range of 180 to 190 mg/dL (10.0-10.5 mmol/L). His current hemoglobin A_{1c} value is 7.5% (58 mmol/mol). He describes night sweats that occur once per week. The patient is happy about his hemoglobin A_{1c} value and is pleased to share he has lost 15 lb (6.8 kg) since initiating semaglutide. His current BMI is 29.5 kg/m^2.

Which of the following is the best next step in this patient's management?

A. Continue current management
B. Discontinue semaglutide
C. Measure fructosamine
D. Perform diagnostic continuous glucose monitoring
E. Recommend 3 to 4 glucose measurement daily (before meals and at bedtime)

3 A 54-year-old man is referred by his primary care provider for further investigation of elevated testosterone. Testosterone was measured because of decreased libido and erectile dysfunction. He has consumed 12 cans of light beer daily for many years and smokes 1 pack of cigarettes daily. He is otherwise well and physically active in his work. He reports normal puberty and normal fertility. He has fathered 2 children, aged 17 and 20 years. He has had no testicular or head injuries. He takes no regular medications or supplements and states that he does not abuse anabolic steroids.

On physical examination, his height is 69 in (175.3 cm) and weight is 180 lb (81.6 kg) (BMI = 26.6 kg/m^2). He has normal body hair and sexual hair and no gynecomastia. His liver edge is smooth and palpable, and his liver span is enlarged (approximately 18 cm). There are no signs of chronic liver disease or stigmata of Cushing syndrome. Testicular volume is 25 mL bilaterally and there are no masses.

Laboratory test results (ordered by his primary care physician):

- Testosterone = 1210 ng/dL (300-900 ng/dL) (SI: 42.0 nmol/L [10.4-31.2 nmol/L])
- LH = 6.0 mIU/mL (1.0-9.0 mIU/mL) (SI: 6.0 IU/L [1.0-9.0 IU/L])
- Serum cortisol (8 AM) = 38 μg/dL (5-25 μg/dL) (SI: 1048.3 nmol/L [137.9-689.7 nmol/L])
- Thyroid function, normal
- HIV testing, negative

Current laboratory test results (total testosterone measured with a different assay platform using validated liquid chromatography–tandem mass spectrometry; sample drawn at 8 AM, while fasting):

- Serum testosterone = 1325 ng/dL (SI: 46.0 nmol/L)
- LH = 4.8 mIU/mL (SI: 4.8 IU/L)
- FSH = 5.5 mIU/mL (SI: 5.5 IU/L)
- ALT = 88 U/L (10-40 U/L) (SI: 1.47 μkat/L [0.17-0.67 μkat/L])
- AST = 110 U/L (20-48 U/L) (SI: 1.84 μkat/L [0.33-0.80 μkat/L])
- γ-Glutamyltransferase = 84 U/L (2-30 U/L) (SI: 1.40 μkat/L [0.03-0.50 μkat/L])
- Serum electrolytes and albumin, normal

Which of the following is the best investigation to perform next?

A. Dexamethasone-suppression test (1 mg)
B. Genetic testing of the gene encoding the androgen receptor
C. Iron studies
D. Pituitary-directed MRI
E. SHBG measurement

4 A 48-year-old man attends the endocrine clinic 6 months after transsphenoidal surgery to remove a nonsecretory pituitary adenoma. Histopathologic examination of the resected tumor confirmed an SF-1–positive pituitary adenoma, with focal FSH staining and a Ki-67 (MIB-1) proliferation index of 0.9%.

Following surgery, he reported an immediate improvement in his vision. At a recent ophthalmology visit, his visual acuity was 20/25 (6/7.5) in both eyes, with normal color vision and visual fields bilaterally. He describes occasional tiredness after significant physical exertion but no other symptoms. He takes no regular medications.

On physical examination, his blood pressure is 142/78 mm Hg and pulse rate is 72 beats/min. His height is 75 in (190.5 cm), and weight is 217 lb (98.4 kg) (BMI = 27.1 kg/m^2). He has normal secondary sexual characteristics, and there are no stigmata of endocrine dysfunction.

Laboratory test results (at 8 AM after overnight fast):

- Prolactin = 27 ng/mL (4-23 ng/mL) (SI: 1.17 nmol/L [0.17-1.00 nmol/L])
- TSH = 1.52 mIU/L (0.5-5.0 mIU/L)
- Free T_4 = 1.30 ng/dL (0.8-1.8 ng/dL) (SI: 16.73 pmol/L [10.30-23.17 pmol/L])
- Cortisol (8 AM) = 12.9 μg/dL (5-25 μg/dL) (SI: 355.9 nmol/L [137.9-689.7 nmol/L])
- IGF-1 = 130 ng/mL (91-246 ng/mL) (SI: 17.0 nmol/L [11.9-32.2 nmol/L])
- FSH = 3.1 mIU/mL (1.0-13.0 mIU/mL) (SI: 3.1 IU/L [1.0-13.0 IU/L])
- LH = 2.9 mIU/mL (1.0-9.0 mIU/mL) (SI: 2.9 IU/L [1.0-9.0 IU/L])
- Total testosterone = 341 ng/dL (300-900 ng/dL) (SI: 11.8 nmol/L [10.4-31.2 nmol/L])

MRI of the sella is shown (*see images*).

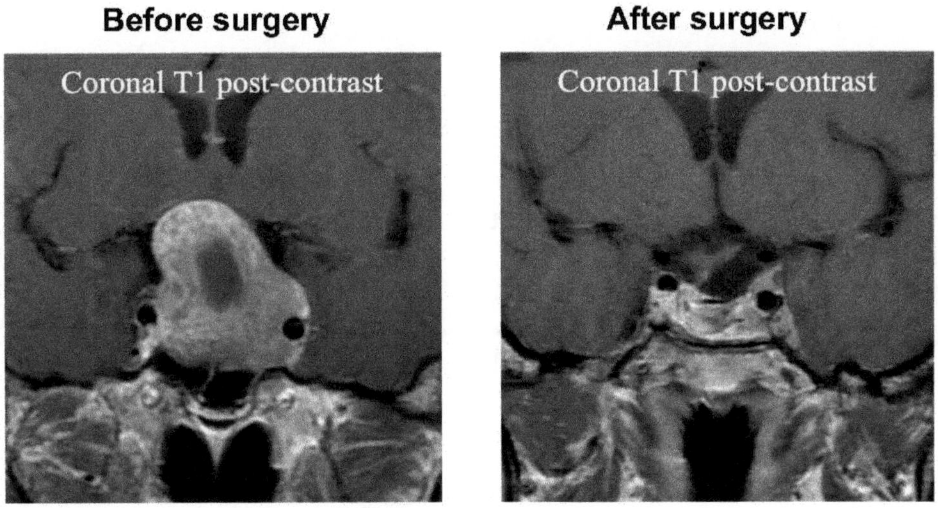

Which of the following is the most appropriate next step in the management of this patient's pituitary tumor?

A. Perform MRI again in 12 months
B. Refer for pituitary radiotherapy
C. Refer for a second transsphenoidal surgery
D. Start dopamine agonist therapy
E. Start first-generation somatostatin receptor ligand therapy

5 A 59-year-old woman with a history of cigarette smoking has been diagnosed with osteoporosis (T-score–2.9 in the lumbar spine and –3.1 in the femoral neck). She has no history of fractures. A FRAX score was calculated with 10-year risks of 14% for major osteoporotic fracture and 7.3% for hip fracture. She works part time and does not have access to health insurance. She has difficulty affording food and medications. She has little dietary calcium intake and does not take supplemental vitamin D. A recent 25-hydroxyvitamin D concentration was 21 ng/mL (52.4 nmol/L), but other routine laboratory test results were normal. In addition to vitamin D and calcium supplements, her primary care provider recommends starting an osteoporosis medication. The patient is concerned that she will be unable to afford treatment.

Which of the following osteoporosis medications is the most appropriate choice for this patient?

A. Alendronate
B. Denosumab
C. Ibandronate
D. Risedronate
E. Zoledronic acid

6 A 44-year-old woman with type 2 diabetes mellitus presents for follow-up. Her diabetes has been well controlled for the past few years on a regimen of multiple daily insulin injections. She takes 6 units of insulin lispro at the start of meals, with a correction scale of 1 unit for every 50 mg/dL (2.8 mmol/L) when blood glucose values are greater than 150 mg/dL (>8.3 mmol/L). She takes 34 units of insulin glargine at bedtime. She expresses dismay at her treatment burden, as multiple daily insulin injections and the need for frequent blood glucose checks are often inconvenient. She is also concerned and frustrated about weight gain with insulin therapy, having gained 15 lb (6.8 kg) over the past year. Her blood glucose log demonstrates fair glycemic control but with variable postprandial hyperglycemia.

On physical examination, her blood pressure is 130/82 mm Hg and pulse rate is 76 beats/min. Her height is 66 in (167.6 cm), and weight is 212 lb (96.2 kg) (BMI = 34.2 kg/m^2). She does not have supraclavicular/nuchal adiposity, or abdominal striae.

Laboratory test result:

Hemoglobin A_{1c} = 7.2% (4.0%-5.6%) (55 mmol/mol [20-38 mmol/mol])
Glutamic acid decarboxylase 65 antibodies, undetectable

Which of the following is the best next step in this patient's management?

A. Add glimepiride
B. Increase the insulin lispro dosage
C. Switch insulin glargine to insulin degludec
D. Switch insulin lispro to a GLP-1 receptor agonist
E. Switch insulin lispro to lispro-aabc

7 A 25-year-old transgender man is referred for gender dysphoria and continuation of gender-affirming hormone therapy. He has a history of bilateral hip impingement (status post bilateral hip surgery), hyperlipidemia, impaired fasting glucose, and vitamin D deficiency. He reports unexplained anxiety and feeling unsettled when he was growing up, but he did not realize he was transgender until a few years ago when he was playing a male role in a theater production. Thereafter, he began transitioning with assistance from his primary care physician. His primary care physician is retiring, and he is seeking continuation of care.

His main goals for gender-affirming care are cessation of menses and masculinizing chest surgery. Monthly bleeding triggers extreme dysphoria that has been associated with suicidal ideation in the past. He is interested in fertility with his current cisgender male partner in the next 2 to 3 years (specifically to carry a pregnancy to term) and has sexual activity that involves sperm. He began initiation of gender-affirming hormone therapy with intramuscular testosterone cypionate, 50 mg every other week, and feels comfortable with self-injections. While pleased with the masculinizing changes, he continued to have monthly bleeding on that dosage. After a dosage increase to 60 mg every other week, the monthly bleeding stopped but he noticed dizziness, both at rest and with movement. The dizziness resolved after decreasing to the former testosterone dosage.

Laboratory test results (sample drawn midway between testosterone injections, fasting at 8 AM):

Total testosterone = 547 ng/dL (SI: 19.0 nmol/L)
Estradiol = 48 pg/mL (SI: 176.2 pmol/L)
SHBG = 4.7 μg/mL (SI: 41.8 nmol/L)

On physical examination, his blood pressure is 133/75 mm Hg and pulse rate is 82 beats/min. His height is 59.4 in (151 cm), and weight is 104.5 lb (47.4 kg) (BMI = 20.8 kg/m^2). He is a well-appearing, well-developed, fully masculinized man, with a fully grown beard. He has had masculinizing chest reconstruction surgery.

Which of the following is the best next step to support this patient's gender-affirming goals?

A. Increase the testosterone cypionate dosage
B. Place an etonogestrel implant
C. Prescribe combined oral contraceptive pills
D. Sterilize with salpingectomy
E. Switch to subcutaneous administration of testosterone cypionate

8 A 52-year-old man is referred after indeterminate bilateral adrenal lesions (each <2.5 cm in maximum diameter with Hounsfield units >30) are identified on contrast-enhanced whole-body trauma CT following a motorcycle accident. He has a history of bipolar disorder with recurrent depressive episodes that are well controlled on venlafaxine and lamotrigine.

On physical examination, his blood pressure is 150/85 mm Hg, and pulse rate is 70 beats/min and regular. His height is 74 in (188.0 cm), and weight is 185 lb (83.9 kg) (BMI = 23.7 kg/m^2). The rest of the physical examination findings are unremarkable.

Initial laboratory test results:

- Serum sodium = 138 mEq/L (136-142 mEq/L) (SI: 138 mmol/L [136-142 mmol/L])
- Serum potassium = 4.1 mEq/L (3.5-5.0 mEq/L) (SI: 4.1 mmol/L [3.5-5.0 mmol/L])
- Plasma renin activity = 1.5 ng/mL per h (0.6-4.3 ng/mL per h)
- Serum aldosterone = 8.7 ng/dL (4-21 ng/dL) (SI: 241.3 pmol/L [111.0-582.5 pmol/L])
- Cortisol (8 AM) = 14.9 μg/dL (5-25 μg/dL) (SI: 411.1 nmol/L [137.9-689.7 nmol/L])
- Cortisol following 1-mg dexamethasone-suppression test = 1.1 μg/dL (SI: 30.3 nmol/L)
- Plasma metanephrine = 35 pg/mL (<99 pg/mL) (SI: 0.18 nmol/L [<0.50 nmol/L])
- Plasma normetanephrine = 302 pg/mL (<165 pg/mL) (SI: 1.65 nmol/L [<0.90 nmol/L])

Repeat laboratory test results after discontinuing venlafaxine for 72 hours:

- Plasma metanephrine = 39 pg/mL (<99 pg/mL) (SI: 0.20 nmol/L [<0.50 nmol/L])
- Plasma normetanephrine = 195 pg/mL (<165 pg/mL) (SI: 1.06 nmol/L [<0.90 nmol/L])

Chemical shift adrenal MRI performed 2 months after initial CT is shown (*see images*).

In-phase | Out-of-phase

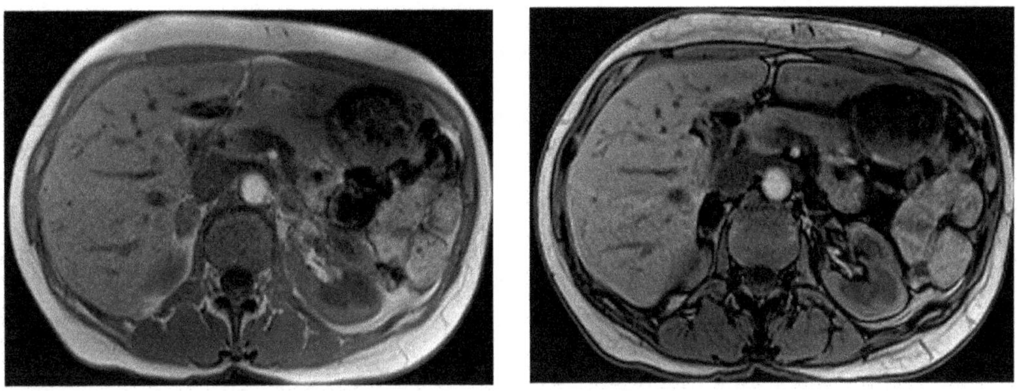

Which of the following is the most likely explanation for the bilateral adrenal lesions?

A. Adenomas
B. Hemorrhage
C. Metastases
D. Myelolipomas
E. Pheochromocytomas

9 A 30-year-old man returns for follow-up of type 1 diabetes mellitus. His treatment regimen consists of insulin glargine, 18 units at bedtime, and premeal insulin aspart, with a carbohydrate ratio of 1 unit for every 12 g of carbohydrates and a correction factor of 1 unit of insulin aspart for every 50 mg/dL (2.8 mmol/L) above a blood glucose concentration of 150 mg/dL (>8.3 mmol/L). He feels comfortable with carbohydrate estimation, as he has a very consistent diet, and reports that he takes all his meal-time and basal insulin doses. He is very fearful of hypoglycemia. He plays basketball daily from 6 to 8 PM. He wears a continuous glucose monitor, and his 90-day report documents the following:

Average glucose = 183 mg/dL (SI: 10.2 mmol/L)
Time in target range: 43.8%
Time above target range = 50.1%
Time below target range = 6.1%
Glucose management indicator = 7.7%

A snapshot of a typical day is shown (*see image*).

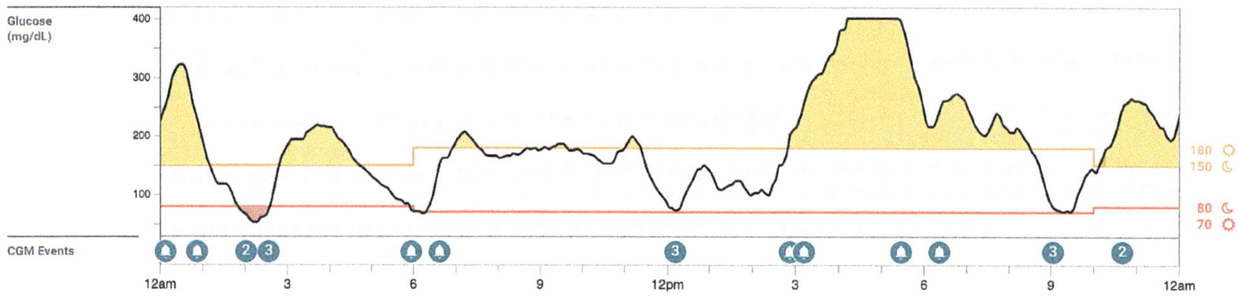

Which of the following is the best next step to improve this patient's time-in-range?

A. Change the carbohydrate ratio to 1 unit for every 10 g carbohydrates
B. Change the correction factor to 1 unit of insulin aspart for every 40 mg/dL (2.2 mmol/L) above a blood glucose concentration of 180 mg/dL (>10.0 mmol/L) at night
C. Switch insulin glargine to insulin degludec
D. Switch to a hybrid closed-loop insulin pump system
E. Switch to a smart insulin pen

10 A 21-year-old woman who is 29 weeks pregnant presents for management of hypoparathyroidism. She has a history of papillary thyroid cancer diagnosed at age 14 years that was treated with surgery and radioactive iodine. She has a long history of frequent paresthesia and muscle cramps, but these symptoms have lessened during recent weeks.

Her current medications are levothyroxine, 150 mcg daily; calcitriol, 0.5 mcg twice daily; and calcium carbonate, as 1000 mg elemental calcium twice daily.

Laboratory test results:

Calcium = 9.5 mg/dL (8.2-10.2 mg/dL) (SI: 2.4 mmol/L [2.1-2.6 mmol/L])
Albumin = 3.2 g/dL (3.5-5.0 g/dL) (SI: 32 g/L [35-50 g/L])
Creatinine = 0.78 mg/dL (0.6-1.1 mg/dL) (SI: 69.0 μmol/L [53.0-97.2 μmol/L])
Intact PTH, undetectable
25-Hydroxyvitamin D = 33 ng/mL (30-80 ng/mL [optimal]) (SI: 82.4 nmol/L [74.9-199.7 nmol/L])
Phosphate = 4.7 mg/dL (2.3-4.7 mg/dL) (SI: 1.5 mmol/L [0.7-1.5 mmol/L])
Magnesium = 1.8 mg/dL (1.5-2.3 mg/dL) (SI: 0.7 mmol/L [0.6-0.9 mmol/L])
Urinary calcium-to-creatinine ratio = 0.47 mg/mg (<0.22 mg/mg) (SI: 1.3 mmol/mmol [<0.61 mmol/mmol])
TSH = 0.38 mIU/L (0.5-5.0 mIU/L)

Which of the following is the best option to address this patient's current status?

A. Add a PTH receptor agonist
B. Add hydrochlorothiazide
C. Change calcium carbonate to calcium citrate
D. Reduce the calcitriol dosage
E. Reduce the levothyroxine dosage

11 A 40-year-old man with severe Graves orbitopathy and postsurgical hypothyroidism starts treatment with teprotumumab. His Graves orbitopathy improves after 4 infusions of teprotumumab with mild residual diplopia. At his follow-up appointment, he feels well except for some tinnitus and hearing loss. He takes levothyroxine, 125 mcg daily, and a daily multivitamin. He has no other notable medical history. His mother has hypothyroidism due to Hashimoto thyroiditis.

On physical examination, his vital signs are stable. His bilateral proptosis, lid lag, and chemosis have improved compared with findings on his last examination. There is a well-healed scar at the base of his neck. The rest of his physical examination findings are unremarkable.

Laboratory test results:

TSH = 2.5 mIU/L (0.5-5.0 mIU/L)
Basic metabolic panel, normal

Which of the following is the best next step in this patient's management?

A. Increase the levothyroxine dosage
B. Perform brain MRI
C. Refer to an oculoplastic surgeon
D. Refer to an otolaryngologist
E. Start selenium

12 A 66-year-old woman with a history of hypertension, chronic kidney disease, and opioid use managed for more than 30 years with methadone undergoes surgery for management of appendicitis. Preoperatively, her course is notable for symptomatic hypoglycemia with a nadir plasma glucose value of 42 mg/dL (2.3 mmol/L) that resolves after administration of intravenous dextrose. Postoperatively, she continues to have hypoglycemia requiring intravenous dextrose infusion despite good recovery and adequate consumption of calories.

On further questioning, she reports a several-month history of episodic blurry vision, slurred speech, confusion, and diaphoresis if she skips meals and does not eat a bedtime snack. Besides this, she has felt well and has no history of significant weight loss, exogenous steroid use, excessive alcohol intake, or use of any illicit substances. Medications before hospitalization were amlodipine, 5 mg daily; hydrochlorothiazide, 12.5 mg daily; and methadone, 115 mg daily.

Laboratory test results at hospital admission:

Serum urea nitrogen = 22 mg/dL (8-23 mg/dL) (SI: 7.9 mmol/L [2.9-8.2 mmol/L])
Creatinine = 2.3 mg/dL (0.6-1.1 mg/dL) (SI: 203.3 µmol/L [53.0-97.2 µmol/L])
Estimated glomerular filtration rate = 28 mL/min per 1.73 m^2 (>60 mL/min per 1.73 m^2) (it was 50 mL/min per 1.73 m^2 1 year prior to admission)

Postoperative laboratory test results:

Cortisol (8-AM) = 24 µg/dL (SI: 662.1 nmol/L)
Insulin antibodies, negative

Toxicology, sulfonylurea, and meglitinide screens are negative except for methadone.

She undergoes a supervised fast, and results are shown (*see table*). The patient's dextrose infusion is suspended, and she develops symptoms of arm numbness and diaphoresis coincident with a low plasma glucose value after just 2 hours.

Analyte	Glucose	Insulin	Proinsulin	C-peptide	β-Hydroxybutyrate
This patient's results	42 mg/dL (SI: 2.3 mmol/L)	10.1 µIU/mL (SI: 70.1 pmol/L)	113.8 pg/mL (SI: 12.9 pmol/L)	1.3 ng/mL (SI: 0.4 nmol/L)	0.1 mmol/L
Values that suggest endogenous hyperinsulinism (or an IGF-1 secreting tumor)	<55 mg/dL (SI: <3.1 mmol/L)	≥3.0 µIU/mL (SI: ≥20.8 nmol/L)	≥44.1 pg/mL (SI: ≥5.0 pmol/L)	≥0.6 ng/mL (SI: 0.2 nmol/L)	≤2.7 mmol/L

Endoscopic ultrasonography (done as first-line imaging given the history of chronic kidney disease) does not reveal a pancreatic mass.

Which of following is the best next step in the management of this patient's hypoglycemia?

A. Discontinue methadone
B. Discontinue thiazide diuretic
C. Prescribe acarbose
D. Prescribe diazoxide
E. Suggest small, frequent meals

13 A 53-year-old man with schizophrenia is concerned about a 3-month history of weight gain, breast enlargement, and low libido. Medications include risperidone, 6 mg daily (initiated 4 months ago after switch from aripiprazole, 7.5 mg daily), and atorvastatin, 10 mg daily.

On physical examination, his blood pressure is 135/85 mm Hg and pulse rate is 90 beats/min. His height is 73 in (185.4 cm), and weight is 250 lb (113.4 kg) (BMI = 33 kg/m^2). He has mild dorsocervical fat accumulation, dry skin, bilateral adipomastia, slight retroareolar gynecomastia, and normal testicular volume.

Laboratory test results (sample drawn in the afternoon):

Prolactin = 100 ng/mL (4-23 ng/mL) (SI: 4.35 nmol/L [0.17-1.00 nmol/L])
Testosterone = 270 ng/dL (300-900 ng/dL) (SI: 9.4 nmol/L [10.4-31.2 nmol/L])
Fasting glucose = 107 mg/dL (70-99 mg/dL) (SI: 5.9 mmol/L [3.9-5.5 mmol/L])
Kidney function, normal
Liver function, normal

MRI of the pituitary gland shows a 1.5-cm pituitary adenoma (*see image*).

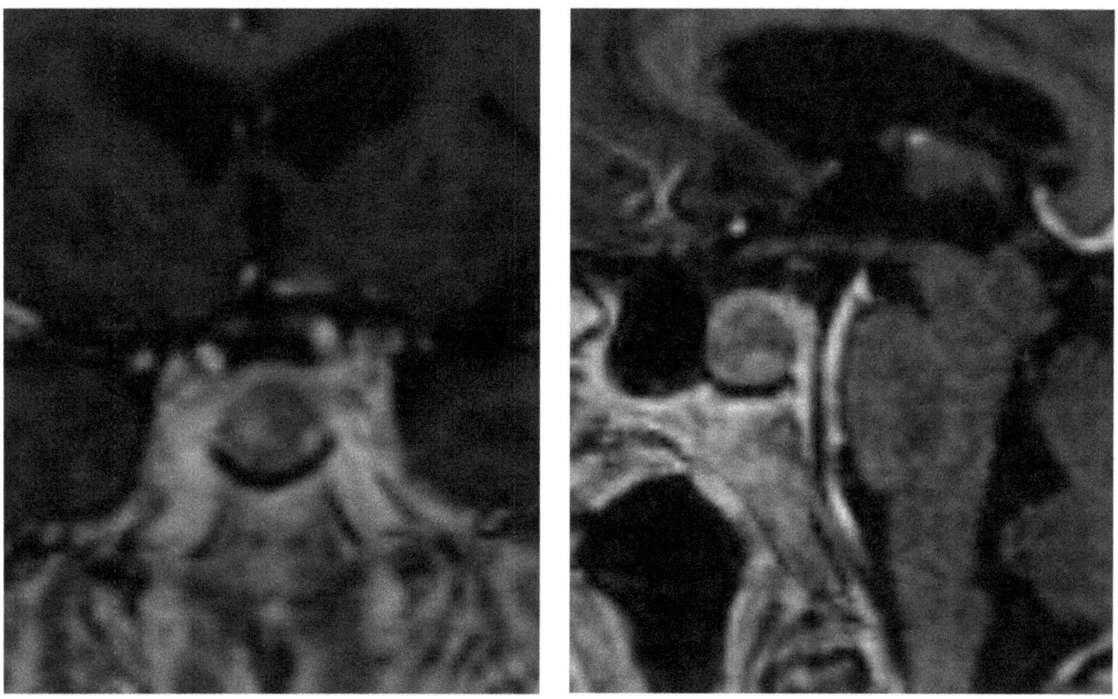

Coronal (left) and sagittal (right) T1 postcontrast images.

Which of the following is the best next step in this patient's management?

A. Measure IGF-1, cortisol, TSH, and free T_4
B. Refer for transsphenoidal surgery
C. Repeat prolactin measurement after replacing risperidone with aripiprazole
D. Start cabergoline, 1 mg twice weekly
E. Start testosterone replacement

14 A 59-year-old man with primary hypothyroidism, gastroesophageal reflux disease, and Barrett esophagus presents for follow-up. Hypothyroidism due to Hashimoto thyroiditis was diagnosed when he was a teenager, and he has since been taking generic levothyroxine tablets for replacement. One year ago, the patient had esophagogastroduodenoscopy demonstrating Barrett esophagus, and he was prescribed oral omeprazole twice daily. He also has a history of tonic-clonic seizures since childhood, which have been well controlled on levetiracetam for the past 2 years.

The patient reports fatigue, dry skin, and constipation over the past 2 to 3 months. He states that he takes his medications as prescribed and has not missed any doses in the past month. He takes levothyroxine, 150 mcg daily, on an empty stomach after waking in the morning (about 30 minutes prior to taking his other prescribed medications) and 60 minutes before breakfast. He does not take any over-the-counter medications or supplements.

On physical examination, his blood pressure is 140/78 mm Hg and pulse rate is 82 beats/min supine. His height is 68 in (172.7 cm), and weight is 186 lb (84.4 kg) (BMI = 28.3 kg/m^2). The thyroid gland is 15 g without nodules. The rest of the examination findings are normal.

Laboratory test results:
TSH = 7.0 mIU/L (0.5-5.0 mIU/L)

2 weeks later:
TSH = 8.4 mIU/L (0.5-5.0 mIU/L)
Free T_4 = 0.9 ng/dL (0.8-1.8 ng/dL) (SI: 11.6 pmol/L [10.30-23.17 pmol/L])

Which of the following is the most appropriate next step in this patient's management?

A. Change levothyroxine administration time to bedtime
B. Change to a branded levothyroxine tablet
C. Change to levothyroxine oral solution
D. Discontinue omeprazole
E. Substitute another anticonvulsant drug for levetiracetam

15 A 46-year-old healthy man presents for advice on decreasing his risk for cardiovascular disease after receiving results of a screening lipid profile and coronary CT. He does not have symptoms of angina or exertional dyspnea, and he engages in regular physical activity by playing tennis at least 3 to 4 days per week. However, he is concerned about his family history of heart disease. His father underwent coronary artery bypass surgery at age 48 years, and his paternal uncle died of a myocardial infarction at age 56 years. He does not smoke cigarettes and is currently not on any medications.

On physical examination, his blood pressure is 132/84 mm Hg and pulse rate is 76 beats/min. His height is 70 in (177.8 cm), and weight is 216 lb (98.0 kg) (BMI = 31 kg/m^2). Examination does not reveal corneal arcus or tendon xanthomas.

Fasting lipid panel:
Total cholesterol = 248 mg/dL (<200 mg/dL) (SI: 6.42 mmol/L [<5.18 mmol/L])
Triglycerides = 265 mg/dL (<150 mg/dL) (SI: 2.99 mmol/L [<1.70 mmol/L])
HDL cholesterol = 35 mg/dL (>60 mg/dL) (SI: 0.91 mmol/L [>1.55 mmol/L])
LDL cholesterol = 160 mg/dL (<100 mg/dL) (SI: 4.14 mmol/L [<2.59 mmol/L])

Coronary CT reveals no evidence of subclinical atherosclerosis with a coronary artery calcium score of zero. The predicted 10-year risk for atherosclerotic cardiovascular disease (ASCVD) is 5.2%.

In addition to advice on weight loss, which of the following is the best next step in this patient's management?

A. Repeat coronary CT in 5 years; start statin therapy at that time if there is detectable coronary artery calcium
B. Repeat lipid panel in 3 to 6 months after intensive lifestyle changes and start moderate-intensity statin therapy if LDL cholesterol is still ≥130 mg/dL (≥3.37 mmol/L)
C. Start moderate-intensity statin therapy
D. Start moderate-intensity statin therapy and repeat coronary CT in 1 to 2 years; consider changing to high-intensity statin therapy if there is detectable coronary artery calcium
E. Start moderate-intensity statin therapy and omega-3 fatty acids

16

Osteoporosis medications change bone turnover (bone formation and resorption) depending on the mechanism of action. Bisphosphonates, teriparatide, and romosozumab each have differing mechanisms.

What are the expected changes in bone formation and bone resorption with these 3 medications, respectively, 3 months after starting therapy?

	Bisphosphonates		**Teriparatide**		**Romosozumab**	
Answer	**Bone formation**	**Bone resorption**	**Bone formation**	**Bone resorption**	**Bone formation**	**Bone resorption**
A.	↑	↓	↓	↓	↑	↑
B.	↓	↑	↑	↑	↑	↑
C.	↓	↓	↑	↓	↑	↑
D.	↑	↓	↑	↑	↑	↓
E.	↓	↓	↑	↑	↑	↓

17

A 78-year-old woman is referred for management of type 2 diabetes mellitus, which was diagnosed more than 20 years ago. Her current treatment regimen is insulin glargine, 10 units at bedtime, and premeal insulin lispro, 4 units before meals. She does not report any hypoglycemia.

Laboratory test results:

- Hemoglobin A_{1c} = 7.2% (4.0%-5.6%) (55 mmol/mol [20-38 mmol/mol])
- Hemoglobin = 8.6 g/dL (12.1-15.1 g/dL) (SI: 86 g/L [121-151 g/L])
- Estimated glomerular filtration rate = 9 mL/min per 1.73 m^2 (>60 mL/min per 1.73 m^2)

Her 90-day continuous glucose monitoring report is shown (*see image*).

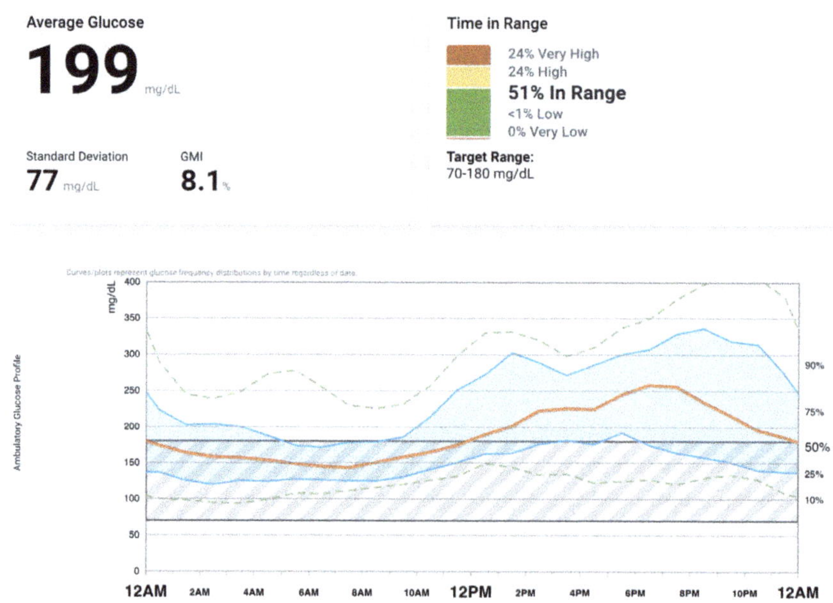

Which of the following is the best interpretation of these data?

A. Hemoglobin A_{1c} and glucose management indicator are inaccurate
B. Hemoglobin A_{1c} is above goal and time-in-range is below goal
C. Hemoglobin A_{1c} is at goal with no hypoglycemia on continuous glucose monitoring
D. Hemoglobin A_{1c} is below goal with no hypoglycemia on continuous glucose monitoring
E. Hemoglobin A_{1c} is inaccurate, so glucose management indicator/time-in-range should be used to guide therapy

18 A 33-year-old woman with X-linked hypophosphatemia presents with bone pain in her lower extremities and stiffness. She has pain in her left thigh that is worse when walking. During childhood, she was treated with calcitriol and phosphate salts and required corrective surgery for bowing of her lower limbs. She stopped medical therapy after growth was completed, but she restarted a few years later because of severe hypophosphatemia. She reports increasing PTH levels during adulthood.

Radiographs demonstrate an insufficiency fracture ("pseudofracture") in the proximal left femur.

Her current medications are calcitriol, 0.25 mcg daily, and neutral sodium phosphate, 500 mg of phosphorus in a tablet, 3 times daily.

Laboratory test results:

Calcium = 11.3 mg/dL (8.2-10.2 mg/dL) (SI: 2.8 mmol/L [2.1-2.6 mmol/L])
Albumin = 4.2 g/dL (3.5-5.0 g/dL) (SI: 42 g/L [35-50 g/L])
Creatinine = 0.78 mg/dL (0.6-1.1 mg/dL) (SI: 69.0 µmol/L [53.0-97.2 µmol/L])
Alkaline phosphatase = 104 U/L (50-120 U/L) (SI: 1.74 µkat/L [0.84-2.00 µkat/L])
Intact PTH = 332 pg/mL (10-65 pg/mL) (SI: 332 ng/L [10-65 ng/L])
25-Hydroxyvitamin D = 33 ng/mL (30-80 ng/mL [optimal]) (SI: 82.4 nmol/L [74.9-199.7 nmol/L])
Phosphate = 2.3 mg/dL (2.3-4.7 mg/dL) (SI: 0.7 mmol/L [0.7-1.5 mmol/L])
Magnesium = 1.8 mg/dL (1.5-2.3 mg/dL) (SI: 0.7 mmol/L [0.6-0.9 mmol/L])
Urinary calcium-to-creatinine ratio = 0.25 mg/mg (<0.22 mg/mg) (SI: 0.69 mmol/mmol [<0.61 mmol/mmol])

Which of the following is the best next step in this patient's management?

A. Discontinue calcitriol and phosphate and start burosumab
B. Increase the calcitriol dosage
C. Increase the phosphate dosage
D. Perform parathyroidectomy with multigland resection
E. Start magnesium oxide

19 A 51-year-old transgender man with a history of depression and tobacco use presents for annual follow-up. He socially transitioned at age 18 years when he graduated from high school and then initiated weekly subcutaneous testosterone at age 20 years. His gender-affirming care has included hysterectomy and oophorectomy and use of binders to decrease his chest appearance. He is adherent to his testosterone regimen and is happy with his mood, overall masculinization, and physical appearance. On review of family history, he mentions that his mother and maternal grandmother have a history of ovarian cancer.

On physical examination, his blood pressure is 127/76 mm Hg and pulse rate is 91 beats/min. His height is 66.1 in (168 cm), and weight is 183.5 lb (83.2 kg) (BMI = 29.5 kg/m^2). He is a well-appearing, fully masculinized man. He has Tanner stage 5 breasts and wears a binder. His Ferriman-Gallwey score is 24.

His annual gender hormone laboratory results are reviewed, and his current testosterone regimen is discussed.

In addition to refilling his testosterone prescription, which of the following should be done?

A. *BRCA* genetic screening
B. Clinical breast examination during the office visit
C. Mammography
D. Referral for masculinizing chest reconstruction
E. Referral to gynecology for a Papanicolaou test

20 A 79-year-old woman is referred for evaluation of a 1-cm left adrenal nodule, which was noted incidentally on abdominal CT when she presented with acute abdominal pain. The nodule enhanced homogeneously at –10 Hounsfield units on noncontrast CT images. Her medical history includes type 2 diabetes mellitus, hypertension, dyslipidemia, coronary artery disease, atrial fibrillation, diverticulosis, vitamin D deficiency, and osteopenia. Her personal and family history is negative for malignancies. Her medications include lisinopril, hydrochlorothiazide, metoprolol, rosuvastatin, metformin, sitagliptin, and warfarin. She has a longstanding history of cigarette smoking, and she drinks 2 beers per week.

On physical examination, her blood pressure is 148/85 mm Hg and pulse rate is 72 beats/min. Her height is 66 in (167.6 cm), and weight is 230 lb (104.3 kg) (BMI = 37.2 kg/m^2). She has poor dentition and inflamed gums. She has uniformly distributed excess adiposity, and pale, thin striae on her lower abdomen. She has no plethora or bruises. Muscle strength is within normal limits. There is no spine tenderness and no edema.

Laboratory test results:

Serum cortisol (8 AM) = 12 µg/dL (5-25 µg/dL) (SI: 331.1 nmol/L [137.9-689.7 nmol/L])
ACTH (8 AM) = 14 pg/mL (10-60 pg/mL) (SI: 3.1 pmol/L [2.2-13.2 pmol/L])
Serum aldosterone = 4.2 ng/dL (4-21 ng/dL) (SI: 116.5 pmol/L [111.0-582.5 pmol/L])
Plasma renin activity = 1.3 ng/mL per h (0.6-4.3 ng/mL per h)
DHEA-S = 25 µg/dL (15-157 µg/dL) (SI: 0.68 µmol/L [0.41-4.25 µmol/L])
Plasma metanephrines, normal
Midnight salivary cortisol = 0.19 µg/dL (<0.13 µg/dL) (SI: 5.2 nmol/L [<3.6 nmol/L])

Laboratory values following a 1-mg dexamethasone-suppression test (8 AM):

Serum cortisol = 1.2 µg/dL (SI: 33.1 nmol/L)
ACTH = <5 pg/mL (<1.1 pmol/L)

Which of the following is the best management approach for this patient?

A. Measure 24-hour urinary cortisol excretion
B. Recommend left adrenalectomy
C. Recommend no further workup or follow-up
D. Start mifepristone
E. Start osilodrostat

21 A 56-year-old woman with a history of hypertension, chronic obstructive pulmonary disease, obstructive sleep apnea, and primary hypothyroidism presents to the emergency department for evaluation of progressive weakness and lethargy. The patient reports that she fell out of bed 5 days ago and struck her head, resulting in a large ecchymosis surrounding her left eye. Prior to the fall she had been experiencing increasing fatigue, generalized weakness, and excessive daytime sleepiness. She has been living in a shelter for the past month because of homelessness and has been unable to obtain her medications. She has a history of cigarette smoking but quit 2 years ago. She does not drink alcohol or use illicit drugs. Review of systems is notable for constipation.

On physical examination, her temperature is 97.5°F (36.4°C), blood pressure is 149/94 mm Hg, and pulse rate is 40 beats/min. Her height is 64 in (162.6 cm), and weight is 240 lb (108.9 kg) (BMI = 41.2 kg/m^2). Oxygen saturation is 95% on room air. Findings on thyroid examination are normal without enlargement or nodules. On cardiac examination, she has bradycardia and no murmurs. She has 1+ bilateral lower-extremity edema. Deep tendon reflexes are 1+. Speech is slowed. The patient is somnolent but arousable. She is oriented to person, place, and time. The rest of the examination findings are normal.

Laboratory test results:

TSH = 179.0 mIU/L (0.5-5.0 mIU/L)
Free T_4 = 0.23 ng/dL (0.8-1.8 ng/dL) (SI: 2.96 pmol/L [10.30-23.17 pmol/L])
Random serum cortisol = 6 µg/dL (5-25 µg/dL) (SI: 165.5 nmol/L [137.9-689.7 nmol/L])
Sodium = 135 mEq/L (136-142 mEq/L) (SI: 135 mmol/L [136-142 mmol/L])
Potassium = 3.9 mEq/L (3.5-5.0 mEq/L) (SI: 3.9 mmol/L [3.5-5.0 mmol/L])
Chloride = 101 mEq/L (96-106 mEq/L) (SI: 101 mmol/L [96-106 mmol/L])
Carbon dioxide = 31 mEq/L (22-28 mEq/L) (SI: 31 mmol/L [22-28 mmol/L])
Creatinine = 1.22 mg/dL (0.6-1.1 mg/dL) (SI: 107.8 µmol/L [53.0-97.2 µmol/L])
Calcium = 9.2 mg/dL (8.2-10.2 mg/dL) (SI: 2.3 mmol/L [2.1-2.6 mmol/L])
Magnesium = 2.4 mg/dL (1.5-2.3 mg/dL) (SI: 1.0 mmol/L [0.6-0.9 mmol/L])
Glucose = 172 mg/dL (70-99 mg/dL) (SI: 9.5 mmol/L [3.9-5.5 mmol/L])
Venous blood gas:
pH = 7.28 (7.35-7.45)
Pco_2 = 69 mm Hg (35-45 mm Hg) (SI: 9.2 kPa [4.7-6.0 kPa])
Complete blood cell count, normal
Troponin I, negative
NT-proB-type natriuretic peptide = 25 pg/mL
Urine toxicology screen, negative

Electrocardiography demonstrates a QT interval of 526 and no acute QT or T-wave changes.

Chest x-ray demonstrates bilateral pleural effusions and pulmonary edema.

In addition to prescribing broad-spectrum antibiotic therapy and evaluating for underlying infection, which of the following is the most appropriate treatment to recommend now?

A. Hydrocortisone, 100 mg intravenously, followed by levothyroxine, 300 mcg intravenously
B. Hydrocortisone, 100 mg intravenously, followed by liothyronine, 75 mcg intravenously
C. Levothyroxine, 125 mcg intravenously
D. Levothyroxine, 175 mcg orally
E. Levothyroxine, 200 mcg intravenously, and liothyronine, 10 mcg intravenously

22 A 24-year-old woman is seen in the endocrine clinic due to concerns about her behavior following a recent medication change. Six months ago, she started treatment with cabergoline for a prolactinoma that was discovered during evaluation of secondary amenorrhea and primary infertility. Pituitary MRI before treatment revealed a 6-mm microadenoma. Despite cabergoline dosage escalation to 750 mcg twice weekly, she reports continuing amenorrhea. More recently she has developed impulsive behaviors, including purchasing multiple personal electronic devices, which her partner reports to be completely out of character. She has no medical or psychiatric history of note and takes no other regular medications. She smokes 10 to 12 cigarettes daily and drinks 10 to 15 units of alcohol most weekends.

On physical examination, her blood pressure is 105/65 mm Hg and resting pulse rate is 78 beats/min and regular. Her height is 70 in (177.8 cm), and weight is 165 lb (74.8 kg) (BMI = 23.7 kg/m^2). She has normal secondary sexual characteristics. There is no galactorrhea. Visual fields are normal to confrontation.

Laboratory test results:

Prolactin = 91 ng/mL (4-30 ng/mL) (SI: 3.96 nmol/L [0.17-1.30 nmol/L])
FSH = 0.4 mIU/mL (2.0-12.0 mIU/mL [follicular]) (SI: 0.4 IU/L [2.0-12.0 IU/L])
LH = 0.3 mIU/mL (1.0-18.0 mIU/mL [follicular]) (SI: 0.3 IU/L [1.0-18.0 IU/L])
Estradiol = 25 pg/mL (10-180 pg/mL [follicular]) (SI: 91.8 pmol/L [36.7-660.8 pmol/L])
Serum cortisol (8 AM) = 16.5 µg/dL (5-25 µg/dL) (SI: 455.2 nmol/L [137.9-689.7 nmol/L])

Free T_4 = 1.4 ng/dL (0.8-1.8 ng/dL) (SI: 18.02 pmol/L [10.30-23.17 pmol/L])
TSH = 2.7 mIU/L (0.5-5.0 mIU/L)

Pituitary MRI shows no change in the appearance of the 6-mm microadenoma, which is located just to the left of midline, with minimal deviation of the infundibulum and no cavernous sinus extension.

Which of the following is the most appropriate management for this patient?

A. Reduce the cabergoline dosage to 250 mcg twice weekly
B. Stop cabergoline and refer for pituitary radiotherapy
C. Stop cabergoline and refer for pituitary surgery
D. Stop cabergoline and start bromocriptine
E. Stop cabergoline and start oral estrogen/progesterone replacement

23 A 53-year-old woman is referred for further investigation of primary aldosteronism. She was initially diagnosed with hypertension 3 years ago following a routine medical assessment. At that time, laboratory workup revealed an elevated aldosterone-to-renin ratio and mild, unprovoked, hypokalemia while taking no medications. Following discussion with her primary care physician, she declined further investigation and elected to proceed with medical therapy. However, she is now keen to explore the possibility of adrenal surgery. Her current treatment regimen is amlodipine, 10 mg daily; eplerenone, 50 mg daily; and potassium chloride, 1 tablet (containing 470 mg [12 mmol] potassium per tablet) twice daily. Her medical history is otherwise unremarkable, and there is no relevant family history.

On physical examination, her blood pressure is 148/90 mm Hg and pulse rate is 76 beats/min and regular. Her height is 68 in (172.7 cm), and weight is 194 lb (88.0 kg) (BMI = 29.5 kg/m^2). Physical examination findings are otherwise unremarkable.

Laboratory test results:

Serum potassium = 3.8 mEq/L (3.5-5.0 mEq/L) (SI 3.8 mmol/L [3.5-5.0 mmol/L])
Plasma renin activity = 0.5 ng/mL per h (0.6-4.3 ng/mL per h)
Serum aldosterone = 42.5 ng/dL (4-21 ng/dL) (SI: 1179.0 pmol/L [111-582.5 pmol/L])
Serum cortisol following 1-mg dexamethasone-suppression test = 1.2 µg/dL (SI: 33.1 nmol/L)

Unenhanced adrenal CT is shown (*see image*).

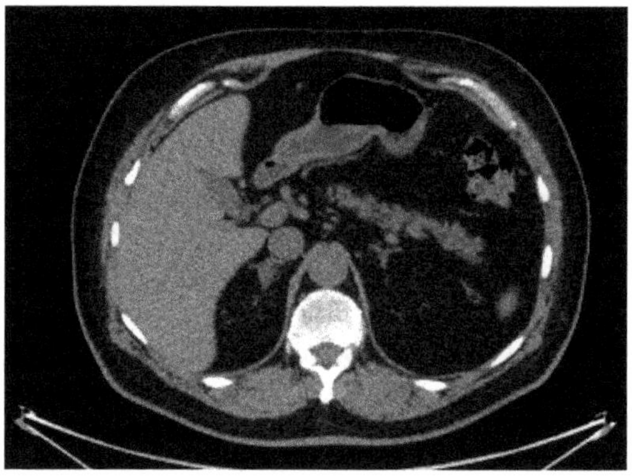

Which of the following is the most appropriate next step in this patient's management?

A. Increase dosage of eplerenone
B. Perform seated saline-suppression test
C. Proceed to adrenal vein sampling
D. Refer for right adrenalectomy
E. Switch eplerenone to doxazosin before proceeding to adrenal vein sampling

24 A 63-year-old man returns for follow-up care. He would like to ensure he is doing everything he can to remain healthy. He does not smoke cigarettes and drinks 1 to 2 alcoholic beverages per week. He follows a vegan diet and exercises 4 days per week.

On physical examination, his blood pressure is 120/68 mm Hg and BMI is 28 kg/m^2.

A recent hemoglobin A_{1c} value is 6.3% (45 mmol/mol).

This patient is at the highest risk to develop which of the following?

A. Cardiovascular disease and cognitive impairment
B. Cardiovascular disease and peripheral neuropathy
C. Chronic kidney disease and cognitive impairment
D. Diabetic retinopathy and cognitive impairment
E. Diabetic retinopathy and peripheral neuropathy

25 A 70-year-old man has been referred by his hematologist for evaluation of hot flushes. He was initially referred to hematology for unexplained normochromic anemia. Results from bone marrow aspiration and trephine biopsy are normal. He reports that over the last 6 months, he noted gradual appearance of the hot flushes, which he describes as brief episodes of "suddenly feeling hot," and his wife says that he appears flushed on occasion. Sometimes, especially overnight, these flushes are associated with drenching night sweats. He has noticed fatigue and low mood, which he attributes to sleep disturbance from hot flushes and to worries about a possible underlying undiagnosed hematological malignancy, as his hematologist is planning to repeat bone marrow biopsy in 3 months. His primary care provider recently prescribed mirtazapine to improve his sleep and low mood, but he has not found this to be helpful. His only other medication is a proton-pump inhibitor for gastroesophageal reflux disease. He takes no over-the-counter medications and has no relevant medical history.

On physical examination, his height is 67 in (170.2 cm) and weight is 170 lb (77.1 kg) (BMI = 26.6 kg/m^2). His blood pressure is 139/68 mm Hg without a postural drop, and pulse rate is 82 beats/min and regular. His thyroid gland is of normal size and has no palpable nodules. Findings on cardiopulmonary examination are normal. Body and sexual hair are normal, muscle bulk is normal, there is no gynecomastia, and testicular size is 15 mL bilaterally with no masses.

Laboratory test results:

Hemoglobin = 12.1 g/dL (13.8-17.2 g/dL) (SI: 121 g/L [138-172 g/L])
Mean corpuscular volume = 86 μm^3 (80-100 μm^3) (SI: 86 fL [80-100 fL])
White blood cell count, normal
Platelet count, normal
Electrolytes, normal
Liver function, normal
Iron studies, normal
Thyroid function, normal

CT of the chest, abdomen, and pelvis performed by his hematologist shows a 2-cm adrenal adenoma with a density of −10 Hounsfield units.

Which of the following should be measured next in this patient's evaluation?

A. 5-Hydroxyindoleacetic acid (24-hour urine collection)
B. Plasma free metanephrines
C. Serum calcitonin
D. Serum chromogranin A
E. Serum total testosterone

26 A 28-year-old man has established care with a new primary care provider. The patient has had a sensorineural hearing impairment since birth and wears hearing aids. Other history includes stage III chronic kidney disease, as he was told by his parents that he was born with an abnormal left kidney. He takes no medications, has no allergies, does not smoke cigarettes, and consumes about 5 servings of alcohol weekly. His family history is notable for his father having a hearing impairment. The patient has no siblings.

Physical examination findings include a positive Chvostek sign and normal-appearing hands. He appears phenotypically normal. His height is 69 in (175.3 cm).

Laboratory test results:

Calcium = 7.8 mg/dL (8.2-10.2 mg/dL) (SI: 2.0 mmol/L [2.1-2.6 mmol/L])
Creatinine = 1.3 mg/dL (0.7-1.3 mg/dL) (SI: 114.9 µmol/L [61.9-114.9 µmol/L])
25-Hydroxyvitamin D = 28 ng/mL (30-80 ng/mL [optimal]) (SI: 69.9 nmol/L [74.9-199.7 nmol/L])

Because of his low serum calcium concentration, the patient is referred to an endocrinologist. Further questioning reveals that he occasionally has perioral paresthesias when he vigorously exercises. He does not have cramping. He has never had a seizure, neck surgery, or neck radiation. He consumes 2 to 3 servings of dairy daily and takes a daily multivitamin.

Laboratory test results:

Calcium = 7.5 mg/dL (8.2-10.2 mg/dL) (SI: 1.9 mmol/L [2.1-2.6 mmol/L])
Albumin = 3.8 g/dL (3.5-5.0 g/dL) (SI: 38 g/L [35-50 g/L])
Intact PTH = 32 pg/mL (10-65 pg/mL) (SI: 32 ng/L [10-65 ng/L])
Creatinine = 1.4 mg/dL (0.7-1.3 mg/dL) (SI: 123.8 µmol/L [61.9-114.9 µmol/L])
Phosphate = 4.9 mg/dL (2.3-4.7 mg/dL) (SI: 0.4 mmol/L [0.7-1.5 mmol/L])
Magnesium = 1.6 mg/dL (1.5-2.3 mg/dL) (SI: 0.7 mmol/L [0.6-0.9 mmol/L])
25-Hydroxyvitamin D = 28 ng/mL (30-80 ng/mL [optimal]) (SI: 69.9 nmol/L [74.9-199.7 nmol/L])
Urinary calcium = 220 mg/24 h (100-300 mg/24 h) (SI: 5.5 mmol/d [2.5-7.5 mmol/d])

This patient is most like to have a pathogenic variant in which of the following genes?

A. *GATA3* (GATA binding protein 3)
B. *GNA11* (G protein subunit alpha 11)
C. *GNAS* (GNAS complex locus)
D. *RET* (ret proto-oncogene)
E. *TBX1* (T-box transcription factor 1)

27 A 58-year-old man is seen for optimization of lipid-lowering therapy after recent angioplasty and stent placement. He underwent coronary artery bypass surgery at age 52 years following an ST-elevation myocardial infarction. He has been experiencing exertional angina for the last year, and angiography shows recurrent graft stenosis. He does not have diabetes and quit cigarette smoking after his heart attack. Family history is relevant for myocardial infarction in his father at age 55 years. His current medications are atorvastatin, 80 mg daily; ezetimibe, 10 mg daily; evolocumab, 140 mg every 2 weeks; metoprolol; aspirin; and clopidogrel. He avoids high-fat foods and limits intake of refined sugar, but he has limited physical activity because of angina.

On physical examination, his height is 73 in (185.4 cm) and weight is 167 lb (75.7 kg) (BMI = 22 kg/m^2). He has a faint corneal arcus but no tendon xanthomas.

Fasting lipid panel:

Total cholesterol = 122 mg/dL (<200 mg/dL) (SI: 3.16 mmol/L [<5.18 mmol/L])
Triglycerides = 90 mg/dL (<150 mg/dL) (SI: 1.02 mmol/L [<1.70 mmol/L])
HDL cholesterol = 38 mg/dL (>60 mg/dL) (SI: 0.98 mmol/L [>1.55 mmol/L])
LDL cholesterol = 66 mg/dL (<100 mg/dL) (SI: 1.71 mmol/L [<2.59 mmol/L])

Before recommending any treatment changes for further cardiovascular risk reduction, which of the following would be beneficial to measure?

A. Apolipoprotein B
B. High-sensitivity C-reactive protein
C. LDL particle number by nuclear magnetic resonance
D. Lipoprotein (a)
E. Plasma phytosterol

28 A 32-year-old woman (G1P0) presents for routine antenatal care. She has a paternal aunt with primary hypothyroidism and a maternal cousin with type 1 diabetes mellitus. She underwent a 2-step approach for gestational diabetes mellitus screening, and the results are shown (*see table*).

Test	Fasting glucose	1-Hour glucose	2-Hour glucose	3-Hour glucose
50-g glucose	...	143 mg/dL (SI: 7.9 mmol/L)	...	...
100-g glucose	96 mg/dL (SI: 5.3 mmol/L)	191 mg/dL (SI: 10.6 mmol/L)	166 mg/dL (SI: 9.2 mmol/L)	139 mg/dL (SI: 7.7 mmol/L)

This patient's child is at greatest risk to develop which of the following?

A. Chronic kidney disease
B. Delayed puberty
C. Metabolic syndrome
D. Primary hypothyroidism
E. Type 1 diabetes mellitus

29 A 19-year-old woman with type 1 diabetes mellitus presents for a follow-up appointment. She also has hypothyroidism and anxiety. Type 1 diabetes was diagnosed at age 9 years when she experienced polyuria and polydipsia. She has been on insulin pump therapy for 10 years. Other medications include levothyroxine, 100 mcg daily, a combined estrogen-progestin oral contraceptive, and a multivitamin. She is a freshman collegiate tennis player. She reports ongoing fatigue, which she attributes to her highly demanding training and academic schedules. She has lost 5 lb (2.3 kg) over the past 6 months.

On physical examination, her blood pressure is 100/65 mm Hg and pulse rate is 98 beats/min. Her height is 64 in (162.6 cm), and weight is 110 lb (49.9 kg) (BMI = 18.9 kg/m^2). She has no proptosis, lid lag, or chemosis. Her skin is tan, without plethora, striae, rashes, or bruises. Her neck is supple, and her thyroid gland is small, without palpable nodules. No lymphadenopathy is present. There is no tremor of her outstretched hands. Her chest is clear to auscultation bilaterally. Her heart has a regular rhythm, without murmurs. Her lower extremities are warm, without edema. She has no focal abnormalities on neurologic examination.

Laboratory test results:

Complete blood cell count, normal
Metabolic panel, normal
Hemoglobin A_{1c} = 7.1% (4.0%-5.6%) (54 mmol/mol [20-38 mmol/mol])
TSH = 3.1 mIU/L (0.5- 5.0 mIU/L)
Serum cortisol (8 AM) = 10 µg/dL (5-25 µg/dL) (SI: 275.9 nmol/L [137.9-689.7 nmol/L])

Which of the following is the best next step in this patient's management?

A. Increase the levothyroxine dosage to 112 mcg daily
B. Measure free T_4
C. Measure plasma ACTH
D. Screen for celiac disease
E. Screen for depression

30 A 60-year-old man with a 20-year history of type 2 diabetes mellitus presents for a follow-up appointment. His outpatient regimen consists of insulin glargine, 25 units daily, and insulin aspart, 7 units with each meal. He also takes insulin aspart as correctional support with 1 unit for every 50 mg/dL (2.8 mmol/L) above 150 mg/dL (>8.3 mmol/L), targeting glucose values of 100 mg/dL (5.6 mmol/L). His medical history is notable for chronic kidney disease stage G3b, advanced liver cirrhosis, hypertension, dyslipidemia, diabetic neuropathy, and diabetic retinopathy.

Laboratory test results:

Hematocrit = 37.2% (41%-51%) (SI: 0.372 [0.41-0.51])
Hemoglobin = 10.6 g/dL (13.8-17.2 g/dL) (SI: 106 g/L [138-172 g/L])
Creatinine = 1.7 mg/dL (0.7-1.3 mg/dL) (SI: 150.3 μmol/L [61.9-114.9 μmol/L])
Albumin = 2.9 g/dL (3.5-5.0 g/dL) (SI: 29 g/L [35-50 g/L])
Hemoglobin A_{1c} = 9.1% (4.0%-5.6%) (SI: 76 mmol/mol [20-38 mmol/mol])

The patient did not bring his glucose meter to the office visit. However, he reports that his point-of-care glucose measurements range from 90 to 140 mg/dL (5.0-7.8 mmol/L). Due to the discrepancy between the glucose values and his hemoglobin A_{1c} value, fructosamine is measured, and the following concentration is reported: 4.8 mg/dL (3.2-5.0 mg/dL) (SI: 265 mmol/L [175-280 mmol/L]).

Which of the following is the best next step in this patient's management?

A. Increase the basal insulin glargine dosage
B. Initiate empagliflozin
C. Initiate semaglutide
D. Proceed with continuous glucose monitoring evaluation
E. Reduce the basal insulin glargine dosage

31

A 32-year-old woman (G2P1) at 10 weeks' gestation presents for management of Graves disease, which was diagnosed prior to this pregnancy. She takes propylthiouracil, 100 mg twice daily, and a daily prenatal vitamin. She feels tired but has no other concerns. She has no Graves orbitopathy or dermopathy. Her mother has rheumatoid arthritis and takes methotrexate and folic acid.

On physical examination, her blood pressure is 120/60 mm Hg and pulse rate is 100 beats/min and regular. Her thyroid gland is 40 g with no nodularity. Her abdomen is gravid and soft. There is no hand tremor or leg edema.

Laboratory test results:

TSH = 0.5 mIU/L (0.5-5.0 mIU/L)
Total T_4 = 9.2 μg/dL (5.5-12.5 μg/dL) (SI: 118.40 nmol/L [94.02-213.68 nmol/L])
Total T_3 = 140 ng/dL (70-200 ng/dL) (SI: 2.16 nmol/L [1.08-3.08 nmol/L])

Which of the following is the best next step in this patient's management?

A. Continue the current propylthiouracil dosage
B. Discontinue propylthiouracil
C. Increase the propylthiouracil dosage
D. Measure thyroid-stimulating immunoglobulin
E. Perform thyroid ultrasonography

32

A 39-year-old woman presents to discuss weight management. She reports weighing 160 lb (72.7 kg) at age 18 years. Her maximum adult weight was 240 lb (109.1 kg) at age 28 years. She has lost weight with calorie restriction, accompanied by careful tracking of her food intake and a structured physical activity regimen. However, over the past few months, she has gained weight and acknowledges that she is not always able to fully adhere to lifestyle changes because of time constraints.

She has steatohepatitis based on MRI with elastography that showed a stiffness reading equivalent to stage 3 to 4 fibrosis (early cirrhosis). Polycystic ovary syndrome has also been diagnosed; however, fertility is not a goal at this time. She has Barrett esophagus under active surveillance and takes a proton-pump inhibitor daily. Her current medications are metformin, 1000 mg twice daily; spironolactone, 100 mg daily; and pantoprazole, 40 mg twice daily.

On physical examination, her blood pressure is 128/72 mm Hg and pulse rate is 82 beats/min. Her height is 66.1 in (167.9 cm), and weight is 200 lb (90.9 kg) (BMI = 32.2 kg/m^2). She has symmetric weight distribution between her upper and lower body. Her abdomen is soft, and there are no stigmata of chronic liver disease.

Laboratory test results:
Serum triglycerides = 482 mg/dL (<150 mg/dL) (SI: 5.45 mmol/L [<1.70 mmol/L])
Hemoglobin A_{1c} = 5.0% (4.0%-5.6%) (31 mmol/mol [20-38 mmol/mol])

Which of the following is the best next step in this patient's management?

A. Recommend a ketogenic or very low-carbohydrate diet
B. Recommend a Mediterranean-style diet, minimizing simple carbohydrates
C. Refer for sleeve gastrectomy
D. Start phentermine/topiramate, 3.75/23 mg daily
E. Start pioglitazone, 30 mg daily

33

A 35-year-old woman is seen for hypocalcemia, hypothyroidism, and hypogonadism. Hypocalcemia was diagnosed at age 8 years after she had a seizure. In infancy, multiple small subcutaneous calcifications were noted in her scalp and other locations, and she has short metacarpals. She recently had a calcified lesion removed from behind her knee because of pain and limitations in joint movement. Pathologic examination demonstrated focal osseus metaplasia. She currently has no symptoms of hypocalcemia and has no history of kidney stones. Kidney ultrasonography shows no nephrocalcinosis.

Her mother also has multiple small subcutaneous calcifications, but her serum calcium and PTH concentrations are within their respective reference ranges.

The patient's current medications are calcitriol, 0.25 mcg twice daily; calcium carbonate, 1000 mg twice daily; cholecalciferol, 1000 IU daily; levothyroxine, 137 mcg daily; and ethinyl estradiol with levonorgestrel daily.

Laboratory test results:
Calcium = 8.8 mg/dL (8.2-10.2 mg/dL) (SI: 2.2 mmol/L [2.1-2.6 mmol/L])
Albumin = 3.9 g/dL (3.5-5.0 g/dL) (SI: 39 g/L [35-50 g/L])
Creatinine = 0.72 mg/dL (0.6-1.1 mg/dL) (SI 63.6 μmol/L [53-97.2 μmol/L])
Alkaline phosphatase = 52 U/L (50-120 U/L) (SI: 0.87 μkat/L [0.84-2.00 μkat/L])
Intact PTH = 440 pg/mL (10-65 pg/mL) (SI: 440 ng/L [10-65 ng/L])
25-Hydroxyvitamin D = 29 ng/mL (30-80 ng/mL [optimal]) (SI: 72.4 nmol/L [74.9-199.7 nmol/L])
Phosphate = 4.2 mg/dL (2.3-4.7 mg/dL) (SI: 1.4 mmol/L [0.7-1.5 mmol/L])
Magnesium = 2.1 mg/dL (1.5-2.3 mg/dL) (SI: 0.86 mmol/L [0.6-0.9 mmol/L])
TSH = 0.56 mIU/L (0.5-5.0 mIU/L)
Urinary calcium = 64 mg/24 h (100-300 mg/24 h) (SI: 1.6 mmol/d [2.5-7.5 mmol/d])

Which of the following is the best next step in this patient's management?

A. Add a thiazide diuretic
B. Decrease the calcium dosage
C. Increase the calcitriol dosage
D. Perform parathyroidectomy with multigland resection
E. Recommend no change in any medication dosages

34

A 40-year-old woman (G2P2) presents for evaluation of oligomenorrhea. Menses were regular until 2 years ago. Review of systems is notable for fatigue, weight gain, and increased perspiration. She underwent bilateral carpal tunnel release 3 years ago. Her medical history is otherwise unremarkable.

On physical examination, her blood pressure is 140/89 mm Hg and pulse rate is 90 beats/min. Her height is 65 in (165.1 cm), and weight is 181 lb (82.1 kg) (BMI = 30.1 kg/m^2). Mild hirsutism is present on her chin. There are no striae and no increased supraclavicular fat deposits.

The patient does not desire another pregnancy. Findings on a recent pelvic examination are normal.

Laboratory test results:

TSH = 2.0 mIU/L (0.5-0.5 mIU/L)
Prolactin = 40 ng/mL (4-30 ng/mL) (SI: 1.74 nmol/L [0.17-1.30 nmol/L])
FSH = 5.0 mIU/mL (2.0-12.0 mIU/mL) (SI: 5.0 IU/L [2.0-12.0 IU/L])
LH = 8.0 mIU/mL (1.0-18.0 mIU/mL) (SI: 8.0 IU/L [1.0-18.0 IU/L])
Testosterone = 42 ng/dL (8-60 ng/dL) (SI: 1.5 nmol/L [0.3-2.1 nmol/L])
Estradiol = 78 pg/mL (SI: 286.4 pmol/L)

Which of the following is the best next step in this patient's management?

A. Measure IGF-1
B. Measure morning fasting prolactin again; if normal, recommend no further endocrine workup
C. Perform ovarian ultrasonography
D. Perform pituitary-directed MRI
E. Start a combined oral contraceptive pill

35

A 32-year-old man with classic congenital adrenal hyperplasia due to 21-hydroxylase deficiency presents for evaluation of infertility. He has been married for 3 years, but he and his wife have been unsuccessful in conceiving a child. His wife has regular periods, and she has a child from a previous marriage. The patient reports feeling well, and his medical history is otherwise unremarkable. He is physically active. He takes hydrocortisone, 10 mg in the morning and 5 mg at 2 PM; prednisolone, 1 mg at bedtime; and fludrocortisone, 0.1 mg daily.

On physical examination, his blood pressure is 102/75 mm Hg and pulse rate is 90 beats/min. His height is 67 in (170.2 cm), and weight is 187 lb (84.8 kg) (BMI = 29.3 kg/m^2). He is well virilized and muscular. His skin is warm, dry, and tan, without plethora, striae, or bruises. His testes are firm and heterogeneous, with a volume of 26 mL bilaterally.

Laboratory test results (sample collected at 8 AM):

Complete blood cell count, normal
Metabolic panel, normal
Hemoglobin A_{1c} = 5.3% (4.0%-5.6%) (34 mmol/mol [20-38 mmol/mol])
TSH = 2.6 mIU/L (0.5-5.0 mIU/L)
Free T_4 = 1.1 ng/dL (0.8-1.8 ng/dL) (SI: 14.2 pmol/L [10.30-23.17 pmol/L])
Total testosterone = 703 ng/dL (300-900 ng/dL) (SI: 24.4 nmol/L [10.4-31.2 nmol/L])

Which of the following is the best next step in this patient's management?

A. Measure gonadotropins and order semen analysis
B. Measure 17-hydroxyprogesterone
C. Perform abdominal MRI
D. Perform testicular ultrasonography
E. Recommend infertility evaluation for his wife

36

A 34-year-old man presents for evaluation of type 2 diabetes mellitus. Diabetes was diagnosed at age 30 years, and he is currently treated with metformin, glimepiride, and pioglitazone. His hemoglobin A_{1c} value is 7.5% (58 mmol/mol), and he does not report any hypoglycemia. He has no evidence of retinopathy or neuropathy. He otherwise feels well and has no relevant cardiovascular history. Multiple family members have type 2 diabetes and chronic kidney disease.

On physical examination, his blood pressure is 135/88 mm Hg and BMI is 31 kg/m^2. His laboratory data over the last 5 years are shown (*see table*).

Measurement	At diagnosis	1 Year after diagnosis	2 Years after diagnosis	3-Years after diagnosis	Present
Hemoglobin A_{1c}	10.0% (86 mmol/mol)	6.5% (48 mmol/mol)	8.2% (66 mmol/mol)	7.9% (63 mmol/mol)	7.5% (58 mmol/mol)
Estimated glomerular filtration rate	61 mL/min per 1.73 m^2	55 mL/min per 1.73 m^2	48 mL/min per 1.73 m^2	40 mL/min per 1.73 m^2	34 mL/min per 1.73 m^2
Urine albumin-to-creatinine ratio	28 mg/g creat	32 mg/g creat	31 mg/g creat	38 mg/g creat	45 mg/g creat
Urinalysis	Negative for white blood cells, red blood cells, bacteria, epithelial cells, casts, and crystals				

Which of the following best explains this patient's kidney function?

A. Genetic predisposition
B. Heart failure
C. Metformin toxicity
D. Suboptimal glycemic control
E. Undiagnosed hypertension

37 A 68-year-old woman with interstitial lung disease received a lung transplant 1 year ago. She has a long history of glucocorticoid treatment. Other medical history includes deep vein thrombosis, pulmonary embolus, hypertension, moderate gastroesophageal reflux, hiatal hernia, and stage 3 chronic kidney disease. She has lost 2 in (5.1 cm) in height. Before lung transplant, she had a right femoral neck stress fracture treated surgically, as well as a toe fracture.

Recent DXA (1 year after lung transplant) indicates a lumbar spine T-score of –2.1, left total hip T-score of –3.1, and left femoral neck T-score of –2.3. Recent chest x-ray identified new moderate compression fractures at T11 and T12.

Current medications include prednisone, 5 mg daily; tacrolimus, 2 mg daily; calcium citrate, 700 mg twice daily; cholecalciferol, 1000 units daily; and furosemide, 20 mg daily.

Laboratory test results:

Calcium = 9.7 mg/dL (8.2-10.2 mg/dL) (SI: 2.4 mmol/L [2.1-2.6 mmol/L])
Albumin = 4.4 g/dL (3.5-5.0 g/dL) (SI: 44 g/L [35-50 g/L])
Creatinine = 1.3 mg/dL (0.6-1.1 mg/dL) (SI: 137.0 μmol/L [53-97.2 μmol/L])
Estimated glomerular filtration rate = 40 mL/min per 1.73 m^2 (>60 mL/min per 1.73 m^2)
Alkaline phosphatase = 114 U/L (50-120 U/L) (SI: 1.90 μkat/L [0.84-2.00 μkat/L])
Intact PTH = 54 pg/mL (10-65 pg/mL) (SI: 54 ng/L [10-65 ng/L])
25-Hydroxyvitamin D = 45 ng/mL (30-80 ng/mL [optimal]) (SI: 112.3 nmol/L [74.9-199.7 nmol/L])
Phosphate = 2.7 mg/dL (2.3-4.7 mg/dL) (SI: 0.9 mmol/L [0.7-1.5 mmol/L])
Magnesium = 1.8 mg/dL (1.5-2.3 mg/dL) (SI: 0.7 mmol/L [0.6-0.9 mmol/L])
TSH = 1.3 mIU/L (0.5-5.0 mIU/L)
Urinary calcium-to-creatinine ratio = 0.08 mg/mg (<0.22 mg/mg) (SI: 0.22 mmol/mmol [<0.6 mmol/mmol])

Which of the following is the best next management step for this patient?

A. Anabolic therapy with a PTH receptor agonist
B. Calcitonin
C. Oral bisphosphonate therapy
D. Reduction in the glucocorticoid dosage
E. Resistance exercises

38 A 34-year-old woman is referred for endocrine evaluation following identification of a sellar mass on MRI performed by her neurologist for investigation of headaches. She describes retro-orbital headaches most days, which have become more troublesome over the last 3 months. There are no associated visual aura or focal neurological features. Her medical history is otherwise unremarkable. She has a monthly withdrawal bleed on her current combined oral contraceptive preparation. She does not take any other medications or over-the-counter preparations.

On physical examination, her blood pressure is 150/92 mm Hg and pulse rate is 75 beats/min. Her height is 69 in (175.3 cm), and weight is 201 lb (91.2 kg) (BMI = 29.7 kg/m^2).

Laboratory test results:

Prolactin = 24 ng/mL (4-30 ng/mL) (SI: 1.04 nmol/L [0.17-1.30 nmol/L])
TSH = 1.21 mIU/L (0.5-5.0 mIU/L)
Free T_4 = 1.15 ng/dL (0.8-1.8 ng/dL) (SI: 14.8 pmol/L [10.30-23.17 pmol/L])
Cortisol (8 AM) = 23.6 µg/dL (5-25 µg/dL) (SI: 651.1 nmol/L [137.9-689.7 nmol/L])
Cortisol following 1-mg dexamethasone-suppression test = 6.1 µg/dL (SI: 168.3 nmol/L)
IGF-1 = 275 ng/mL (106-277 ng/mL) (SI: 36.0 nmol/L [13.9-36.3 nmol/L])
FSH = <0.3 mIU/mL (2.0-12.0 mIU/mL) (SI: <0.3 IU/L [2.0-12.0 IU/L])
LH = <0.3 mIU/mL (1.0-18.0 mIU/mL) (SI: <0.3 IU/L [1.0-18.0 IU/L])

MRI of the sella is shown (*see images*).

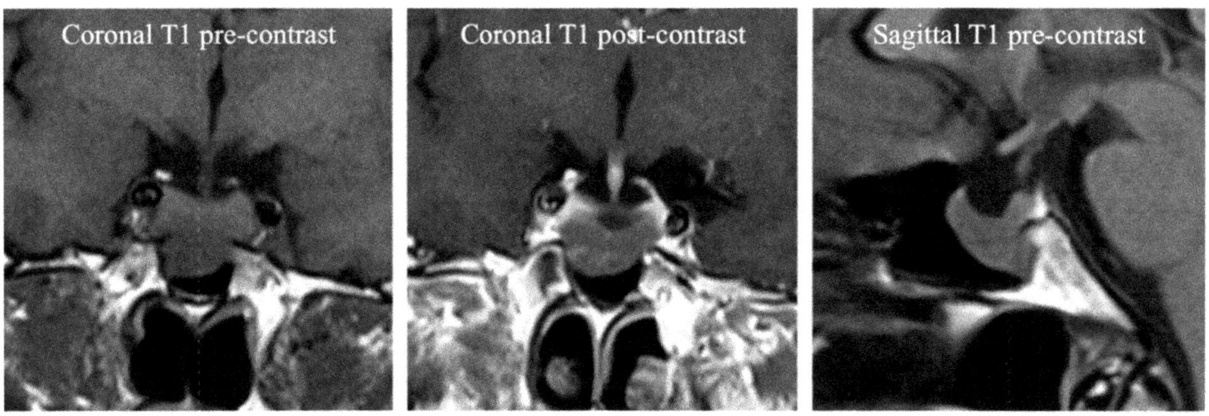

Which of the following investigations is most likely to confirm this patient's underlying diagnosis?

A. Bilateral inferior petrosal sinus sampling
B. Late-night salivary cortisol measurement
C. Oral glucose tolerance test with serum GH measurement
D. Serum cortisol measurement following 48-hour (0.5 mg every 6 hours) dexamethasone-suppression test
E. Serum prolactin measured in dilution

39 A 68-year-old woman with a history of type 2 diabetes mellitus presents to the diabetes clinic for evaluation and management of hyperglycemia. She was previously treated with a basal-bolus insulin regimen. Her insulin regimen was discontinued 6 months ago by her last medical provider because she developed worsening kidney failure and her glycemic control was becoming "very tight." She regularly undergoes hemodialysis and takes no medications for diabetes management. She describes a history of treatment nonadherence. Her medical history is notable for hypertension, dyslipidemia, diabetic neuropathy, and diabetic retinopathy.

Download from her glucose meter shows that she checks glucose values 2 to 3 times daily. Her average 90-day glucose value is 182 mg/dL (10.1 mmol/L). Her hemoglobin A_{1c} measurement is 8.0% (63 mmol/mol).

On physical examination, her height is 64 in (162.6 cm) and weight is 125 lb (56.7 kg) (BMI = 21.5 kg/m^2).

Which of the following medications should be initiated as the best next step in this patient's management?

A. Basal-bolus insulin
B. Empagliflozin
C. Linagliptin
D. Semaglutide
E. No medication (her glycemic control is on target)

40 A 52-year-old man with a history of infertility is referred to determine whether testosterone therapy is still indicated. He started testosterone treatment 20 years ago, and in recent years, his regimen has consisted of testosterone enanthate, 200 mg intramuscularly monthly. He thinks his pubertal development might have been "a little behind the other boys." He has no history of orchitis, testicular trauma, or head trauma. He had an ST-elevation myocardial infarction 5 months ago, with placement of a drug-eluting stent to the left anterior descending artery. He is adopted and is unfamiliar with his family history. He has never smoked cigarettes. He does not have hypertension, and his lipid panel results are unremarkable. His cardiologist stopped testosterone treatment and referred the patient for endocrine consultation. His current medications are aspirin, clopidogrel, metoprolol, and atorvastatin. His wife conceived 1 son (now 21 years old) with donor sperm, and the patient has no plans for future paternity.

Laboratory test results 4 months after stopping testosterone treatment:

Total testosterone = 100 ng/dL (300-900 ng/dL) (SI: 3.5 nmol/L [10.4-31.2 nmol/L])
LH = 30.0 mIU/mL (1.0-9.0 mIU/mL) (SI: 30.0 IU/L [1.0-9.0 IU/L])
FSH = 30.0 mIU/mL (1.0-13.0 mIU/mL) (SI: 30.0 IU/L [1.0-13.0 IU/L])

Test results 1 month later:

Testosterone = 80 ng/dL (SI: 2.8 nmol/L)
LH = 38.0 mIU/mL (SI: 38.0 IU/L)
Karyotype = 46,XY
Hemoglobin = 12.5 g/dL (13.8-17.2 g/dL) (SI: 125 g/L [138-172 g/L])
25-Hydroxyvitamin D = 24 ng/mL (30-80 ng/mL [optimal]) (SI: 59.9 nmol/L [74.9-199.7 nmol/L])

On physical examination, his blood pressure is 120/70 mm Hg and pulse rate is 58 beats/min and regular. His height is 70 in (177.8 cm), and weight is 172 lb (78 kg) (BMI = 24.6 kg/m^2). There is no gynecomastia. Body hair and muscle bulk are mildly reduced. Pubic hair is normal. Testes are 4 mL bilaterally and soft to palpation, with no masses.

Since his myocardial infarction, he has had worsening fatigue, low libido, and erectile dysfunction. Muscle weakness has been noted during cardiac rehabilitation. DXA documents osteopenia, with his lowest T-score being −2.3 at the lumbar spine.

Which of the following medications should be started as the best next step in this patient's management?

A. Aromatase inhibitor
B. Cholecalciferol
C. Clomiphene
D. Phosphodiesterase-5 inhibitor
E. Topical testosterone replacement

41 A 22-year-old man is referred for evaluation of hypertension. Two years ago, his blood pressure was documented to be elevated (181/92 mm Hg) during an annual visit with his primary care physician. Since then, he has been prescribed several antihypertensive agents. He currently takes lisinopril, 20 mg daily; amlodipine, 10 mg daily; and labetalol, 200 mg twice daily. Hydrochlorothiazide was stopped recently after he was found to have severe hypokalemia.

Laboratory test results (sample drawn at a recent afternoon office visit with his primary care physician):

Direct renin mass = <2 pg/mL (4-44 pg/mL) (SI: <0.05 pmol/L [0.1-1.0 pmol/L])
Plasma aldosterone = 7 ng/dL (4-21 ng/dL) (SI: 194.2 pmol/L [111.0-582.5 pmol/L])
Serum potassium = 3.7 mEq/L (3.5-5.0 mEq/L) (SI: 3.7 mmol/L [3.5-5.0 mmol/L])

On physical examination, his blood pressure is 172/90 mm Hg, and pulse rate is 76 beats/min. His height is 71 in (180.3 cm), and weight is 250 lb (113.4 kg) (BMI = 34.9 kg/m^2). He has normal facies, no dorsocervical adiposity, and no supraclavicular fullness. He has a few thin, pale striae on his thighs, but no plethora or bruises. Findings on cardiovascular and respiratory examination are unremarkable. He has no edema. Findings on neurologic examination are normal. His muscle strength is 5/5 throughout and is symmetric.

Laboratory test results (sample drawn at 8 AM):

Serum potassium = 3.6 mEq/L (3.5-5.0 mEq/L) (SI: 3.6 mmol/L [3.5-5.0 mmol/L])
Serum sodium = 138 mEq/L (136-142 mEq/L) (SI: 138 mmol/L [136-142 mmol/L])
Serum creatinine = 1.0 mg/dL (0.7-1.3 mg/dL) (SI: 88.4 µmol/L [61.9-114.9 µmol/L])
Aldosterone = 27 ng/dL (4-21 ng/dL) (SI: 749.0 pmol/L [111.0-582.5 pmol/L])
Direct renin mass concentration = <2 pg/mL (4-44 pg/mL) (SI: <0.05 pmol/L [0.1-1.0 pmol/L])
ACTH = 14 pg/mL (10-60 pg/mL) (SI: 3.1 pmol/L [2.2-13.2 pmol/L])
Cortisol = 12 µg/dL (5-25 µg/dL) (SI: 331.1 nmol/L [137.9-689.7 nmol/L])

Which of the following tests would be best to confirm this patient's suspected diagnosis?

A. Captopril challenge test
B. Dexamethasone-suppression test
C. Genetic testing
D. 24-Hour urinary cortisol measurement
E. Oral salt-loading test

42 A 26-year-old woman (G0P0) is referred for evaluation of secondary amenorrhea. Menarche was at age 14 years, and she reports that her menses were irregular from the outset with cycles occurring unpredictably every 4 to 8 weeks. She typically experienced moderate to severe abdominal cramping and acne flares with her menses. To help regulate her menstrual cycle, combined hormonal contraception was prescribed and she has been on that regimen for 5 years. She reports that her symptoms of abdominal cramping and acne resolved, and she was experiencing menses every 28 days. However, 7 months ago, she discontinued combined hormonal contraception because she was no longer sexually active. She has not had a menstrual cycle since.

She has no virilization, new terminal hair growth, clitoromegaly, headaches, vision changes, galactorrhea, change in thirst or urination pattern, nausea or emesis, skin hyperpigmentation, central obesity, violaceous striae, or dorsocervical fat pad. There is no family history of fertility issues or autoimmune diseases.

She reports feeling very stressed about graduate school and shares that she watches her carbohydrate, fat, and protein intake. She describes daily physical activity consisting of running 30 to 60 minutes and using resistance bands and lifting weights for 1.5 hours. She states she does not binge and purge and that she has no history of an eating disorder. Her maximum weight was 143.3 lb (65 kg) 3 years ago.

On physical examination, her blood pressure is 109/68 mm Hg and pulse rate is 61 beats/min. Her height is 65 in (165.1 cm), and weight is 114.5 lb (52 kg) (BMI = 19.1 kg/m^2). She has no thyromegaly. Visual fields are full to confrontation. She has no violaceous striae, dorsocervical or supraclavicular fat pads, hirsutism, acne, hyperpigmentation of oral mucosa, or surgical scars.

Laboratory test results:

Complete blood cell count, normal
Complete metabolic panel, normal
Erythrocyte sedimentation rate, normal
TSH = 3.87 mIU/L (0.5-5.0 mIU/L)
Free T_4 = 0.95 ng/dL (0.8-1.8 ng/dL) (SI: 12.2 pmol/L [10.30-23.17 pmol/L])

FSH = 6.1 mIU/mL (2.0-12.0 mIU/mL [follicular]) (SI: 6.1 IU/L [2.0-12.0 IU/L])
LH = 1.2 mIU/mL (1.0-18.0 mIU/mL [follicular]) (SI: 1.2 mIU/mL [1.0-18.0 mIU/mL])
Estradiol = 33 pg/mL (10-180 pg/mL [follicular]) (SI: 121.1 pmol/L [26.7-660.8 pmol/L])
Prolactin = 7.9 ng/mL (4-30 ng/mL [nonlactating female]) (SI: 0.34 nmol/L [0.17-1.30 nmol/L])
Serum cortisol (8 AM) = 16.4 µg/dL (5-25 µg/dL) (SI: 452.4 nmol/L [137.9-689.7 nmol/L])
ACTH = 30.6 pg/mL (10-60 pg/mL) (SI: 452.4 pmol/L [2.2-13.2 pmol/L])
β-hCG = <1.0 mIU/mL (<3.0 mIU/mL) (SI: <1.0 IU/L [<3.0 IU/L])
Celiac disease screen, negative
17-Hydroxyprogesterone = 48 ng/dL (<80 ng/dL [follicular]) (SI: 1.45 nmol/L [<2.42 nmol/L])
Total testosterone = 26 ng/dL (8-60 ng/dL) (SI: 0.90 nmol/L [0.3-2.1 nmol/L])
Antimullerian hormone = 6.8 ng/mL (0.9-9.5 ng/mL) (SI: 48.6 pmol/L [6.4-67.9 pmol/L])

A 7-day progestin withdrawal challenge with medroxyprogesterone acetate does not induce a menstrual bleed. Pelvic ultrasonography shows mild polycystic ovarian morphology, but findings are otherwise normal.

Which of the following is the most likely explanation for this patient's secondary amenorrhea?

A. Functional hypothalamic amenorrhea
B. Pituitary adenoma
C. Polycystic ovary syndrome
D. Primary ovarian insufficiency
E. Uterine outflow tract obstruction

43

A 58-year-old man returns for continued management of latent autoimmune diabetes of adulthood. He is insulin-dependent and is currently on a basal-bolus treatment regimen. He takes lispro-aabc, 3 units at meals, and insulin glargine, 8 units at bedtime. His hemoglobin A_{1c} values have consistently been around 9.0% (75 mmol/mol). He has a history of psychosis for which he takes a dopamine antagonist (quetiapine) at 8 PM daily. His glycemic control is fair during the day and at bedtime, but blood glucose concentrations rise considerably throughout the night while he sleeps. His morning blood glucose values are often 250 mg/dL or higher (≥13.9 mmol/L), requiring a correction dose of lispro-aabc. He brings his continuous glucose monitor for download (*see image*).

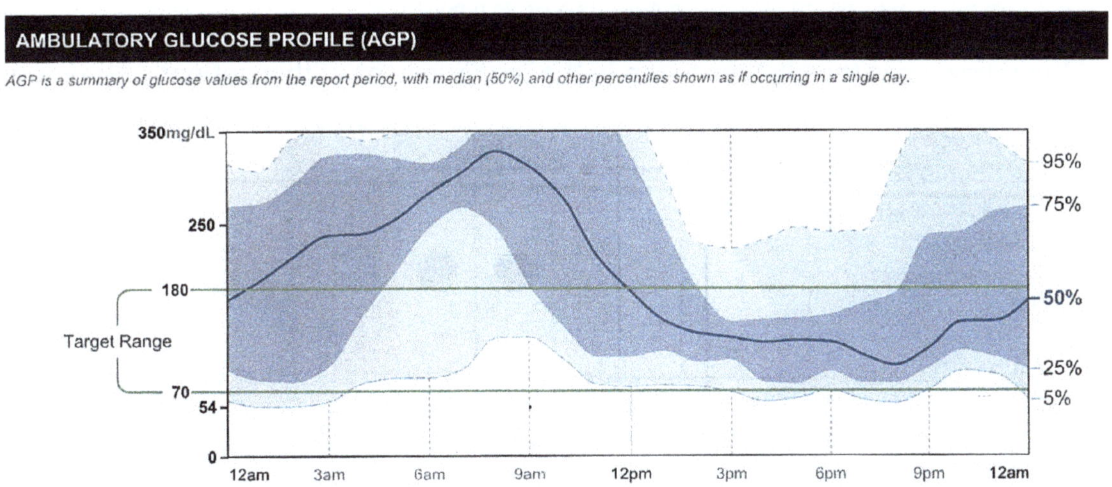

On physical examination, his blood pressure is 118/72 mm Hg and pulse rate is 68 beats/min. His height is 70 in (177.8 cm), and weight is 155 lb (70.3 kg) (BMI = 22.2 kg/m²). No lipohypertrophy is noted at the usual sites of insulin administration.

Laboratory test results:

Electrolytes, normal
Creatinine = 1.3 mg/dL (0.7-1.3 mg/dL) (SI: 114.9 µmol/L [61.9-114.9 µmol/L])
Hemoglobin A_{1c} = 9.1% (4.0%-5.6%) (76 mmol/mol [20-38 mmol/mol])
Glutamic acid decarboxylase 65 antibodies, detectable
C-peptide, undetectable
Glucose = 187 mg/dL (70-99 mg/dL) (SI: 10.4 mmol/L [3.9-5.5 mmol/L])

Which of the following interventions is the best next step in this patient's management?

A. Administer a dose of insulin lispro-aabc at bedtime
B. Administer a dose of NPH insulin at bedtime and continue insulin glargine
C. Administer a dose of NPH insulin at bedtime and stop insulin glargine
D. Increase the dosage of insulin glargine
E. Start glipizide extended release

44 A 62-year-old man with a history of type 2 diabetes mellitus, hypertension, dyslipidemia, and gastroesophageal reflux is admitted to the hospital with congestive heart failure. He has been tired and short of breath with minimal exertion for the last 3 months. His home medications include metformin, degludec, sitagliptin, atorvastatin, losartan, amlodipine, and omeprazole. He is being treated with furosemide during this admission.

On physical examination, his blood pressure is 149/82 mm Hg and pulse rate is 90 beats/min. His height is 67 in (170.2 cm), and weight is 205 lb (93.0 kg) (BMI = 32.1 kg/m²). His thyroid gland is not palpable. There are bibasilar crackles with wheezing. His heart is regular in rate and rhythm. There is 2+ pitting leg edema.

Laboratory test results:

Sodium = 135 mEq/L (136-142 mEq/L) (SI: 135 mmol/L [136-142 mmol/L])
Potassium = 3.2 mEq/L (3.5-5.0 mEq/L) (SI: 3.2 mmol/L [3.5-5.0 mmol/L])
Creatinine = 1.96 mg/dL (0.7-1.3 mg/dL) (SI: 173.3 µmol/L [61.9-114.9 µmol/L])
TSH = 0.30 mIU/L (0.5-5.0 mIU/L)
Free T_4 = 0.70 ng/dL (0.8-1.8 ng/dL) (SI: 9.0 pmol/L [10.30-23.17 pmol/L])
Free T_3 = 2.1 pg/mL (2.3-4.2 pg/mL) (SI: 3.22 pmol/L [3.53-6.45 pmol/L])

Which of the following is the best next step in the management of this patient's abnormal thyroid function test results?

A. Perform pituitary MRI
B. Perform thyroid laboratory tests in 3 months
C. Perform thyroid ultrasonography
D. Start levothyroxine
E. Start liothyronine

45 A 44-year-old woman presents for evaluation of abnormal results following routine bloodwork. After undergoing Roux-en-Y gastric bypass approximately 10 years ago, she lost about 40% of her body weight, eventually reaching a nadir weight of 150 lb (75 kg). She maintained that weight for several years. However, following an accident and consequent orthopedic injuries, she has gained some weight due to less physical activity.

She currently takes 5000 units of ergocalciferol daily, an iron-containing multivitamin, calcium citrate, and monthly vitamin B_{12} injections. Other medications include levothyroxine, 50 mcg daily, and topiramate, 75 mg daily.

On physical examination, her height is 65.7 in (167 cm) and weight is 284 lb (128.8 kg) (BMI = 46.3 kg/m²). She has symmetric weight distribution between the upper and lower body. She walks with a cane. Her abdomen is soft with well-healed laparoscopic scars.

Laboratory test results:

25-Hydroxyvitamin D = 27 ng/mL (30-80 ng/mL [optimal]) (SI: 67.4 nmol/L [74.9-199.7 nmol/L])
PTH = 94 pg/mL (10-65 pg/mL) (SI: 94 ng/L [10-65 ng/L])
Serum calcium = 9.5 mg/dL (8.2-10.2 mg/dL) (SI: 2.4 mmol/L [2.1-2.6 mmol/L])
Serum albumin = 4.2 g/dL (3.5-5.0 g/dL) (SI: 42 g/L [35-50 g/L])
Serum creatinine = 0.9 mg/dL (0.6-1.1 mg/dL) (SI: 79.6 μmol/L [53.0-97.2 μmol/L])

Results of which of the following tests would best help explain her biochemical profile?

A. Bone alkaline phosphatase measurement
B. 1,25-Dihydroxyvitamin D measurement
C. 24-Hour urinary calcium and creatinine excretion
D. Parathyroid sestamibi scan
E. Serum magnesium measurement

46 A 30-year-old man with 16-year history of type 1 diabetes mellitus has been admitted to the hospital after presenting with nausea, vomiting, and abdominal pain. His diabetes-related complications include mild nonproliferative diabetic retinopathy and microalbuminuria. Over the last 3 years, his hemoglobin A_{1c} values have ranged from 7.2% to 8.2% (55-66 mmol/mol). His home medications include lisinopril, insulin glargine, and insulin lispro. His medical and family histories are unremarkable. He smokes 1 pack of cigarettes every 2 weeks, consumes 4 to 6 alcoholic beverages per week, and uses marijuana several times per week. He states he does not use illicit substances.

Over the last 6 months, he has been hospitalized 4 times for presumed diabetic ketoacidosis. The previous episodes were similar to his current one: he recalls awakening with nausea that progresses to abdominal pain and vomiting that lasts several hours. Hyperglycemia and large ketones in the urine have prompted him to seek medical attention each time. He reports no localizing symptoms to suggest an infection and has no chest pain or shortness of breath. He has had no difficulty accessing medications. He misses doses of bolus insulin about once weekly but never misses basal insulin.

On physical examination, his blood pressure is 110/70 mm Hg, respiratory rate is 12 breaths/min, oxygen saturation is 96% on pulse room air, and temperature is 98.7°F (37.1°C). He appears ill. Notable findings include dry mucous membranes; normal active bowel sounds; and diffuse, mild tenderness of the abdomen without hepatosplenomegaly, masses, or abdominal bruits. Chest is clear to auscultation, and findings on cardiac examination are unremarkable. Findings on diabetic foot exam are normal.

Laboratory test results (sample drawn at hospital admission):

Kidney function, normal
Complete blood cell count, normal
Liver function, normal
Blood glucose = 260 mg/dL (70-99 mg/dL) (SI: 14.4 mmol/L [3.9-5.5 mmol/L])
Serum bicarbonate = 20 mEq/L (21-28 mEq/L) (SI: 20 mmol/L [21-28 mmol/L])
Serum sodium = 140 mEq/L (136-142 mEq/L) (SI: 140 mmol/L [136-142 mmol/L])
Serum potassium = 4.0 mEq/L (3.5-5.0 mEq/L) (SI: 4.0 mmol/L [3.5-5.0 mmol/L])
Serum chloride = 100 mEq/L (96-106 mEq/L) (SI: 100 mmol/L [96-106 mmol/L])
Calculated anion gap = 20 mEq/L (3-11 mEq/L) (SI: 20 mmol/L [3-11 mmol/L])
Blood pH = 7.38 (7.35-7.45)
Hemoglobin A_{1c} = 7.8% (4.0%-5.6%) (62 mmol/mol [20-38 mmol/mol])
Urinary ketones, positive
Urine toxicology screen, positive for cannabinoids but no other illicit substances

Given the elevated anion gap and presence of urine ketones, he is treated with intravenous normal saline and intravenous insulin. Previous upper endoscopy and abdominal ultrasonography did not show any abnormalities except for gastritis.

Which of the following is the best next step in addressing this patient's recurrent hospitalizations for hyperglycemia with ketosis?

A. Examine pharmacy dispensation of insulin for possible nonadherence
B. Perform a gastric-emptying study
C. Perform CT of the abdomen and pelvis
D. Prescribe a proton-pump inhibitor
E. Recommend discontinuation of cannabis

47

A 56-year-old transgender woman is referred to endocrinology for gender-affirming hormone therapy. Her sex assigned at birth was male. She reports feeling female since childhood, is recently divorced, and would like to initiate hormone therapy. She has a letter from her mental health provider confirming the diagnosis of gender dysphoria. The patient is counseled regarding realistic therapy goals, including cessation of erections, breast growth, and change in body fat distribution. She does not smoke cigarettes, has no history of thromboembolic disease or chronic kidney disease, and has no personal or family history of cardiovascular disease.

She is prescribed estradiol, 1 mg orally daily for 1 month, with a gradual increase to 4 mg daily. Spironolactone is also started at a dosage of 100 mg daily. After 6 months of medication adjustments, she is very happy with breast growth and cessation of morning erections.

Which of the following is most likely to occur with long-term hormonal therapy in this patient?

A. Decreased risk of venous thromboembolic disease
B. Decreased serum triglycerides
C. Increased bone mineral density
D. Increased risk of breast cancer
E. Increased risk of prostate cancer

48

A 57-year-old man presents for routine follow-up of type 2 diabetes mellitus. He also has hypertension, hyperlipidemia, and obesity. His current treatment regimen is metformin, 1000 mg twice daily; empagliflozin, 25 mg daily; insulin degludec, 40 units daily; olmesartan, 40 mg daily; and atorvastatin, 80 mg daily at bedtime. He is up to date on screening for retinopathy, neuropathy, and nephropathy. He has no history of chest pain, shortness of breath, or cardiovascular events. He does not smoke cigarettes or drink alcohol. His blood pressure is 128/83 mm Hg, and BMI is 32 kg/m^2.

Laboratory test results from 1 month ago:

Hemoglobin = 15.8 g/dL (13.8-17.2 g/dL) (SI: 158 g/L [138-172 g/L])
Platelet count = 238 × 10^3/µL (150-450 × 10^3/µL) (SI: 238 × 10^9/L [150-450 × 10^9/L])
Creatinine = 1.2 mg/dL (0.7-1.3 mg/dL) (SI: 106.1 µmol/L [61.9-114.9 µmol/L])
Hemoglobin A_{1c} = 7.1% (4.0%-5.6%) (54 mmol/mol [20-38 mmol/mol])
Total cholesterol = 209 mg/dL (<200 mg/dL) (SI: 5.41 mmol/L [<5.18 mmol/L])
Triglycerides = 312 mg/dL (<150 mg/dL) (SI: 3.53 mmol/L <1.70 mmol/L])
HDL cholesterol = 38 mg/dL (>60 mg/dL) (SI: 0.98 mmol/L [>1.55 mmol/L])
LDL cholesterol = 109 mg/dL (<100 mg/dL) (SI: 2.82 mmol/L [<2.59 mmol/L])
AST = 72 U/L (20-48 U/L) (SI: 1.20 µkat/L [0.33-0.80 µkat/L])
ALT = 58 U/L (10-40 U/L) (SI: 0.97 µkat/L [0.17-0.67 µkat/L])
Urinary albumin-to-creatinine ratio = <30 mg/g creat (<30 mg/g creat)

Which of the following is the best next step in this patient's management?

A. Calculate his Fibrosis-4 (FIB-4) score
B. Decrease the atorvastatin dosage to 20 mg daily
C. Perform MRI of the liver
D. Recommend 150 minutes of exercise daily
E. Refer for nutrition counseling

49 A 26-year-old man presents for evaluation of obesity. He reports being overweight as a child and was placed on his first "diet" in kindergarten. He describes constantly feeling hungry, and his weight has progressively increased over time despite attempts at lifestyle change. His medical history is notable for congenital unilateral hydronephrosis and legal blindness due to retinitis pigmentosa.

On physical examination, his height is 65.7 in (167 cm) and weight is 254 lb (115.2 kg) (BMI = 41.4 kg/m^2). Blood pressure is 136/80 mm Hg. He has truncal obesity, with no stigmata of hypercortisolism. He has polydactyly of the right hand.

Laboratory test results:

Fasting plasma glucose = 109 mg/dL (70-99 mg/dL) (SI: 6.0 mmol/L [3.9-5.5 mmol/L])
TSH = 5.5 mIU/L (0.5-5.0 mIU/L)
Total testosterone = 210 mg/dL (300-900 ng/dL) (SI: 7.3 nmol/L [10.4-31.2 nmol/L])

Which of the following treatments is most appropriate to address obesity in this patient?

A. Recombinant leptin
B. Semaglutide
C. Setmelanotide
D. Somatropin
E. Testosterone

50 A 47-year-old woman with stage IIIc melanoma metastatic to inguinal lymph nodes was previously treated with nivolumab (2 cycles). She received her first cycle of combination therapy with nivolumab/ipilimumab 4 weeks ago. Today she presents to the emergency department after experiencing nausea with occasional vomiting, diarrhea, tachycardia, and anxiety over the past week. There is no family history of thyroid disease.

On physical examination, her temperature is 99.1°F (37.3°C), blood pressure is 100/66 mm Hg, and pulse rate is 110 beats/min. Her height is 63 in (160.0 cm), and weight is 160 lb (72.6 kg) (BMI = 28.3 kg/m^2). Findings on eye examination are notable for lid lag, but no chemosis or proptosis. The thyroid gland is nontender and without nodules. A fine tremor of the upper extremities is present. Deep tendon reflexes are 3+. The rest of her examination findings are normal.

Laboratory test results:

Measurement	3 months ago	3 weeks ago	Today	Reference range
TSH	1.43 mIU/L	0.21 mIU/L	0.01 mIU/L	0.5-5.0 mIU/L
Free T_4	...	...	2.08 ng/dL (SI: 26.77 pmol/L)	0.8-1.8 ng/dL (SI: 10.30-23.17 pmol/L)
Total T_3	...	...	144 ng/dL (SI: 2.22 nmol/L)	70-200 ng/dL (SI: 1.08-3.08 nmol/L)
Cortisol (9 AM)	...	...	21 µg/dL (SI: 579.3 nmol/L)	5-25 µg/dL (SI: 137.9-689.7 nmol/L)
Complete metabolic panel	...	...	Normal	

Which of the following is the most appropriate initial management to recommend for this patient?

A. Discontinue nivolumab/ipilimumab
B. Prescribe propranolol
C. Prescribe propranolol and methimazole
D. Prescribe propranolol and prednisone
E. Refer for radioactive iodine therapy

51 A 61-year-old woman with postmenopausal osteoporosis has sustained multiple low-trauma vertebral fractures. She was previously healthy and had no prior fractures. There is no family history of osteoporosis or fractures. Menopause was at age 50 years, and she has not taken hormone therapy. On physical examination, she has moderate kyphosis. Other secondary causes of osteoporosis are ruled out during her evaluation.

DXA demonstrates a spine T-score of −3.3, left femoral neck T-score of −2.3, and left total hip T-score of −2.1.

Given this patient's findings, which treatment sequence is most appropriate to optimize her bone mineral density, taking into account the drugs' mechanisms of action?

A. Abaloparatide > denosumab > drug holiday
B. Alendronate > abaloparatide > drug holiday
C. Denosumab > teriparatide > zoledronate
D. Romosozumab > drug holiday > zoledronate
E. Romosozumab > zoledronate > drug holiday

52 A 26-year-old man with an 11-year history of type 1 diabetes mellitus has difficulty with hypoglycemia during exercise. He has no known microvascular complications. Over the last 4 years, his hemoglobin A_{1c} values have ranged from 6.7% to 7.5% (50-58 mmol/mol), and his most recent values have been less than 7.0% (<53mmol/mol). He uses an insulin pump with continuous glucose monitoring with the predictive low-glucose suspend feature. He is motivated to lose 15 lb (6.8 kg) and has started to engage in regular exercise. He typically does yoga twice weekly and jogs 3 times weekly. He aims to jog for 30 to 60 minutes but is frustrated that he almost always develops hypoglycemia 15 to 30 minutes after starting to run. He typically jogs in the morning before eating or in the late afternoon about 4 to 5 hours after lunch. He has tried reducing his basal insulin rate during the period of exercise but experiences hyperglycemia after his workouts.

Which of the following suggestions would be most appropriate to help this patient avoid hypoglycemia during aerobic exercise?

A. Consume 45 to 60 g of carbohydrates just before exercise
B. Engage in resistance exercise before starting aerobic exercise
C. Increase protein and fat consumption in the meal before exercise
D. Reduce basal insulin by 50% at the beginning of exercise
E. Reduce preexercise meal bolus by 30% to 50%

53 A 38-year-old man presents with fatigue, new striae, decreased muscle mass, and anxiety. He reports going through a difficult marital separation. He no longer plays soccer with his friends and drinks 6 to 10 servings of beer most evenings. His medical history is remarkable for 2 episodes of symptomatic nephrolithiasis in the past 5 years.

On physical examination, his blood pressure is 150/82 mm Hg and pulse rate is 92 beats/min. His weight is 145.5 lb (66 kg) without significant changes (BMI = 24 kg/m^2). His face is plethoric and more rounded compared with his appearance in photos taken 6 months ago. He has centripetal fat distribution, discolored, wide abdominal striae, easy bruising, thin skin, and 4/5 bilateral proximal muscle weakness.

Laboratory test results:

Testosterone (fasting morning sample) = 198 ng/dL (300-900 ng/dL) (SI: 6.9 nmol/L [10.4-31.2 nmol/L])
FSH = 2.0 mIU/mL (1.0-13.0 mIU/mL) (SI: 2.0 IU/L [1.0-13.0 IU/L])
LH = 3.0 mIU/mL (1.0-9.0 mIU/mL) (SI: 3.0 IU/L [1.0-9.0 IU/L])
ACTH = 70 pg/mL (10-60 pg/mL) (SI: 15.4 pmol/L [2.2-13.2 pmol/L])
Serum cortisol after 1-mg dexamethasone administration at bedtime = 6 μg/dL (SI: 165.5 nmol/L)
Urinary free cortisol = 90 μg/24 h (4-50 μg/24 h) (SI: 248.4 nmol/d [11-138 nmol/d])
Urinary creatinine = 2.6 g/24 h (1.0-2.0 g/24 h) (SI: 23.0 mmol/d [8.8-17.7 mmol/d])
Urine volume = 5100 mL/24 h

MRI of the pituitary gland shows a 4-mm hypodense abnormality.

Which of the following is the best next step in this patient's management?

A. High-dose dexamethasone-suppression test
B. Inferior petrosal sinus sampling
C. Referral to neurosurgery for transsphenoidal removal of the pituitary adenoma
D. Referral to psychology for counseling on alcohol overuse
E. Testosterone replacement

54 A 32-year-old woman with Addison disease diagnosed at age 24 years presents for annual follow-up. She reports several weeks of tiredness, lethargy, and weight loss, which she attributes to recently being diagnosed with tuberculosis following a 3-month trip to visit her family in India. She has also experienced nocturnal sweating episodes, but these have improved significantly since starting treatment with isoniazid, rifampicin, pyrazinamide, ethambutol, and pyridoxine 6 weeks ago. She reports no other symptoms. Her regular medications are hydrocortisone, 20 mg daily (in 3 divided doses), and fludrocortisone, 150 mcg daily.

On physical examination, her blood pressure is 105/55 mm Hg and pulse rate is 96 beats/min and regular. Her height is 65 in (165.1 cm), and weight is 179 lb (81.2 kg) (BMI = 29.8 kg/m^2). She has bilateral cervical lymphadenopathy and a small, symmetric goiter. The rest of the examination findings are unremarkable.

Laboratory test results:

Hemoglobin = 11.2 g/dL (12.1-15.1 g/dL) (SI: 112 g/L [121-151 g/L])
Mean corpuscular volume = 96 mm^3 (80-100 mm^3) (SI: 96 fL [80-100 fL])
Serum sodium = 134 mEq/L (136-142 mEq/L) (SI: 134 mmol/L [136-142 mmol/L])
Serum potassium = 4.6 mEq/L (3.5-5.0 mEq/L) (SI: 4.6 mmol/L [3.5-5.0 mmol/L])
Serum creatinine = 1.0 mg/dL (0.6-1.1 mg/dL) (SI: 88.4 μmol/L [53.0-97.2 μmol/L])
Hemoglobin A_{1c} = 6.0% (4.0%-5.6%) (SI: 42 mmol/mol [28-38 mmol/mol])
Free T_4 = 1.0 ng/dL (0.8-1.8 ng/dL) (SI: 12.87 pmol/L [10.30-23.17 pmol/L])
TSH = 0.3 mIU/L (0.5-5.0 mIU/L)
TRAb = 0.5 IU/L (≤1.75 IU/L)
TPO antibodies = 5.0 IU/mL (<2.0 IU/mL) (SI: 5.0 kIU/L [<2.0 kIU/L])

Which of the following is most likely to explain this patient's current symptoms?

A. Drug-induced hemolytic anemia
B. Hyperglycemia
C. Hypoadrenalism
D. Subclinical T_3 thyrotoxicosis
E. Vitamin B_{12} insufficiency

55 A 27-year-old woman (G0P0) with a history of anxiety and insomnia presents for evaluation of infertility. Menarche was at age 11 years, and she had regular menses every 28 days until a levonorgestrel intrauterine device was placed at age 24 years. The device was removed 1.5 years ago with the goal of preparing her body for conception. Since the device was removed, menses have occurred every 3 to 4 months, and she has been trying to conceive without success. She has also developed night sweats, 4 times per night, bothersome fatigue, low mood, brain fog, and decreased libido.

On physical examination, her blood pressure is 98/61 mm Hg and pulse rate is 60 beats/min and regular. Her height is 63 in (160.0 cm), and weight is 130 lb (59.0 kg) (BMI = 23.0 kg/m^2). Examination findings are unremarkable.

Laboratory test results (menstrual cycle day 3):

TSH = 1.95 mIU/L (0.5-5.0 mIU/L)
Free T_4 = 1.2 ng/dL (0.8-1.8 ng/dL) (SI: 15.4 pmol/L [10.30-23.17 pmol/L])
Estradiol = 15 pg/mL (10-180 pg/mL [follicular]) (SI: 55.1 pmol/L [26.7-660.8 pmol/L])
FSH = 47.1 mIU/mL (2.0-12.0 mIU/mL [follicular]) (SI: 47.1 IU/L [2.0-12.0 IU/L])

LH = 30.0 mIU/mL (1.0-18.0 mIU/mL [follicular]) (SI: 30.0 mIU/mL [(1.0-18.0 mIU/mL])
Prolactin = 11.7 ng/mL (4-30 ng/mL [nonlactating female]) (SI: 0.51 nmol/L [0.17-1.30 nmol/L])
Karyotype = 46,X,del(X)(q25)
Fragile X premutation, negative
Serum adrenal cortical and 21-hydroxylase antibodies, negative

Which of the following therapies is most likely to help this patient conceive?

A. Clomiphene citrate
B. Letrozole
C. Oocyte donation and in vitro fertilization
D. Ovarian drilling
E. Pulsatile GnRH therapy

56 A 66-year-old man is referred for management of type 2 diabetes mellitus. He has had type 2 diabetes for 16 years. His current regimen includes metformin therapy. His glycemic control remains suboptimal with a hemoglobin A_{1c} value of 8.7% (72 mmol/mol). He has tried a GLP-1 receptor agonist, but he stopped it after developing nausea and diarrhea. He then tried an SGLT-2 inhibitor, but he developed nocturia, often 3 times per night. He reports that both of these medications were very expensive on his insurance plan, and he asks about taking a medication that is cheaper. The patient has obesity (BMI = 32 kg/m^2) and is sedentary. His comorbidities include coronary artery disease status post coronary artery bypass grafting 3 years ago, hypertension, hyperlipidemia, and stage 3 chronic kidney disease with microalbuminuria. He has no chest pain or shortness of breath, and he continues to follow-up with his cardiologist annually. The decision is made to initiate sulfonylurea therapy.

Current medications are atorvastatin, lisinopril, amlodipine, and metformin.

Laboratory test results:

Hemoglobin A_{1c} = 8.7% (4.0%-5.6%) (72 mmol/mol [20-38 mmol/mol])
Estimated glomerular filtration rate = 54 mL/min per 1.73 m^2 (>60 mL/min per 1.73 m^2)

Which of the following medications should be initiated as the best next step in this patient's management?

A. Chlorpropamide
B. Glimepiride
C. Glipizide
D. Glyburide
E. Tolbutamide

57 A 52-year-old man would like to discuss his weight. He has watched his weight since he was a young child and remembers being on his first diet at age 10 years. His lowest adult weight was 200 lb (90.9 kg), and his highest adult weight was 305 lb (139 kg). He estimates having gained and lost at least 50 lb (22.7 kg) on multiple occasions over his lifetime.

His current weight is 243 lb (110.2 kg). He has been diligently reducing caloric intake and estimates that he consumes about 1800 kcal daily. He walks his dog several times a week. He is maintaining his weight but desires further weight loss and long-term weight maintenance. He takes no regular medications.

On physical examination, his blood pressure is 120/85 mm Hg. His height is 68.9 in (175 cm) and weight is 243 lb (110.2 kg) (BMI = 36.0 kg/m^2). His weight is distributed preferentially over his lower body. There are no stigmata of hypercortisolism.

Laboratory test results:

Fasting plasma glucose = 90 mg/dL (70-99 mg/dL) (SI: 5.0 mmol/L [3.9-5.5 mmol/L])
TSH = 0.8 mIU/L (0.5-5.0 mIU/L)

His estimated basal energy expenditure (Mifflin-St. Jeor equation) is 1940 kcal per day.

Which of the following interventions would be most helpful for this patient to achieve his weight-loss goals?

A. Dietary review to ensure he is consuming adequate amounts of high-quality protein
B. Referral for bariatric surgery
C. Referral to a psychologist for behavioral modification
D. Starting a moderate-intensity exercise program, aiming for 200 minutes weekly
E. Starting an appetite suppressant to promote additional calorie restriction

58 A 42-year-old woman with no notable medical history presents with neck tenderness 5 days after receiving a COVID-19 mRNA vaccine. She also notes palpitations, heat intolerance, weight loss, and fever (101.5°F [38.6°C]). She has been taking acetaminophen with no improvement in neck tenderness. She takes no other medication or over-the-counter supplements. She has no compressive symptoms, diplopia, or diarrhea. PCR testing is negative for COVID-19 infection. There is no history of radiation exposure or family history of thyroid disorders.

On physical examination, her blood pressure is 120/70 mm Hg and pulse rate is 110 beats/min. Her thyroid gland is mildly enlarged and tender. She has a hand tremor. The rest of the examination findings are unremarkable.

Laboratory test results:

- White blood cell count = 6200/μL (4500-11,000/μL) (SI: 6.2×10^9/L [4.5-11.0 × 10^9/L])
- Hemoglobin = 11.1 g/dL (12.1-15.1 g/dL) (SI: 111 g/L [121-151 g/L])
- TSH = <0.01 mIU/L (0.5-5.0 mIU/L)
- Free T_4 = 4.20 ng/dL (0.8-1.8 ng/dL) (SI: 54.06 pmol/L [10.30-23.17 pmol/L])
- Free T_3 = 7.2 pg/mL (2.3-4.2 pg/mL) (SI: 11.06 pmol/L [3.53-6.45 pmol/L])
- Erythrocyte sedimentation rate = 80 mm/h (0-20 mm/h)

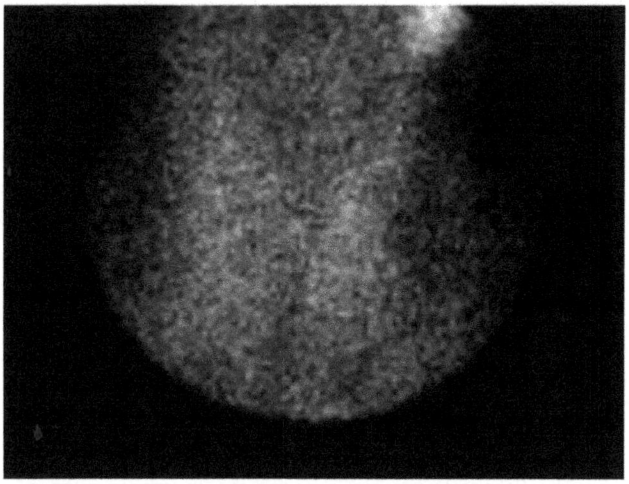

A thyroid scan is shown (*see image*).

In addition to recommending ibuprofen, which of the following is the best next step in this patient's management?

A. Administer radioiodine treatment
B. Measure thyroid-stimulating immunoglobulin
C. Repeat thyroid laboratory tests in 1 week
D. Start a β-adrenergic blocker
E. Start an antithyroid drug

59 A 56-year-old woman was diagnosed with estrogen receptor/progesterone receptor–positive breast cancer 3 years ago. She has completed lumpectomy and radiation therapy and has taken an aromatase inhibitor for 2 years for a planned 10-year treatment course. Screening DXA was performed before starting the aromatase inhibitor, which documented osteopenia with the lowest T-score of –2.2 in the lumbar spine. DXA was recently repeated. She now has a T-score of –2.7 in her lumbar spine, representing a 9.8% decrease in bone mineral density at that location. She is reluctant to start an oral bisphosphonate because she is concerned about adverse effects. The patient is counseled that oral bisphosphonates effectively prevent bone loss in patients on aromatase inhibitors.

Which of the following would be an additional benefit of bisphosphonate treatment benefit for this patient?

A. Increased muscle mass
B. Reduced risk of breast cancer recurrence
C. Reduced risk of osteosarcoma
D. Reduced risk of falls
E. Reduced risk of osteoarthritis symptoms

60 A 60-year-old man with prediabetes is seen for annual follow-up. He has had impaired fasting glucose for the last 5 years and is not on any glucose-lowering therapies. His weight has fluctuated between 187 and 198 lb (85 and 90 kg), and he tries to walk at least 10,000 steps most days of the week. He feels well, but he reports an episode of slurred speech and right-sided weakness for about an hour 1 week ago. He was seen in the local emergency department where findings on head CT were normal and a random blood glucose concentration was 116 mg/dL (6.4 mmol/L). He has been on atorvastatin, 40 mg daily, for the last 4 years (he takes one-half tablet [80 mg], as the full tablet causes leg pain) and was also recently started on amlodipine and aspirin.

On physical examination, he appears well. His blood pressure is 124/80 mm Hg, and pulse rate is 80 beats/min. His height is 67 in (170.2 cm), and weight is 198 lb (89.8 kg) (BMI = 31 kg/m^2). He has no focal neurologic deficits.

Laboratory test results:

Fasting plasma glucose = 118 mg/dL (70-99 mg/dL) (SI: 6.5 mmol/L [3.9-5.5 mmol/L])
Hemoglobin A_{1c} = 6.3% (4.0%-5.6%) (45 mmol/mol [20-38 mmol/mol])
Serum creatinine = 1.2 mg/dL (0.7-1.3 mg/dL) (SI: 106.1 µmol/L [61.9-114.9 µmol/L])
ALT = 52 U/L (10-40 U/L) (SI: 0.87 µkat/L [0.17-0.67 µkat/L])
AST = 35 U/L (20-48 U/L) (SI: 0.58 µkat/L [0.33-0.80 µkat/L])
Total cholesterol = 170 mg/dL (<200 mg/dL) (SI: 4.40 mmol/L [<5.18 mmol/L])
Triglycerides = 220 mg/dL (<150 mg/dL) (SI: 2.49 mmol/L [<1.70 mmol/L])
HDL cholesterol = 46 mg/dL (>60 mg/dL) (SI: 1.19 mmol/L [>1.55 mmol/L])
LDL cholesterol = 80 mg/dL (<100 mg/dL) (SI: 2.07 mmol/L [<2.59 mmol/L])

Which of the following is the best next step in this patient's management?

A. Add ezetimibe, 10 mg daily
B. Add icosapent ethyl, 4 g daily
C. Increase the atorvastatin dosage to 80 mg daily
D. Intensify weight-loss efforts, maintain current medications
E. Start metformin, 500 mg daily, and increase to 2000 mg daily as tolerated

61 A 31-year-old man is seen for consultation regarding type 1 diabetes mellitus and painful neuropathy. Diabetes was diagnosed 3 months ago when the following laboratory values were documented: fasting glucose, 327 mg/dL (18.1 mmol/L); hemoglobin A_{1c}, 12.3% (111 mmol/mol); and elevated glutamic acid decarboxylase 65 antibodies. He has a brother with celiac disease and no family members with diabetes. A basal-bolus insulin regimen was initiated, and he received diabetes education and nutritional counseling. Within 1 month of treatment, his average fingerstick blood glucose value (checked 6 to 7 times daily) was 110 mg/dL (6.1 mmol) with occasional postprandial hypoglycemia leading to insulin dosage reduction.

Five weeks after diabetes was diagnosed, he started to have bilateral pain in the knees, ankles, and wrists, which he describes as a soreness, throbbing, and constant deep discomfort in the joints and surrounding muscles. He has similar but less intense pain in his upper extremities and neck. In addition, he has noticed skin sensitivity in his legs and groin that is worse in late afternoon and is affecting his sleep. He finds even putting on underwear to be painful. As the pain began to worsen and remain unresponsive to marijuana use, oxycodone was prescribed.

Current medications include insulin glargine, 6 units daily; insulin lispro, 2 units with meals (he requires no correction doses for high glucose levels); gabapentin; and oxycodone as needed at night.

On physical examination, his height is 66 in (167.6 cm) and weight is 163 lb (74 kg) (BMI = 26.3 kg/m^2). Vital signs are normal. On motor examination, he has normal muscle bulk and tone, and strength is 5/5 throughout. He has no fasciculations or pronator drift. On sensory examination, he has intact sensation to light touch, pin prick, and vibration. Proprioception is normal. He has reduced sensation to temperature on his calves bilaterally. Coordination is normal as tested by finger-to-nose, gait, and the Romberg test.

Laboratory test results:

Hemoglobin A_{1c} = 6.6% (4.0%-5.6%) (49 mmol/mol [20-38 mmol/mol])
Erythrocyte sedimentation rate = 2 mm/h (0-20 mm/h)
C-reactive protein = <0.5 mg/L (0.8-3.1 mg/L) (SI: <4.76 nmol/L [7.62-29.52 nmol/L])
Serum urea nitrogen = 16 mg/dL (8-23 mg/dL) (SI: 5.7 mmol/L [2.9-8.2 mmol/L])
Serum creatinine = 0.78 mg/dL (0.7-1.3 mg/dL) (SI: 69.0 µmol/L [61.9-114.9 µmol/L])
Serum protein electrophoresis, consistent hypogammaglobulinemia (immunoelectrophoresis shows a normal pattern)
Vitamin B_{12} = 724 pg/mL (180-914 pg/mL) (SI: 534 pmol/L [133-674 pmol/L])
TSH, normal
HIV screening, negative

Which of the following is the most appropriate next step in this patient's management?

A. Change the insulin regimen to insulin detemir and insulin aspart
B. Change the regimen to oral hypoglycemic agents
C. Measure the urine albumin-to-creatinine ratio
D. Recommend no additional evaluation or treatment changes
E. Relax glycemic control to target a hemoglobin A_{1c} value between 8.0% and 8.5% (64-69 mmol/mol)

62 A 34-year-old Black man presents to the emergency department with abdominal pain, nausea, and vomiting. He has had these symptoms on and off for the past month, his appetite has been decreased, and he has lost a few pounds. He has not had diarrhea. He does not smoke cigarettes, he drinks alcohol socially, and he uses marijuana to alleviate his symptoms. His medical history includes hypothyroidism treated with levothyroxine, 100 mcg daily.

On physical examination, his blood pressure is 98/66 mm Hg and pulse rate is 102 beats/min. His height is 69 in (175.3 cm), and weight is 131 lb (59.4 kg) (BMI = 19.3 kg/m^2). He has no proptosis, lid lag, or chemosis. He has no plethora, striae, rashes, or bruises. Patchy hyperpigmentation is noted on his oral mucosae and tongue. His neck is supple, and his thyroid gland is small, without palpable nodules. No lymphadenopathy is present. His heart rate has a regular rhythm, without murmurs. His chest is clear to auscultation bilaterally. His abdomen is soft, nondistended, and diffusely tender on palpation, but there is no rebound tenderness. Lower extremities are warm and without edema. There are no focal abnormalities on neurologic examination. He has no tremor of his outstretched hands.

Laboratory test results:

Complete blood cell count, normal
Glucose = 98 mg/dL (70-99 mg/dL) (SI: 5.4 mmol/L [3.9-5.5 mmol/L])
Serum potassium = 5.5 mEq/L (3.5-5.0 mEq/L) (SI: 5.5 mmol/L [3.5-5.0 mmol/L])
Serum sodium = 134 mEq/L (136-142 mEq/L) (SI: 134 mmol/L [136-142 mmol/L])
Serum chloride = 110 mEq/L (96-106 mEq/L) (SI: 110 mmol/L [96-106 mmol/L])
Serum bicarbonate = 18 mEq/L (21-28 mEq/L) (SI: 18 mmol/L [21-28 mEq/L])
Serum creatinine = 1.2 mg/dL (0.7-1.3 mg/dL) (SI: 106.1 µmol/L [61.9-114.9 µmol/L])
TSH = 0.3 mIU/L (0.5-5.0 mIU/L)

Which of the following is the most likely cause of this patient's symptomatology?

A. Diabetic ketoacidosis
B. Hyperthyroidism
C. Marijuana use
D. Primary adrenal insufficiency
E. Secondary adrenal insufficiency

63 A 42-year-old woman is seeking a second opinion regarding a right-sided thyroid nodule. She has no history of radiation exposure or thyroid disease. There is also no family history of thyroid cancer. She is otherwise healthy and takes a daily multivitamin.

On physical examination, her vital signs are normal. The right thyroid lobe is palpable and hard, and the left thyroid lobe is not palpable. There is no enlarged cervical adenopathy. The rest of her examination findings are normal.

Laboratory test result:

TSH = 1.26 mIU/L (0.5-5.0 mIU/L)

Thyroid ultrasonography shows a 2.8 × 1.8 × 1.5-cm solid thyroid nodule in the right lobe. No other thyroid nodule or cervical adenopathy is identified. Ultrasound-guided FNA biopsy of her right thyroid nodule confirms papillary thyroid cancer.

Based on current American Thyroid Association thyroid cancer guidelines, which of the following is the best next step in this patient's management?

A. Radiofrequency ablation
B. Right lobectomy
C. Total thyroidectomy
D. Total thyroidectomy followed by radioiodine treatment
E. Total thyroidectomy with central neck dissection

64 A 70-year-old woman presents to discuss her diabetes management because she will soon be fasting during the day for Ramadan. She has had type 2 diabetes for 23 years, and insulin was introduced to her regimen a year ago. She is up to date with screening for neuropathy, nephropathy, and retinopathy and has no diabetes-related complications. She monitors fasting blood glucose values 3 times a week but not more frequently because of painful fingers.

When she fasts, she will eat at sunrise and will not consume any food or liquids until sunset. She plans to do this for the 1-month duration of Ramadan. She reports that her meal at sunset will be much more substantial than her meal at sunrise.

Her current treatment regimen for diabetes consists of NPH insulin, 18 units twice daily; metformin, 1000 mg twice daily; and empagliflozin, 25 mg daily.

On physical examination, her height is 60.7 in (152 cm) and weight is 160 lb (72.7 kg) (BMI = 31.5 kg/m^2).

Laboratory test results:

Hemoglobin A_{1c} = 8.1% (4.0%-5.6%) (65 mmol/mol [20-38 mmol/mol])
Fasting plasma glucose = 162 mg/dL (70-99 mg/dL) (SI: 9.0 mmol/L [3.9-5.5 mmol/L])
Serum creatinine = 0.92 mg/dL (0.6-1.1 mg/dL) (SI: 81.3 μmol/L [53.0-97.2 μmol/L])

How should this patient's diabetes regimen be modified when she starts fasting?

Answer	Metformin	Empagliflozin	Insulin
A.	Stop	Stop	Continue NPH insulin, 18 units twice daily
B.	Stop	Continue	Reduce NPH insulin to 18 units once daily
C.	Continue	Stop	Stop NPH insulin; start rapid-acting insulin with evening and morning meals
D.	Continue	Continue	Stop NPH insulin
E.	Stop	Stop	Stop NPH insulin; start rapid-acting insulin as needed for hyperglycemia (ie, correction insulin) 3 times daily

65 A 39-year-old woman with a history of type 1 diabetes mellitus presents to the diabetes clinic for evaluation and management. Her medical history is notable for hypertension and dyslipidemia. Her treatment consists of insulin glargine, 16 units daily; short-acting insulin aspart, 5 units with each meal; and correctional insulin, 1 unit for every 50 mg/dL (2.8 mmol/L) above 150 mg/dL (>8.3 mmol/L). She also uses a continuous glucose monitoring device (*see image*). She wakes at 5:00 AM and has 2 meals per day (lunch between 11:30 AM and 1:00 PM and dinner at 7:00 PM). She is frustrated with her glycemic control and says, "It is impossible to get my hemoglobin A_{1c} below 7.0% (<53 mmol/mol)." Her glucose management indicator is 7.5% (58 mmol/mol), and her hemoglobin A_{1c} value is 7.6% (60 mmol/mol).

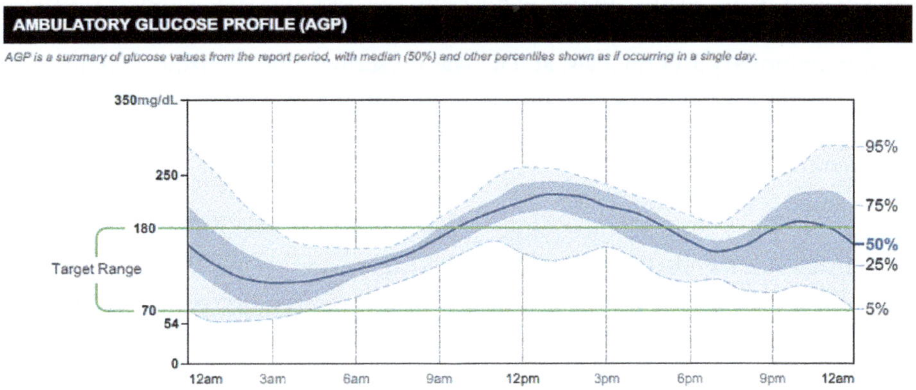

Which of the following is the best next step in this patient's management?

A. Decrease the basal insulin glargine dosage
B. Increase the basal insulin glargine dosage
C. Increase the short-acting prandial insulin doses with meals
D. Recommend insulin pump initiation
E. Recommend no regimen modification (her glycemic control is on target)

66 A 40-year-old man presents with 60-lb (27.2-kg) weight gain, easy bruising, multiple striae on the abdomen and axillae, hypertension, and hypogonadism. Biochemical workup demonstrates ACTH-related hypercortisolism and MRI identifies a 4-mm microadenoma. The patient undergoes transsphenoidal surgery, and pathologic examination confirms an ACTH-secreting adenoma. Proliferation marker MIB1 is identified in less than 3% of cells, and mitoses are not observed. On postoperative day 1, his serum cortisol concentration is 5.2 µg/dL (143.5 nmol/L). He is discharged on hydrocortisone, 20 mg in the morning, which is stopped after 3 weeks when normal morning serum cortisol concentrations are documented. Twelve weeks after surgery, he returns to clinic and reports improved skin manifestations and normal blood pressure while taking fewer medications than he did preoperatively. He continues to experience muscle weakness, and he is concerned about persistently low libido and inability to lose weight. Several first-degree relatives have type 2 diabetes mellitus.

Two late-night salivary cortisol measurements are elevated 2 and 3 times above the upper reference range.

Other laboratory test results:

Urinary free cortisol = 70 µg/24 h (4-50 µg/24 h) (SI: 193.2 nmol/d [11-138 nmol/d])
Urinary creatinine = 1.9 g/24 h (1.0-2.0 g/24 h) (SI: 16.8 mmol/d [8.8-17.7 mmol/d])
Urine volume = 2500 mL/24 h
Hemoglobin A_{1c}, normal
Fasting glucose, normal
Serum testosterone = 150 ng/dL (300-900 ng/dL) (SI: 5.2 nmol/L [10.4-31.2 nmol/L])
TSH, normal
Free T_4, normal

MRI of the pituitary gland indicates postoperative changes without visible residual tumor.

Which of the following is the best next step in this patient's management?

A. Bone densitometry and testosterone replacement
B. Inferior petrosal sinus sampling
C. Medical therapy with the glucocorticoid receptor antagonist mifepristone
D. Medical therapy with the steroidogenesis inhibitor osilodrostat
E. Pituitary gland radiation

67 A 27-year-old man with a history of polycystic kidney disease received a kidney transplant 2 years ago. His immunosuppression regimen consists of prednisone, tacrolimus, and mycophenolate. His course has been complicated by invasive pulmonary aspergillosis, and he was prescribed voriconazole, 200 mg twice daily, 9 months ago. Last month, he reported the development of diffuse bone pain that is worse in the right tibia. He has had no fever, recent trauma, dyspnea, rash, kidney stones, or dietary changes. The only over-the-counter medication he takes is a daily multivitamin.

Laboratory test results:

Calcium = 8.4 mg/dL (8.2-10.2 mg/dL) (SI: 2.1 mmol/L [2.1-2.6 mmol/L])
Albumin = 3.8 g/dL (3.5-5.0 g/dL) (SI: 38 g/L [35-50 g/L])
Creatinine = 1.2 mg/dL (0.6-1.1 mg/dL) (SI: 106.1 μmol/L [53.0-97.2 μmol/L])
Intact PTH = 123 pg/mL (10-65 pg/mL) (SI: 123 ng/L [10-65 ng/L])
Magnesium = 1.7 mg/dL (1.5-2.3 mg/dL) (SI: 0.7 mmol/L [0.6-0.9 mmol/L])
25-Hydroxyvitamin D = 28 ng/mL (30-80 ng/mL [optimal]) (SI: 69.9 nmol/L [74.9-199.7 nmol/L])
Alkaline phosphatase = 528 U/L (50-120 U/L) (SI: 8.82 μkat/L [0.84-2.00 μkat/L])

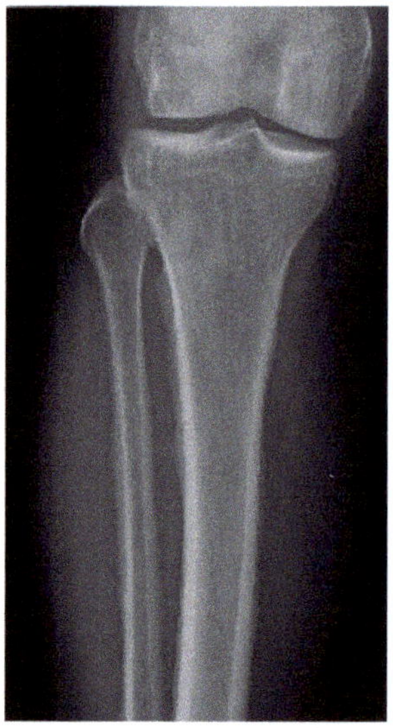

X-ray of the right tibia and fibula shows a thickened cortex and evidence of periostitis.

Serum measurement of which of the following is most likely to be elevated in this patient?

A. Cadmium
B. Fluoride
C. Tryptase
D. Vitamin A
E. Vitamin B_{12}

68 A 67-year-old woman with a history of total thyroidectomy with central neck dissection and radioiodine treatment (100 mCi) for metastatic papillary thyroid cancer to the cervical nodes is evaluated for new nontender lumps in the left side of her neck. There is no recent history of viral illness or vaccination. Neck ultrasonography identifies several abnormal lymph nodes in the left level III, IV, and V. FNA biopsy of 2 cervical nodes confirms metastatic papillary thyroid cancer. She undergoes left modified neck dissection and is discharged home the next day.

Eight weeks later, she presents for a follow-up visit. She feels fine but has dry eyes. She is taking levothyroxine, 150 mcg daily.

On physical examination, her vital signs are normal. There are several healed scars on her neck. There is no tremor in her hands. A photograph of her eyes is shown (*see image*).

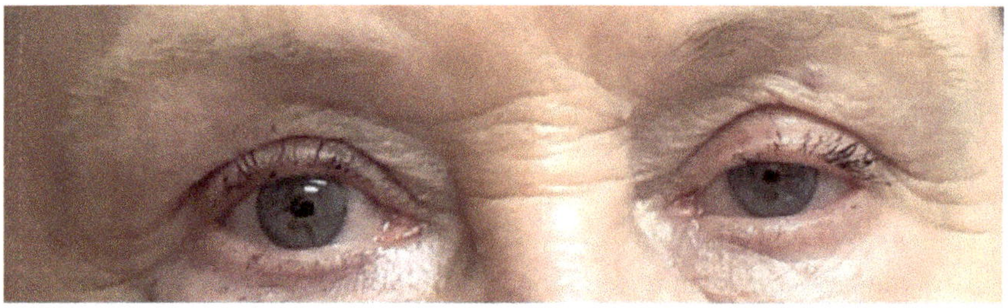

Laboratory test results:

TSH = 0.2 mIU/L (0.5-5.0 mIU/L)

Thyroglobulin = <0.1 ng/mL (3-42 ng/mL) (SI: <0.1 μg/L [3-42 μg/L]) (after surgery and radioactive iodine treatment = <1.0 ng/mL [SI: <1.0 μg/L])

Thyroglobulin antibodies = <1.0 IU/mL (≤4.0 IU/mL) (SI: <1.0 kIU/L [≤4.0 kIU/L])

Which of the following is the best next step in this patient's management?

A. Consider steroids
B. Perform neck CT
C. Perform orbit CT
D. Recommend no change to current therapy
E. Refer to ophthalmology

69 A 51-year-old menopausal woman presents with concerns regarding multiple fractures. She grew normally as a child, but she fractured both wrists and her collarbone when she was a teenager. She had multiple metatarsal fractures in her 20s, some sustained while running, which were slow to heal. Last year she fractured her right proximal femur with a fall from a standing height. She reports dorsal foot pain for the past few days and also notes chronic joint pain that has limited her physical activity in recent years. She has a history of pseudogout. She tried oral bisphosphonates but had gastrointestinal complaints that prevented adherence to therapy. Her father died of complications of myeloma, and her mother has had foot fractures.

DXA documents a spine T-score of −1.5, left femoral neck T-score of −2.1, and left total hip T-score of −1.9. She currently takes no medications or supplements.

Laboratory test results:

Calcium = 9.6 mg/dL (8.2-10.2 mg/dL) (SI: 2.4 mmol/L [2.1-2.6 mmol/L])
Albumin = 3.9 g/dL (3.5-5.0 g/dL) (SI: 39 g/L [35-50 g/L])
Creatinine = 0.78 mg/dL (0.6-1.1 mg/dL) (SI: 69 μmol/L [53.0-97.2 μmol/L])
Alkaline phosphatase = 19 U/L (50-120 U/L) (SI: 0.32 μkat/L [0.84-2.00 μkat/L])
Intact PTH = 18 pg/mL (10-65 pg/mL) (SI: 1.90 pmol/L [1.1-6.8 pmol/L])
25-Hydroxyvitamin D = 48 ng/mL (30-80 ng/mL [optimal]) (SI: 119.8 nmol/L [74.9-199.7 nmol/L])
Phosphate = 4.2 mg/dL (2.3-4.7 mg/dL) (SI: 1.4 mmol/L [0.7-1.5 mmol/L])
Magnesium = 2.1 mg/dL (1.5-2.3 mg/dL) (SI: 0.86 mmol/L [0.6-0.9 mmol/L])
Vitamin B_6 = 376 nmol/L (20-125 nmol/L)
TSH = 1.6 mIU/L (0.5-5.0 mIU/L)
Urinary calcium = 250 mg/24 h (100-300 mg/24 h) (SI: 6.25 mmol/d [2.5-7.5 mmol/d])

Which of the following is the best approach to address her risk of additional fractures?

A. Asfotase alfa
B. Burosumab
C. Calcium and vitamin D
D. Intravenous bisphosphonate
E. Teriparatide

70 A 22-year-old woman (G0P0) with prediabetes and hyperlipidemia seeks further evaluation and treatment of polycystic ovary syndrome. In reviewing her reproductive history, she notes menarche occurred at age 12 or 13 years. She has always had irregular menstrual cycles with menses every 4 to 5 months. At age 19 years, polycystic ovary syndrome was diagnosed, and a combined oral contraceptive pill was initiated. She has been on and off this therapy because of adverse effects (depression, anxiety, nausea). The last time she was on a combined oral contraceptive pill was a year ago. Her last 2 menstrual bleeds were 2 months and 6 months ago. She has never been pregnant.

Her symptoms include hair loss (especially frontal), which she thinks has increased recently. She also notes acne, particularly on her chin. She has increased body hair growth and shaves her chin daily and her upper chest and lower abdomen weekly.

She currently lives with her cisgender female partner and does not engage in sexual activity where sperm meets egg. She smokes 1 pack of cigarettes per day and does not drink alcohol or engage in recreational drug use.

On physical examination, her blood pressure is 139/70 mm Hg and pulse rate is 120 beats/min. However, she mentions that she ran to the clinic. Upon recheck, her pulse rate is 95 beats/min. Her height is 68.0 in (172.5 cm), and weight is 231 lb (104.8 kg) (BMI = 35.1 kg/m^2). Her neck is supple with no evidence of lymphadenopathy or thyromegaly. There is no acanthosis in her axillary region. Terminal hairs are visible above her lip, chin, and lower abdomen. She also has sparse hairs around her nipple areolar complex.

Laboratory test results:

FSH = 6.1 mIU/mL (2.0-12.0 mIU/mL [follicular]) (SI: 6.1 IU/L [2.0-12.0 IU/L])
LH = 14.4 mIU/mL (1.0-18.0 mIU/mL [follicular]) (SI: 14.4 mIU/mL [1.0-18.0 mIU/mL])
Estradiol = 136 pg/mL (10-180 pg/mL [follicular]) (SI: 499.3 pmol/L [26.7-660.8 pmol/L])
Total testosterone = 49 ng/dL (8-60 ng/dL) (SI: 1.7 nmol/L [0.3-2.1 nmol/L])
DHEA-S = 134 µg/dL (44-332 µg/dL) (SI: 3.63 µmol/L [1.19-9.00 µmol/L])
17-Hydroxyprogesterone = 54 ng/dL (<80 ng/dL [follicular]) (SI: 1.64 nmol/L [<2.42 nmol/L])
TSH = 3.31 mIU/L (0.5-5.0 mIU/L)

Findings on transvaginal ultrasonography are consistent with polycystic morphology, with increased small follicles bilaterally. Her endometrial stripe is 7 mm.

In addition to lifestyle measures, which of the following is the best treatment option for this patient?

A. Combined oral contraceptive pill
B. Dexamethasone
C. Laser hair removal
D. Metformin
E. Weight loss and spironolactone

71 A 48-year-old postmenopausal woman presents for further evaluation of type 2 diabetes mellitus diagnosed at age 28 years. She struggles with needle phobia and is overwhelmed by her worsening glycemic control and new diagnosis of metabolic dysfunction-associated steatotic liver disease with stage 2 fibrosis. She has been adhering to her Mediterranean diet and exercise regimen since her last visit and has lost 6% of her body weight but has now plateaued. Her current treatment regimen is metformin, dapagliflozin, and glipizide. Her current hemoglobin A_{1c} value is 7.9% (63 mmol/mol), down from 8.4% (68 mmol/mol) before her weight loss. She would like to improve her glycemic control and prevent cirrhosis.

Which of the following is the best management plan for this patient?

A. Intensify lifestyle changes
B. Start basal insulin
C. Start pioglitazone
D. Start sitagliptin
E. Start vitamin E

72 A 30-year-old man with presumed familial hypercholesterolemia is seen for follow-up. Both of his parents and multiple uncles are known to have significantly elevated cholesterol levels. His father underwent angioplasty with stent placement at age 48 years. The patient's maximum untreated LDL-cholesterol concentration was 460 mg/dL (11.91 mmol/L), and he has been on statin therapy since age 15 years. Current medications include atorvastatin, 80 mg daily; ezetimibe, 10 mg daily; and evolocumab, 140 mg every 2 weeks. He has no symptoms and feels well. He plays basketball 3 days per week, does not smoke cigarettes, and has liberal intake of fruits and vegetables in his diet. His weight has been stable.

On physical examination, his blood pressure is 115/75 mm Hg, and pulse rate is 70 beats/min. His height is 73 in (185.4 cm), and weight is 197 lb (89.4 kg) (BMI = 26 kg/m^2). His right Achilles tendon is thickened.

Fasting lipid panel:

Total cholesterol = 220 mg/dL (<200 mg/dL) (SI: 5.70 mmol/L [<5.18 mmol/L])
Triglycerides = 120 mg/dL (<150 mg/dL) (SI: 1.36 mmol/L [<1.70 mmol/L])
HDL cholesterol = 50 mg/dL (>60 mg/dL) (SI: 1.30 mmol/L [>1.55 mmol/L])
LDL cholesterol = 146 mg/dL (<100 mg/dL) (SI: 3.78 mmol/L [<2.59 mmol/L])

Which of the following is the best next step in this patient's management?

A. Add evinacumab (monoclonal antibody to ANGPTL3)
B. Add inclisiran (siRNA targeting PCSK9)
C. Change atorvastatin to rosuvastatin, 40 mg daily
D. Maintain current medication regimen and encourage continued adherence to healthy lifestyle habits
E. Start biweekly LDL apheresis

73 A 24-year-old overseas student is referred after he fractures his ankle playing badminton. X-ray unexpectedly reveals unfused growth plates, and DXA documents low bone density for age, with Z-scores of −3.2 at the lumbar spine and −2.8 at the femoral neck. He takes no prescription or over-the-counter medications. Further history reveals that his mother, while pregnant with him, exhibited signs of progressive virilization that resolved in the postpartum period. There is a possible history of parental consanguinity.

On physical examination, his height is 75 in (190.5 cm) and weight is 231 lb (104.8 kg) (BMI = 28.9 kg/m^2). He has eunuchoidal body proportions with central adiposity (waist circumference is 40 in [101.6 cm]). Moderate acanthosis nigricans is notable in the axillae. There is no gynecomastia. He is normally virilized, with male-pattern body hair and normal findings on genital examination. Testicular volume is 25 mL bilaterally.

Laboratory test results:

LH = 28.0 mIU/mL (1.0-9.0 mIU/mL) (SI: 28.0 IU/L [1.0-9.0 IU/L])
FSH = 27.0 mIU/mL (1.0-13.0 mIU/mL) (SI: 27.0 IU/L [1.0-13.0 IU/L])
Testosterone = 1200 ng/dL (300-900 ng/dL) (SI: 41.6 nmol/L [10.4-31.2 nmol/L])
SHBG = 3.4 µg/mL (1.1-6.7 µg/mL) (SI: 30 nmol/L [10-60 nmol/L])
Total cholesterol = 250 ng/dL (<200 mg/dL) (SI: 6.48 mmol/L [<5.18 mmol/L])
LDL cholesterol = 150 ng/dL (<100 mg/dL) (SI: 3.88 mmol/L [<2.59 mmol/L])
HDL cholesterol = 30 ng/dL (>60 mg/dL) (SI: 0.78 mmol/L [>1.55 mmol/L])
Glucose = 120 mg/dL (70-99 mg/dL) (SI: 6.7 mmol/L [3.9-5.5 mmol/L])
Insulin = 20.0 µIU/mL (1.4-14.0 µIU/mL) (SI: 138.9 pmol/L [9.7-97.2 pmol/L])
Serum calcium, normal

Which of the following is the best investigation to perform next?

A. ACTH and cortisol measurement and a 1-mg dexamethasone-suppression test
B. Serum DHEA-S measurement
C. Serum estradiol measurement
D. Serum 17-hydroxyprogesterone measurement
E. Serum IGF-1 and GH measurement

74 A 33-year-old woman presents for evaluation of an asymptomatic right thyroid nodule that was detected during workup for primary hyperparathyroidism. The patient had initially presented with hypercalcemia that was incidentally noted on routine laboratory testing. She reports no symptoms and is otherwise healthy with no history of nephrolithiasis or fracture. There is no personal history of head or neck ionizing radiation exposure. There is no family history of thyroid malignancy, but the patient's paternal grandmother had primary hyperparathyroidism.

On physical examination, her blood pressure is 128/74 mm Hg and pulse rate is 78 beats/min. Her height is 66 in (167.6 cm), and weight is 156 lb (70.8 kg) (BMI = 25.2 kg/m^2). Findings on thyroid examination are unremarkable without enlargement or nodules. The rest of her examination findings are normal.

Laboratory test results:

- TSH = 0.8 mIU/L (0.5-5.0 mIU/L)
- Calcium = 10.5 mg/dL (8.2-10.2 mg/dL) (SI: 2.6 mmol/L [2.1-2.6 mmol/L])
- Albumin = 4.0 g/dL (3.5-5.0 g/dL) (SI: 40 g/L [35-50 g/L])
- Creatinine = 0.74 mg/dL (0.6-1.1 mg/dL) (SI: 65.4 μmol/L [53.0-97.2 μmol/L])
- Phosphate = 2.7 mg/dL (2.3-4.7 mg/dL) (SI: 0.9 mmol/L [0.7-1.5 mmol/L])
- PTH = 128 pg/mL (10-65 pg/mL) (SI: 128 ng/L [10-65 ng/L])
- 25-Hydroxyvitamin D = 40 ng/mL (30-80 ng/mL [optimal]) (SI: 99.8 nmol/L [74.9-199.7 nmol/L])
- Urinary calcium = 235 mg/24 h (100-300 mg/24 h) (SI: 5.9 mmol/d [2.5-7.5 mmol/d])
- Urinary creatinine = 0.85 g/24 h (1.0-2.0 g/24 h) (SI: 7.5 mmol/d [8.8-17.7 mmol/d])

Neck ultrasonography demonstrates a 0.9 × 0.4 × 0.5-cm, hypoechoic, solid, hypervascular nodule in the right lower thyroid gland (*see images*). No left thyroid nodules or abnormal lymph nodes are identified.

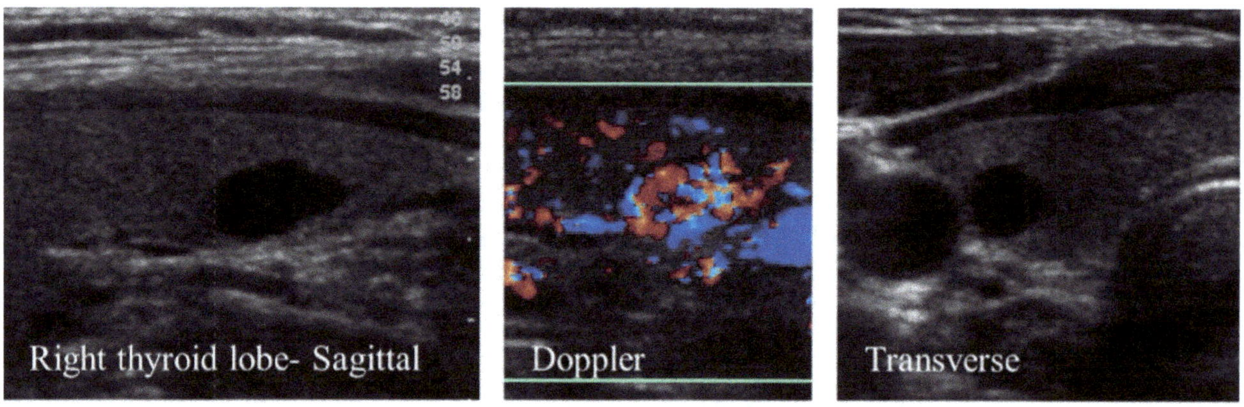

A nuclear medicine parathyroid localization study is also performed. Approximately 2 hours after ^{123}I administration, ^{99m}Tc sestamibi is administered. Initial planar sestamibi images show focal increased activity in the inferior aspect of the right thyroid lobe. Subtraction of the initial pinhole images confirms this impression (*see images*). Delayed planar sestamibi images show persistent focal equivocal increased activity. Subtraction of the delayed pinhole images confirms this impression (*images not shown*). Thyroid ^{123}I images show no significant thyroid abnormalities. The pattern and intensity of sestamibi activity in the area of the tumor do not match ^{123}I activity.

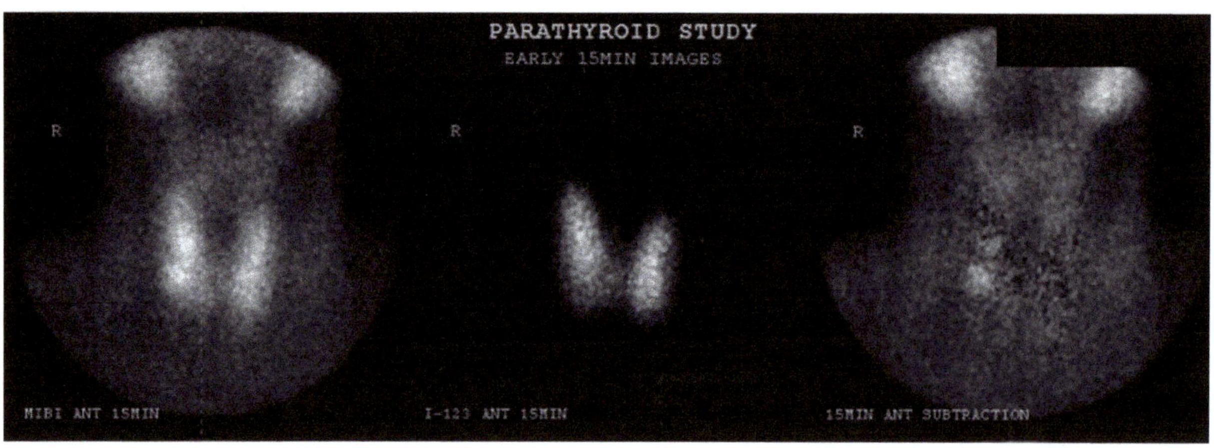

Which of the following is the most appropriate management to recommend next?

A. Measure calcium, albumin, and creatinine in 6 months
B. Perform DXA
C. Perform kidney ultrasonography
D. Perform ultrasound-guided FNA of right thyroid nodule
E. Refer for right thyroid lobectomy

75 A 37-year-old woman is referred for further investigation of oligomenorrhea and primary infertility. Following menarche at age 13 years, her menses were regular, including while taking a combined oral contraceptive preparation until 18 months ago. However, since discontinuing the pill in anticipation of starting a family, she has had only 3 light withdrawal bleeds, and this has coincided with the onset of episodic sweating with heat intolerance, especially at night. More recently she has noticed her clothes no longer fit properly, and she estimates she has lost 10 lb (4.5 kg) in the last 4 months.

On physical examination, her height is 68 in (172.7 cm) and weight is 134 lb (60.8 kg) (BMI = 20.4 kg/m^2). Her resting pulse rate is 108 beats/min and regular, and blood pressure is 110/70 mm Hg seated and 100/70 mm Hg after standing for 2 minutes. She has normal secondary sexual characteristics.

Laboratory test results:

Prolactin = 24 ng/mL (4-30 ng/mL) (SI: 1.04 nmol/L [0.17-1.30 nmol/L])
FSH = 1.1 mIU/mL (2.0-12.0 mIU/mL [follicular]) (SI: 1.1 IU/L [2.0-12.0 IU/L])
LH = 1.3 mIU/mL (1.0-18.0 mIU/mL [follicular]) (SI: 1.3 IU/L [1.0-18.0 IU/L])
Estradiol = 32 pg/mL (10-180 pg/mL [follicular]) (SI: 117.5 pmol/L [36.7-660.8 pmol/L])
SHBG = 16.3 μg/mL (2.2-14.6 μg/mL) (SI: 145 nmol/L [20-130 nmol/L])
Serum cortisol (8 AM) = 6.5 μg/dL (5-25 μg/dL) (SI: 179.3 nmol/L [137.9-689.7 nmol/L])
Free T_4 = 2.1 ng/dL (0.8-1.8 ng/dL) (SI: 27.03 pmol/L [10.30-23.17 pmol/L])
TSH = 1.8 mIU/L (0.5-5.0 mIU/L)

There is no evidence of laboratory assay interference.

Which of the following is the most likely cause of this patient's presentation?

A. Addison disease
B. Graves disease
C. Low body weight
D. Pituitary adenoma
E. Premature ovarian insufficiency

76 A 42-year-old woman returns for continued management of type 2 diabetes mellitus and obesity that was diagnosed at age 29 years. She has made multiple attempts to change her lifestyle and most recently underwent a trial of orlistat to facilitate weight loss. She has lost only 5 lb (2.3 kg) over the past 6 months and expresses her desire to try another antiobesity therapy. She is also contemplating other options, including other medications and gastric bypass surgery. She would like to choose a therapy that would help with all of her weight-related risk factors, including her cancer risk (her mother died of pancreatic cancer and her father died of lung cancer).

Her other medical conditions include hypertension, hyperlipidemia, acute pancreatitis, glaucoma, and a remote history of seizures.

Current medications are insulin glargine, 50 units daily; insulin aspart, 10 units with meals, and correction insulin aspart, 2 units for every 50 mg/dL (2.8 mmol/L) that blood glucose is above 150 mg/dL (>8.3 mmol/L); metformin; lisinopril; rosuvastatin; and carbamazepine.

On physical examination, her blood pressure is 138/92 mm Hg and pulse rate is 78 beats/min. Her height is 65 in (165.1 cm), and weight is 315 lb (142.9 kg) (BMI = 52.4 kg/m^2). No lipohypertrophy is noted at the usual sites of insulin injections. She has no abdominal striae, supraclavicular fat pads, or proximal muscle weakness.

Laboratory test result:

Hemoglobin A_{1c} = 8.2% (4.0%-5.6%) (66.1 mmol/mol [20-38 mmol/mol])

Which of the following should be recommended as the best next step in this patient's management?

A. Bupropion/naltrexone
B. Gastric bypass surgery
C. Phentermine/topiramate
D. Semaglutide
E. Tirzepatide

77 A 58-year-old woman presents for evaluation of osteoporosis and a recent L2 vertebral compression fracture. She has a history of type 1 diabetes mellitus complicated by stage 5 chronic kidney disease. Two months ago, she experienced sudden low back pain after standing, which prompted evaluation in a local emergency department. Lumbar spine x-ray demonstrated an L2 compression fracture. This was followed by lumbar spine MRI, which revealed findings consistent with an acute vertebral compression fracture. She was prescribed pain medications and a short-term course of intranasal calcitonin. Her primary care provider ordered DXA, which documented osteoporosis with a T-score of −3.7 in L3-L4 and −2.9 in the femoral neck. The patient's chronic kidney disease is managed by a nephrologist who prescribes calcitriol, 0.5 mcg daily, to control secondary hyperparathyroidism. The nephrologist agrees that the patient should be referred to an endocrinologist to discuss osteoporosis treatment options.

Laboratory test results:

Calcium = 8.3 mg/dL (8.2-10.2 mg/dL) (SI: 2.1 mmol/L [2.1-2.6 mmol/L])
Albumin = 3.5 g/dL (3.5-5.0 g/dL) (SI: 35 g/L [35-50 g/L])
Phosphate = 4.9 mg/dL (2.3-4.7 mg/dL) (SI: 4.9 mmol/L [0.7-1.5 mmol/L])
Creatinine = 5.1 mg/dL (0.6-1.1 mg/dL) (SI: 450.8 µmol/L [53.0-97.2 µmol/L])
Glomerular filtration rate (estimated) = 13 mL/min per 1.73 m^2 (>60 mL/min per 1.73 m^2)
Intact PTH = 63 pg/mL (10-65 pg/mL) (SI: 63 ng/L [10-65 ng/L])
Magnesium = 2.3 mg/dL (1.5-2.3 mg/dL) (SI: 0.9 mmol/L [0.6-0.9 mmol/L])
25-Hydroxyvitamin D = 28 ng/mL (30-80 ng/mL [optimal]) (SI: 69.9 nmol/L [74.9-199.7 nmol/L])

Which of the following is the best next step in this patient's management?

A. Increase the calcitriol dosage to 1 mcg orally daily
B. Measure bone-specific alkaline phosphatase
C. Measure serum C-telopeptide
D. Measure serum 1,25-dihydroxyvitamin D
E. Prescribe cinacalcet

78 A 53-year-old man is interested in bariatric surgery. He reports that he can lose weight when he follows a structured diet and physical activity routine, but he regains weight when he does not follow the plan consistently. He describes himself as an emotional eater. Several times a month, he engages in a "binge," when he eats large quantities of food. He feels he has no control over his food intake during these episodes and feels guilty afterwards. He has not spoken about these episodes with anyone but worries that continued weight gain will adversely affect his health.

On physical examination, his blood pressure is 142/82 mm Hg, and pulse rate is 70 beats/min. His height is 63.5 in (161.3 cm), and weight is 234 lb (106.1 kg) (BMI = 40.8 kg/m^2). There is no peripheral edema. He has increased abdominal girth, relatively lean extremities, and no dorsocervical fat pad.

His current medication regimen consists of lisinopril, 20 mg daily; atorvastatin, 20 mg daily; mirtazapine, 30 mg at bedtime for insomnia; and famotidine, 10 mg as needed for heartburn.

In addition to a psychological assessment, which of the following is the best next step?

A. Discontinue mirtazapine
B. Refer for Roux-en-Y gastric bypass
C. Refer for sleeve gastrectomy
D. Start bupropion
E. Start lisdexamfetamine

79 A 67-year-old man with a 25-year history of type 2 diabetes mellitus presents for a follow-up appointment. His medical history is notable for obesity, coronary artery disease (status post coronary artery bypass graft surgery 4 months ago), chronic obstructive pulmonary disease treated with home oxygen, hypertension, dyslipidemia, diabetic neuropathy, and mild diabetic retinopathy. His medication regimen consists of U500 insulin, 75 units subcutaneous 3 times daily, and metformin, 500 mg twice daily (which is the highest dosage the patient can tolerate). His hemoglobin A_{1c} value today is 8.5% (69 mmol/mol). He self-checks blood glucose 2 to 3 times daily and says that his values are consistently in the "200s." His BMI is 39 kg/m^2.

Which of the following is the best next step in this patient's management?

A. Increase the dosage of U500 insulin
B. Initiate phentermine/topiramate
C. Initiate saxagliptin
D. Initiate semaglutide
E. Refer for bariatric surgery

80 A 26-year-old woman (G0P0) presents with irregular menstrual cycles. She experienced menarche at age 11 years and had regular cycles until this past year. Over the past year, she experienced greater variability, with menses occurring every 1 to 4 months. She has no history of weight fluctuation, eating disorders, excessive exercise, hirsutism, bothersome acne, clitoromegaly, hot flashes, systemic illness, or uterine instrumentation. However, she has been chronically underweight for a decade. She has had no diplopia or change in peripheral vision, but she does note frequent headaches occurring at night 2 to 3 times per week starting 2 months ago. She is currently sexually active with a cisgender man and does not want to conceive until her 30s. She does not use any form of contraception. She does not use tobacco, alcohol, or recreational drugs.

On physical examination, her blood pressure is 95/50 mm Hg and pulse rate is 95 beats/min. Her height is 64 in (162.5 cm), and weight is 99 lb (45 kg) (BMI = 17.0 kg/m^2). Her thyroid gland is symmetric without enlargement or nodules. She has no acanthosis nigricans and no hirsutism. Her visual fields are full to confrontation.

Laboratory test results:

Complete metabolic panel, normal
Complete blood cell count, normal
Hemoglobin A_{1c}, normal
LH = 1.7 mIU/mL (1.0-18.0 mIU/mL [follicular]) (SI: 1.7 IU/L [(1.0-18.0 IU/L])
FSH = 2.0 mIU/mL (2.0-12.0 mIU/mL [follicular]) (SI: 2.0 IU/L [2.0-12.0 IU/L])
Estradiol = 35 pg/mL (10-180 pg/mL [follicular]) (SI: 128.5 pmol/L [26.7-660.8 pmol/L])
TSH = 1.32 mIU/L (0.5-5.0 mIU/L)
Prolactin = 51 ng/mL (4-30 ng/mL [nonlactating female]) (SI: 2.13 nmol/L [0.17-1.30 nmol/L])

Pituitary MRI reveals a normal-sized gland with a 2-mm nonenhancing focus with an intrinsic T1 hyperintense rim, most likely representing a microadenoma with old blood products lining the rim.

Which of the following is the best next management approach for this patient?

A. Bromocriptine
B. Cabergoline
C. Combined oral contraceptive pill (ethinyl estradiol-norelgestromin)
D. Norethindrone
E. Progestogen challenge with medroxyprogesterone acetate

81 A 36-year-old man with type 3 osteogenesis imperfecta presents for a routine visit. Treatment has included recent intravenous bisphosphonate therapy. He reports more than 80 fractures in his lifetime. Most recently, he sustained 1 radius fracture 8 months ago. He has deformities of his forearms and a history of severe scoliosis. He uses a wheelchair but is able to transfer himself. He notes gradual onset and increase of dyspnea with minimal exertion. He does not have orthopnea, but he is on continuous positive airway pressure at night for obstructive sleep apnea. His activity is limited. He has no chest or rib pain, fevers, cough, or other associated symptoms. He does not have diabetes, hypertension, or high cholesterol. He does not smoke cigarettes. His father had a myocardial infarction at age 63 years.

His medications include zoledronic acid infusion (last dose 6 months ago); calcium carbonate, 600 mg daily; and vitamin D, 2000 units daily.

On physical examination, he has short stature (height Z-score, −3.2), gray sclerae, dentinogenesis imperfecta, severe kyphoscoliosis, shortened upper arms, bowing deformities of forearms and lower extremities, and hypermobile fingers. There are no rales or wheezing on auscultation. His pulse rate is 74 beats/min, with a regular rhythm and no murmurs. He has no peripheral edema or areas of tenderness in his lower extremities.

Findings on electrocardiography are normal.

Which of the following assessments is most likely to reveal the cause of this patient's new symptoms?

A. Cardiac stress test
B. Chest radiography
C. Echocardiography
D. Pulmonary function tests
E. Venous Doppler study

82 A 38-year-old woman with a recent diagnosis of Graves disease (suppressed TSH and free T_4 value of 3.6 ng/dL [46.3 pmol/L]) presents for a follow-up visit. She has taken methimazole, 20 mg daily, for the last 8 weeks. She has nausea and severe epigastric pain and generally feels unwell. She has gastroesophageal reflux disease and takes omeprazole, 20 mg daily.

On physical examination, her blood pressure is 100/60 mm Hg and pulse rate is 80 beats/min and regular. Her thyroid gland is mildly enlarged, there is no proptosis, and there is no tremor in her outstretched hands. She has tenderness in the epigastric area. The rest of her examination findings are unremarkable.

Laboratory test results:

TSH = <0.01 mIU/L (0.5-5.0 mIU/L)
Free T_4 = 2.0 ng/dL (0.8-1.8 ng/dL) (SI: 25.74 pmol/L [10.30-23.17 pmol/L])
Thyroid-stimulating immunoglobulin = 200% (≤120% of basal activity)
Lipase = 320 U/L (10-73 U/L) (SI: 5.34 μkat/L [0.17-1.22 μkat/L])
AST = 36 U/L (20-48 U/L) (SI: 0.60 μkat/L [0.33-0.80 μkat/L])
ALT = 24 U/L (10-40 U/L) (SI: 0.40 μkat/L [0.17-0.67 μkat/L])
Serum alkaline phosphatase = 100 U/L (50-120 U/L) (SI: 1.67 μkat/L [0.84-2.00 μkat/L])
White blood cell count = 10,600/μL (4500-11,000/μL) (SI: 10.6 × 10^9/L [4.5-11.0 × 10^9/L])
Triglycerides = 100 mg/dL (<150 mg/dL) (SI: 1.13 mmol/L [<1.70 mmol/L])

Which of the following is the best next step in this patient's management?

A. Decrease the methimazole dosage
B. Discontinue methimazole
C. Increase the omeprazole dosage
D. Perform abdominal CT
E. Perform upper endoscopy

83

A 31-year-old woman of Asian descent is concerned about impaired glucose tolerance. A fasting plasma glucose value of 106 mg/dL (5.9 mmol/L) was documented on a comprehensive metabolic panel as part of routine annual laboratory testing ordered by her primary care physician. The rest of the complete metabolic panel was normal. Her hemoglobin A_{1c} measurement was 5.6% (4.0%-5.6%) (37.7 mmol/mol [20-38 mmol/mol]).

Her primary care physician advised her to reduce carbohydrate intake and undergo a 75-g oral glucose tolerance test after 1 month. This test demonstrated a fasting glucose value of 98 mg/dL (5.4 mmol/L) and a 2-hour value of 198 mg/dL (11.0 mmol/L).

Medications include esomeprazole and drospirenone/ethinyl estradiol, 0.02/0.451 mg daily.

She is asymptomatic. Family history is unknown because she was adopted. Social history is noncontributory.

On physical examination, her height is 65 in (165.1 cm) and weight is 148 lb (67.1 kg) (BMI = 24.6 kg/m^2). There is no acanthosis. She has no physical stigmata of cortisol excess such as preauricular fullness, wide pigmented striae, or proximal weakness.

Which of the following is the best next step in the evaluation of this patient's impaired glucose tolerance?

A. Measure C-peptide
B. Measure fructosamine
C. Recommend self-assessment of blood glucose at home
D. Repeat oral glucose tolerance testing, with consumption of 150 g carbohydrate per day for 3 days before testing
E. Screen for type 1 diabetes risk by measuring glutamic acid decarboxylase 65 and islet-cell antigen antibodies

84

A 55-year-old woman with a medical history of hypertension and hyperlipidemia is admitted to the hospital for chest pain, shortness of breath, and hypertensive urgency. She has felt fatigued for the last year and has gained 30 lb (13.6 kg) in the past 6 months. She has hypokalemia and a non-ST elevation myocardial infarction. During her hospitalization, new-onset diabetes mellitus is also diagnosed (hemoglobin A_{1c} = 7.6% [60 mmol/mol]). A 1.1-cm left adrenal nodule is detected on chest CT angiography. The nodule's density is 37 Hounsfield units after contrast administration.

Medications include amlodipine, 10 mg daily; benazepril, 40 mg daily; spironolactone, 100 mg daily; potassium chloride, 10 mEq twice daily; atorvastatin, 40 mg daily; isosorbide dinitrate, 20 mg twice daily; and metformin, 500 mg twice daily.

On physical examination at a follow-up appointment, her blood pressure is 170/92 mm Hg and pulse rate is 85 beats/min. Her height is 64 in (162.6 cm), and weight is 232 lb (105.2 kg) (BMI = 39.8 kg/m^2). She is unable to stand from a chair without support and has multiple bruises on her arms and legs.

Laboratory test results:

Random serum cortisol = 50 µg/dL (SI: 1379.4 nmol/L)
ACTH = 450 pg/mL (10-60 pg/mL) (SI: 99.0 pmol/L [2.2-13.2 pmol/L])

Pituitary-directed MRI identifies a 1.3-cm adenoma (*see image*).

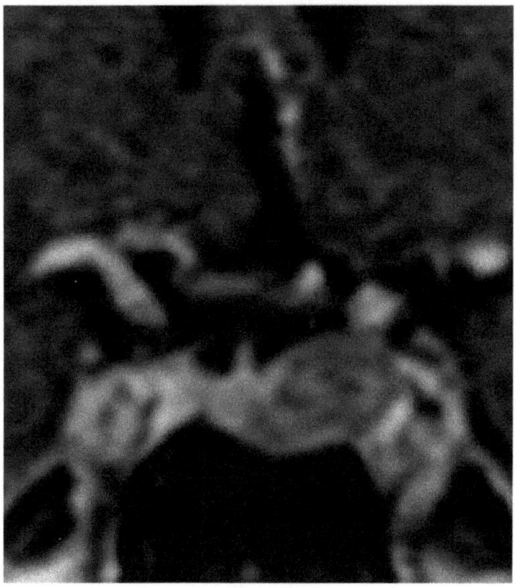

Repeated workup after hospital discharge documents 24-hour urinary free cortisol measurements of 500 and 663 µg/24 h (1380 and 1830 nmol/d) on 2 occasions. Plasma normetanephrine and metanephrine concentrations are normal.

The patient undergoes a 2-day dexamethasone-suppression test combined with corticotropin-releasing hormone stimulation with the following results:

Time of measurement	Cortisol concentration	ACTH concentration	Dexamethasone concentration
Baseline #1	27.1 µg/dL (SI: 747.6 nmol/L)	262 pg/mL (SI: 57.6 pmol/L)	491 ng/dL
Baseline #2	28.2 µg/dL (SI: 778.0 nmol/L)	276 pg/mL (SI: 60.7 pmol/L)	...
15 minutes after CRH	26.1 µg/dL (SI: 720.0 nmol/L)	230 pg/mL (SI: 50.6 pmol/L)	...
30 minutes after CRH	27.6 µg/dL (SI: 761.4 nmol/L)	262 pg/mL (SI: 57.6 pmol/L)	...
45 minutes after CRH	26.6 µg/dL (SI: 733.8 nmol/L)	249 pg/mL (SI: 54.8 pmol/L)	...
60 minutes after CRH	27.6 µg/dL (SI: 761.4nmol/L)	278 pg/mL (SI: 61.2 pmol/L)	...

CRH, corticotropin-releasing hormone.

Which of the following is the best next step in this patient's management?

A. Chest and abdominal CT with and without contrast
B. High-dose dexamethasone-suppression test
C. Inferior petrosal sinus sampling
D. Laparoscopic removal of the left adrenal gland
E. Transsphenoidal resection of the pituitary adenoma

85 A 23-year-old woman is referred for investigation of weight gain (18 lb [8.2 kg]) over a 6-month interval). She also reports that her menses have been irregular since discontinuing an oral contraceptive pill 4 months ago. Her medical history is otherwise unremarkable.

On physical examination, her blood pressure is 165/90 mm Hg and pulse rate is 76 beats/min and regular. Her height is 67 in (170.2 cm), and weight is 212 lb (96.1 kg) (BMI = 33.2 kg/m^2). She has facial plethora, central obesity with purple/red abdominal striae, and bruises of different ages over her forearms and lower legs. She has difficulty rising from a chair. There is no skin pigmentation or cutaneous nodules, and the rest of the examination findings are normal.

Laboratory test results:

Serum cortisol (8 AM) = 22.2 µg/dL (5-25 µg/dL) (SI: 612.5 nmol/L [137.9-689.7 nmol/L])
Cortisol following 1-mg dexamethasone-suppression test = 20.1 µg/dL (SI: 554.5 nmol/L)
Cortisol (salivary), midnight: 0.51 µg/dL (<0.13 µg/dL) (SI: 14.1 nmol/L [<3.6 nmol/L])
Urinary free cortisol = 145 µg/24 h (4-50 µg/24 h) (SI: 400.2 nmol/d [11-138 nmol/d])
Plasma ACTH = <5 pg/mL (10-60 pg/mL) (SI: <1.1 pmol/L [2.2-13.2 pmol/L])
Serum DHEA-S = 15 µg/dL (44-332 µg/dL) (SI: 0.41 µmol/L [(1.19-9.00 µmol/L])

On abdominal CT, both adrenal glands appear normal with no nodules or hyperplasia.

Which of the following is the most appropriate next step in this patient's management?

A. Adrenal vein sampling
B. Chemical shift adrenal MRI
C. Combined low- and high-dose dexamethasone-suppression test (Liddle test)
D. ^{68}Ga-DOTATATE PET/CT scan
E. 24-Hour urinary steroid profile

86 A 28-year-old man is referred for further evaluation of low testosterone. He presented to his primary care provider with fatigue and low mood in the context of losing his job during the COVID-19 pandemic. At his evaluation 2 months ago, his serum total testosterone concentration was 89 ng/dL (3.1 nmol/L). He now has a new job, and his fatigue and mood have improved. He reports good libido and no erectile dysfunction, hot flushes, or muscle weakness. He recalls normal puberty, but he has not attempted paternity. Findings on review of systems are otherwise normal. He takes no prescribed or over-the-counter medications. He attends the gym twice weekly, performing a mixture of aerobic and resistance exercise, and states that he has never taken anabolic steroids. He takes no over-the-counter supplements or internet-sourced products.

On physical examination, his blood pressure is 122/68 mm Hg and pulse rate is 68 beats/min and regular. His height is 67 in (175 cm), and weight is 179 lb (81 kg) (BMI = 26.4 km/m^2). Physical examination findings are otherwise normal, including male-pattern body hair, muscle bulk, and genitalia. Testicular volume is 25 mL bilaterally, without masses.

Current laboratory test results:

Total testosterone by immunoassay = 80.7 ng/dL (300-900 ng/dL) (SI: 2.8 nmol/L [10.4-31.2 nmol/L])
Total testosterone 2 weeks later by liquid chromatography–tandem mass spectrometry = 98.0 ng/dL (SI: 3.4 nmol/L)
LH = 4.8 mIU/mL (1.0-9.0 mIU/mL) (SI: 4.8 IU/L [1.0-9.0 IU/L])
FSH = 3.5 mIU/mL (1.0-13.0 mIU/mL) (SI: 3.5 IU/L [1.0-13.0 IU/L])
Full blood examination and differential, normal
Serum prolactin, normal

Which of the following laboratory tests should be done next?

A. 24-Hour urinary cortisol measurement
B. Serum estradiol measurement
C. Serum 17-hydroxyprogesterone measurement
D. Serum SHBG measurement
E. Urinary anabolic steroid testing

87 A 63-year-old woman presents to her primary care provider reporting a 4-week history of extreme fatigue, dizziness, polyuria, and polydipsia. Her medical history includes gastroesophageal reflux disease treated with omeprazole and hypertension treated with metoprolol. She does not smoke cigarettes or consume alcohol. Her last mammogram was 4 years ago and findings were normal.

Laboratory test results:

Calcium = 13.1 mg/dL (8.2-10.2 mg/dL) (SI: 3.3 mmol/L [2.1-2.6 mmol/L])
Albumin = 4.1 g/dL (3.5-5.0 g/dL) (SI: 41 g/L [35-50 g/L])
Creatinine = 2.1 mg/dL (0.6-1.1 mg/dL) (SI: 185.6 µmol/L [53.0-97.2 µmol/L])

She is sent to a local emergency department for evaluation and management of hypercalcemia, and laboratory tests are repeated:

Calcium = 13.4 mg/dL (8.2-10.2 mg/dL) (SI: 3.4 mmol/L [2.1-2.6 mmol/L])
Albumin = 3.9 g/dL (3.5-5.0 g/dL) (SI: 39 g/L [35-50 g/L])
Calcium (ionized) = 5.85 mg/dL (4.60-5.08 mg/dL) (SI: 1.46 mmol/L [1.2-1.3 mmol/L])
Creatinine = 2.4 mg/dL (0.6-1.1 mg/dL) (SI: 212.2 µmol/L [53.0-97.2 µmol/L])

Phosphate = 5.1 mg/dL (2.3-4.7 mg/dL) (SI: 1.6 mmol/L [0.7-1.5 mmol/L])
Magnesium = 1.6 mg/dL (1.5-2.3 mg/dL) (SI: 0.7 mmol/L [0.6-0.9 mmol/L])

She receives intravenous hydration and is admitted to the hospital. With hydration, her serum calcium concentration decreases to 10.5 mg/dL (2.6 mmol/L) the next day. Additional laboratory tests are ordered:

Intact PTH = 6 pg/mL (10-65 pg/mL) (SI: 6 ng/L [10-65 ng/L])
25-Hydroxyvitamin D = 25 ng/mL (30-80 ng/mL [optimal]) (SI: 62.4 nmol/L [74.9-199.7 nmol/L])
1,25-Dihydroxyvitamin D = 28 pg/mL (16-65 pg/mL) (SI: 72.8 pmol/L [41.6-169.0 pmol/L])
PTHrP = 0.5 pmol/L (<2.0 pmol/L)

An x-ray skeletal survey is performed, and the findings are reported as abnormal. A cross-sectional image from spine CT is shown (*see image right*).

A nuclear medicine bone scan is also performed (*see image far right*).

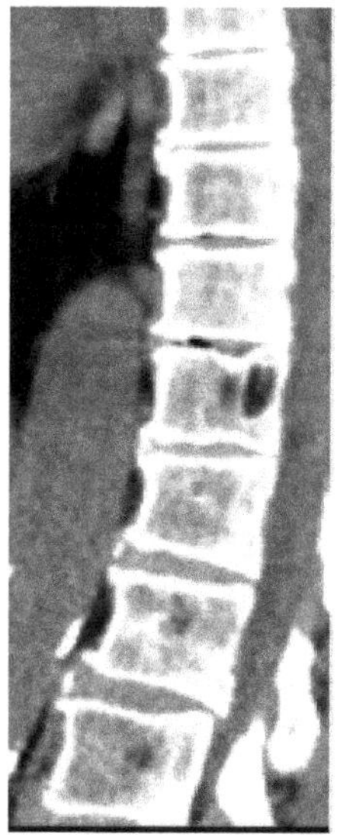

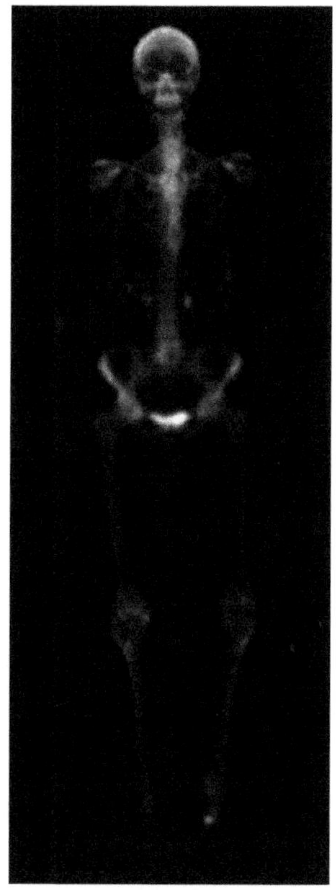

Which of the following is the most likely cause of this patient's hypercalcemia?

A. Metastatic breast cancer
B. Metastatic lung cancer
C. Metastatic renal cell carcinoma
D. Multiple myeloma
E. NonHodgkin lymphoma

88

A 32-year-old previously healthy woman is referred for evaluation and management of hypercholesterolemia.

Fasting lipid panel results:

Measurement	Two years ago	Current
Total cholesterol	197 mg/dL (SI: 5.10 mmol/L)	872 mg/dL (SI: 3.78 mmol/L)
Triglycerides	122 mg/dL (SI: 1.38 mmol/L)	77 mg/dL (SI: 0.87 mmol/L)
HDL cholesterol	77 mg/dL (SI: 1.99 mmol/L)	134 mg/dL (SI: 3.47 mmol/L)
LDL cholesterol	96 mg/dL (SI: 2.49 mmol/L)	723 mg/dL (SI: 18.7 mmol/L)

Reference ranges: total cholesterol, <200 mg/dL (SI: <5.18 mmol/L); triglycerides, <150 mg/dL (SI: <1.70 mmol/L); HDL cholesterol, >60 mg/dL (SI: >1.55 mmol/L); LDL cholesterol, <100 mg/dL (SI: <2.59 mmol/L).

She currently takes rosuvastatin, 5 mg 3 times weekly, because she cannot tolerate a higher dosage. She also takes levothyroxine, 50 mcg daily, for primary hypothyroidism.

She has been extremely cautious about her diet, scrupulously avoiding most starchy foods, and she primarily consumes eggs, spinach, and leafy vegetables. She reports no recent change in weight. Review of symptoms is notable for amenorrhea, constipation, and cold intolerance. She has no angina or exertional dyspnea.

On physical examination, her blood pressure is 90/72 mm Hg and pulse rate is 92 beats/min. Her height is 64 in (162.6 cm), and weight is 88 lb (39.9 kg) (BMI = 15.1 kg/m²). She has no corneal arcus or tendon xanthomas.

Additional laboratory results:

Fasting plasma glucose = 90 mg/dL (70-99 mg/dL) (SI: 5.0 mmol/L [3.9-5.5 mmol/L])
Serum creatinine = 0.5 mg/dL (0.6-1.1 mg/dL) (SI: 44.2 µmol/L [53.0-97.2 µmol/L])
ALT = 22 U/L (10-40 U/L) (SI: 0.37 µkat/L [0.17-0.67 µkat/L])
AST = 24 U/L (20-48 U/L) (SI: 0.40 µkat/L [0.33-0.80 µkat/L])
Total bilirubin = 0.9 mg/dL (0.3-1.2 mg/dL) (SI: 15.4 µmol/L [5.1-20.5 µmol/L])
TSH = 4.8 mIU/L (0.5-5.0 mIU/L)
Free T_4 = 1.1 ng/dL (0.8-1.8 ng/dL) (SI: 14.16 pmol/L [10.30-23.17 pmol/L])
Free T_3 = 1.0 pg/mL (2.3-4.2 pg/mL) (SI: 1.54 pmol/L [3.53-6.45 pmol/L])
Cortisol (8 AM) = 39 µg/dL (5-25 µg/dL) (SI: 1075.9 nmol/L [137.9-689.7 nmol/L])
Urine analysis, normal

Which of the following is the best next step in this patient's management?

A. Add a PCSK9 inhibitor
B. Add ezetimibe
C. Increase the levothyroxine dosage to 75 mcg daily
D. Initiate LDL apheresis
E. Recommend psychiatric evaluation for anorexia nervosa

89 A 37-year-old woman presents for further evaluation of an asymptomatic right thyroid nodule that was initially noted on routine clinical neck examination several months ago. At the time, neck ultrasonography revealed a 1.7 × 1.5 × 0.8-cm right mid pole thyroid nodule, no left thyroid nodules, and no abnormal lymph nodes (*see images*). Her serum TSH concentration was 1.0 mIU/L. The patient has no personal history of head or neck ionizing radiation exposure or family history of thyroid malignancy.

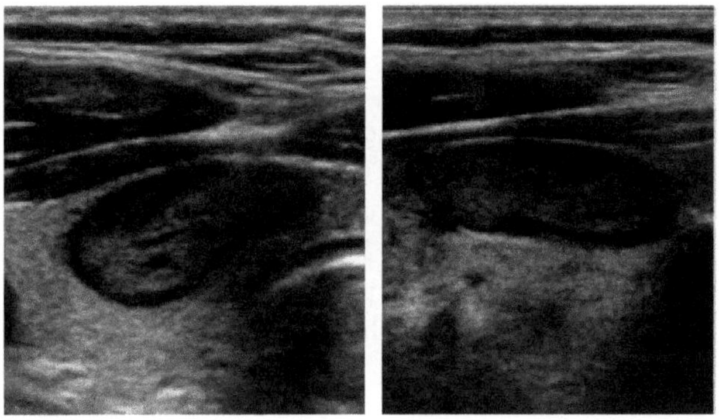

Ultrasound-guided FNA of the right thyroid nodule with a total of 3 separate needle passes was performed. Material from 2 of the passes was submitted for cytologic assessment using a liquid-based medium. One pass was collected for molecular analysis and the sample was frozen as per the manufacturer's instructions. Cytopathology findings were interpreted as nondiagnostic (Bethesda I) because of an insufficient quantity of thyroid follicular cells.

The patient presents today to discuss the next management steps.

On physical examination, her blood pressure is 110/66 mm Hg, and pulse rate is 70 beats/min. Her height is 62 in (157.5 cm), and weight is 140 lb (63.5 kg) (BMI = 25.6 kg/m²). There is a palpable nodule in the right thyroid lobe. There is no cervical lymphadenopathy. The rest of the examination findings are normal.

Which of the following is the most appropriate management to recommend next?

A. Perform neck ultrasonography in 12 months
B. Perform ultrasound-guided FNA with rapid on-site evaluation of cytology specimens
C. Perform ultrasound-guided FNA with 5 separate needle passes
D. Refer for right thyroid lobectomy
E. Send specimen collected during previous FNA for molecular analysis

90 A 68-year-old man is referred for evaluation of an adrenal mass. The patient has a history of stage IV nodal marginal zone lymphoma, initially diagnosed a decade ago when he presented with headaches, night sweats, and weight loss. He was treated with rituximab and bendamustine, and he was in remission for several years. He was recently hospitalized for severe headaches. Chest CT showed recurrent lymphoma and a partially visible right adrenal mass. Subsequent abdominal CT with and without contrast (*see image*) shows an enlarging noncalcified right adrenal nodule, now 2.7 cm (previously 2.2 cm 2 years ago and 1.7 cm 5 years ago).

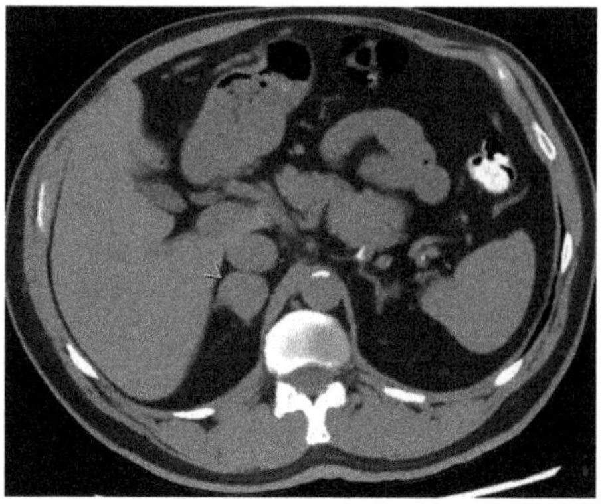

Imaging characteristics:

- Precontrast = 45 Hounsfield units
- 60-second postcontrast = 90 Hounsfield units
- 10-minute delayed = 64 Hounsfield units

The left adrenal gland is normal.

His additional medical history includes type 2 diabetes mellitus, hypertension, gastroesophageal reflux disease, and dyslipidemia. He takes a baby aspirin, candesartan, atorvastatin, pantoprazole, insulin glargine, and insulin aspart.

Laboratory test results:

Plasma metanephrine = 99 pg/mL (<99 pg/mL) (SI: 0.50 nmol/L [<0.50 nmol/L])
Plasma normetanephrine = 1032.1 pg/mL (<165 pg/mL) (SI: 5.64 nmol/L [<0.90 nmol/L])
Estimated glomerular filtration rate = 81 mL/min per 1.73 m^2 (>60 mL/min per 1.73 m^2)
Aldosterone = 12.7 ng/dL (4-21 ng/dL) (SI: 352.3 pmol/L [111.0-582.5 pmol/L])
Plasma renin = 9.4 pg/mL (4-44 pg/mL) (SI: 0.2 pmol/L [0.1-1.0 pmol/L])
ACTH = 14 pg/mL (10-60 pg/mL) (SI: 3.1 pmol/L [2.2-13.2 pmol/L])
Cortisol = 8.0 µg/dL (5-25 µg/dL) (SI: 220.7 nmol/L [137.9-689.7 nmol/L])

Which of the following is the best next step in this patient's evaluation?

A. ^{68}Ga-DOTATATE scan
B. Measurement of chromogranin A
C. Measurement of 24-hour urinary metanephrines
D. Measurement of plasma catecholamines
E. MIBG scintigraphy

91 A 54-year-old man presents for management of type 2 diabetes mellitus, which was diagnosed 10 years ago. His hemoglobin A_{1c} has been well controlled on sitagliptin therapy, and his most recent measurement is 6.8% (51 mmol/mol). Coronary artery disease was diagnosed 5 years ago when he had a myocardial infarction, and he has since had 4 coronary artery bypass grafts. He currently has no symptoms of chest pain or shortness of breath. He recently underwent transthoracic echocardiography, and his left ventricular ejection fraction is 35%.

He has a 30 pack-year history of cigarette smoking, but he quit 5 years ago. He has hypertension, hyperlipidemia, and chronic kidney disease. His medications include sitagliptin, metoprolol extended release, olmesartan, atorvastatin, and furosemide.

On physical examination, his blood pressure is 134/64 mm Hg and pulse rate is 58 beats/min. His height is 70 in (178 cm), and weight is 220 lb (99.8 kg) (BMI = 31.6 kg/m^2).

Laboratory test results:

Hemoglobin A_{1c} = 6.8% (4.0%-5.6%) (51 mmol/mol [20-30 mmol/mol])
Total cholesterol = 195 mg/dL (<200 mg/dL [optimal]) (SI: 5.05 mmol/L [<5.18 mmol/L])
LDL cholesterol = 55 mg/dL (<100 mg/dL [optimal]) (SI: 1.42 mmol/L [<2.59 mmol/L])
HDL cholesterol = 25 mg/dL (>60 mg/dL [optimal]) (SI: 0.65 mmol/L [>1.55 mmol/L])
Triglycerides = 132 mg/dL (<150 mg/dL [optimal]) (SI: 1.49 mmol/L [<1.70 mmol/L])
Estimated glomerular filtration rate = 28 mL/min per 1.73 m^2 (>60 mL/min per 1.73 m^2)
Urinary albumin-to-creatinine ratio = 220 mg/g creat (<30 mg/g creat)
Potassium = 5.4 mEq/L (3.5-5.0 mEq/L) (SI: 5.4 mmol/L [3.5-5.0 mmol/L])

Which of the following medications should be added as the best next step to reduce this patient's cardiovascular risk?

A. Dapagliflozin
B. Eplerenone
C. Metformin
D. Ramipril
E. Semaglutide

92 A 47-year-old woman (G1P2) presents with hot flashes, disturbed sleep (waking 2 to 3 times per night), impaired cognition (feeling more forgetful), increased irritability, and new-onset anxiety. She has gained 5 lb (2.3 kg) that is more notable in her abdominal area despite an increase in aerobic physical activity. Her last menstrual period was 4.5 months ago, and she notes that over the past 2 years she has had fluctuations in the length of her consecutive menstrual cycles. She also notes a decrease in the number of bleeding days. She is currently sexually active with a cisgender man and does not use any form of barrier or hormonal contraception.

She has no history of breast or uterine cancer, cerebrovascular attack, heart disease, venous thromboembolism, or tobacco use. Her primary care physician checked her thyroid function, which is normal. The goal of her visit today is to start menopausal hormone therapy because she cannot bear her symptoms any longer.

On physical examination, her blood pressure is 125/84 mm Hg and pulse rate is 71 beats/min. Her height is 65 in (165 cm), and weight is 155 lb (70.3 kg) (BMI = 25.8 kg/m^2). She appears well and is in no acute distress. She has no dorsocervical fat pad or violaceous striae. The rest of her examination findings are unremarkable.

Which of the following is the best next step in this patient's management?

A. β-Estradiol patch and oral micronized progesterone
B. Combined oral contraceptive pill
C. Conjugated estrogens and medroxyprogesterone acetate in oral formulation
D. Estradiol acetate vaginal ring
E. Levonorgestrel-releasing intrauterine system

93 A 44-year-old woman with a history of thyroid cancer comes for a follow-up visit. She underwent total thyroidectomy with central neck dissection followed by 150 mCi of radioiodine treatment last year. She had a second radioiodine treatment (100 mCi) 4 months ago, and a posttherapy scan revealed no foci of radioiodine uptake in her neck or anywhere else. She currently takes levothyroxine, 150 mcg daily, and recent laboratory testing documented undetectable thyroglobulin with no thyroglobulin antibodies. At today's appointment, she reports constipation, dry mouth, and swelling with mild pain under her right jaw for the last several months. She particularly notices this swelling after eating. She has tried massage, warm compresses, oral hydration, and nonsteroidal anti-inflammatory agents with very little relief. She also mentions she had 2 more tooth fillings last month.

On physical examination, she is in no acute distress and her vital signs are normal. Oral mucosa is dry. Multiple dental amalgams are present. There is a palpable, mildly tender right submandibular gland.

Laboratory test results:

TSH = 7.2 mIU/L (0.5-5.0 mIU/L)
Basic metabolic panel, normal

In addition to adjusting her levothyroxine dosage, which of the following is the best next step in the management of this patient's symptoms?

A. Apply warm compresses twice daily
B. Initiate amoxicillin-clavulanate twice daily
C. Perform FNA biopsy
D. Refer to an otolaryngologist
E. Try sour drops/candies

94 A 65-year-old woman returns to clinic for follow-up of type 2 diabetes mellitus. She is frustrated by the recent need for medication despite ongoing weight loss. Diabetes was diagnosed 10 years ago and metformin, 500 mg daily, was initiated 6 years ago. When her hemoglobin A_{1c} level rose to 8.5% (69 mmol/mol) 6 months ago, her metformin dosage was titrated to its maximum and a low-carbohydrate diet was initiated. Three months ago, despite weight loss of 6 lb (2.7 kg) (from 179 to 173 lb [81.2 to 78.5 kg]), her hemoglobin A_{1c} had risen further to 10.3% (89 mmol/mol). Glipizide XL was started, and the dosage has been titrated to 10 mg daily.

At today's visit, she has lost another 8 lb (3.6 kg) (down to 165 lb [74.8 kg]). Her point-of-care hemoglobin A_{1c} value is 8.0% (64 mmol/mol), and a glucose meter shows a 14-day average value of 155 mg/dL (8.6 mmol/L) (28 readings).

Her medical history is notable for Graves disease, postablative hypothyroidism, and mild intermittent asthma.

Current medications are glipizide XL, 10 mg daily; metformin ER, 1000 mg twice daily; rosuvastatin; ezetimibe; icosapent ethyl; aspirin; and levothyroxine.

Her family history is notable for chronic obstructive pulmonary disease, breast cancer, and diabetes in her mother and esophageal cancer in her father.

Her hemoglobin A_{1c} trend is shown:

10 Years ago	5 Years ago	4 Years ago	2.5 Years ago	2 Years ago	1 Year ago	Current
6.7% (50 mmol/mol)	6.1% (43 mmol/mol)	6.0% (42 mmol/mol)	6.6% (49 mmol/mol)	8.5% (69 mmol/mol)	10.3% (89 mmol/mol)	8.0% (64 mmol/mol)

Laboratory test results 1 year ago:

TSH = 0.65 mIU/L (0.5-5.0 mIU/L)
Total cholesterol = 91 mg/dL (<200 mg/dL [optimal]) (SI: 2.36 mmol/L [<5.18 mmol/L])
LDL cholesterol = 31 mg/dL (<100 mg/dL [optimal]) (SI: 0.80mmol/L [<2.59 mmol/L])
HDL cholesterol = 43 mg/dL (>60 mg/dL [optimal]) (SI: 1.11 mmol/L [>1.55 mmol/L])
Triglycerides = 84 mg/dL (<150 mg/dL [optimal]) (SI: 0.95 mmol/L [<1.70 mmol/L])
Fructosamine = 298 μmol/L (0-285 μmol/L)
Glutamic acid decarboxylase 65 antibodies = <5.0 U/mL (0-5.0 U/mL)
Islet antigen 2 antibodies = <5.0 U/mL (0-5.0 U/mL)
Complete blood cell count, normal
Comprehensive metabolic panel, normal
Glucose = 199 mg/dL (70-99 mg/dL) (SI: 11.0 mmol/L [3.9-5.5 mmol/L])

On physical examination, blood pressure is 126/63 mm Hg and pulse rate is 88 beats/min. Her height is 64 in (162.6 cm), and weight is 173.1 lb (78.5 kg) (BMI = 29.7 kg/m^2). She does not have acanthosis nigricans or striae.

Which of the following steps is most important to pursue in this patient's evaluation and management?

A. Continuation of the current treatment regimen
B. CT of the abdomen/pelvis
C. Serum C-peptide measurement
D. Serum glucagon measurement
E. Zinc transporter 8 antibody testing

95 A 52-year-old man presents with concerns about inability to lose weight, decreased exercise endurance, and fatigue. He has a history of a large nonfunctioning pituitary adenoma diagnosed at age 34 years, status post surgery and radiation. He would like to discuss hormone optimization, the effect of GH replacement on cardiovascular and metabolic health, and tumor progression. His father died of a myocardial infarction at age 55 years, his mother had type 2 diabetes mellitus, and his sister had a vertebral fracture at age 65 years.

Medications include hydrocortisone, 15 mg in the morning and 5 mg in the afternoon; levothyroxine, 200 mcg daily; and testosterone, 200 mg every 2 weeks.

On physical examination, he appears tired. Blood pressure is 155/80 mm Hg and pulse rate is 82 beats/min. His height is 72 in (183 cm), and weight is 264.5 lb (120 kg) (BMI = 36 kg/m^2). He has generalized fat distribution and a large neck circumference. Examination findings are otherwise unremarkable.

Laboratory test results (sample drawn 10 days after the last testosterone injection):

Hemoglobin = 15.9 g/dL (13.8-17.2 g/dL) (SI: 159 g/dL [138-172 g/dL])
Hematocrit = 46% (41%-51%) (SI: 0.46 [0.41-0.51])
Fasting glucose = 110 mg/dL (70-99 mg/dL) (SI: 6.1 mmol/L [3.9-5.5 mmol/L])
Hemoglobin A_{1c} = 6.0% (4.0%-5.6%) (42 mmol/mol [20-28 mmol/mol])
LDL cholesterol = 120 mg/dL (<100 mg/dL) (SI: 3.11 mmol/L [<2.59 mmol/L])
Cortisol (1 hour after taking the morning dose of hydrocortisone) = 23.5 μg/dL (SI: 648.3 nmol/L)
Free T_4 = 1.55 ng/dL (0.8-1.8 ng/dL) (SI: 19.95 pmol/L [10.30-23.17 pmol/L])
TSH = 0.02 mIU/L (0.5-5.0 mIU/L)
IGF-1 = 73 ng/mL (84-233 ng/mL) (SI: 9.6 nmol/L [11.0-30.5 nmol/L])
Total testosterone = 500 ng/dL (300-900 ng/dL) (SI: 17.4 nmol/L [10.4-31.2 nmol/L])

MRI shows postoperative changes without a visible tumor. Findings on DXA done 1 year ago indicate osteopenia with lowest T-score of −1.9 at the lumbar spine.

Which of the following is the best next step in this patient's management?

A. Decrease the hydrocortisone dosage to 10 mg in the morning
B. Increase the testosterone dosage
C. Perform a GH-stimulation test with glucagon administration
D. Refer for overnight polysomnography
E. Start GH replacement, 0.2 mg daily

96 An 81-year-old woman is referred for evaluation of a 5.3-cm right adrenal mass, which was noted incidentally on abdominal CT without contrast *(see image)* that was performed for acute right flank pain. Her medical history includes type 2 diabetes mellitus, osteoporosis, hypertension, dyslipidemia, coronary artery disease, and chronic obstructive pulmonary disease.

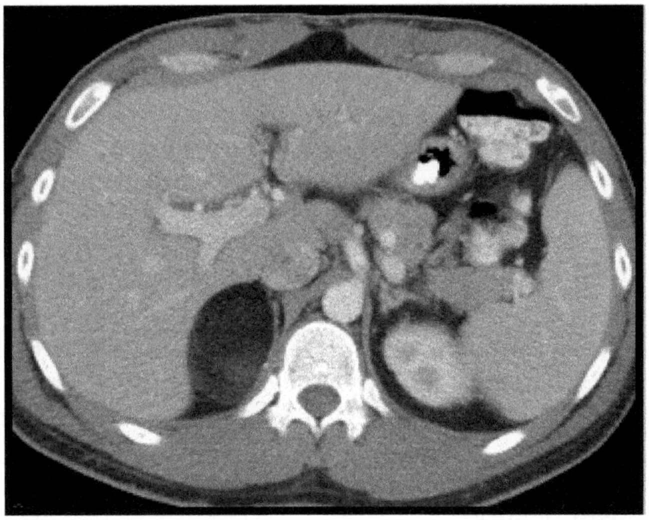

On physical examination, her blood pressure is 142/78 mm Hg and pulse rate is 82 beats/min. Her height is 65.3 in (166 cm), and weight is 210 lb (95.3 kg) (BMI = 34.6 kg/m^2). Excess adiposity is distributed predominantly centrally. She has mild hirsutism on her chin. She has light-colored striae on her abdomen but no plethora or bruises. Muscle strength is normal. She has no edema.

Laboratory test results:

Serum potassium = 4.5 mEq/L (3.5-5.0 mEq/L) (SI: 4.5 mmol/L [3.5-5.0 mmol/L])
Serum sodium = 139 mEq/L (136-142 mEq/L) (SI: 139 mmol/L [136-142 mmol/L])
Serum creatinine = 1.1 mg/dL (0.6-1.1 mg/dL) (SI: 97.3 μmol/L [53.0-97.2 μmol/L])
Serum cortisol = 10 μg/dL (5-25 μg/dL) (SI: 275.9 nmol/L [137.9-689.7 nmol/L])
ACTH = 13 pg/mL (10-60 pg/mL) (SI: 2.9 pmol/L [2.2-13.2 pmol/L])
Serum aldosterone = 5.8 ng/dL (4-21 ng/dL) (SI: 160.9 pmol/L [111.0-582.5 pmol/L])
Plasma renin activity = 1.3 ng/mL per h (0.6-4.3 ng/mL per h)

Following a 1-mg dexamethasone-suppression test, her morning serum cortisol concentration is 1.2 µg/dL (33.1 nmol/L) and ACTH concentration is less than 5 pg/mL (<1.1 pmol/L).

Which of the following is the best next step in this patient's management?

A. FDG PET-CT
B. Follow-up CT in 12 months
C. Right adrenalectomy
D. Measurement of plasma metanephrines
E. Measurement of serum DHEA-S

97 A competitive male weightlifter is referred to an endocrinologist after a positive hCG result on routine urine screening (B sample). He is asymptomatic and states that he does not use illicit drugs or exogenous hCG. Additional comprehensive testing at a laboratory accredited by the World Anti-Doping Agency shows no evidence that he is using exogenous anabolic steroids or any other performance-enhancing drugs.

Confirmatory laboratory test results:

hCG = 66.0 mIU/mL (<2.0 mIU/mL) (SI: 66.0 IU/L [<2.0 IU/L])
LH = <0.2 mIU/mL (1.0-9.0 mIU/mL) (SI: <0.2 IU/L [1.0-9.0 IU/L])
FSH = <0.2 mIU/mL (1.0-13.0 mIU/mL) (SI: <0.2 IU/L [1.0-13.0 IU/L])
Testosterone = 965 ng/dL (300-900 ng/dL) (SI: 33.5 nmol/L [10.4-31.2 nmol/L])
Thyroid function, normal

On physical examination, he has a muscular physique and mild gynecomastia.
Findings on testicular assessment, including those on ultrasonography, are unremarkable.

Which of the following is the best investigation to perform next?

A. CT of the chest, abdomen, and pelvis
B. ^{68}Ga DOTA-octreotate (GaTate) PET-CT
C. Serum α-fetoprotein measurement
D. Serum α-subunit measurement
E. Serum estradiol measurement

98 A 55-year-old woman with a history of type 2 diabetes mellitus is admitted to the hospital for evaluation of right foot osteomyelitis, which was confirmed on recent MRI. She has had uncontrolled diabetes for many years, and her most recent hemoglobin A_{1c} value, just prior to admission, was 11.2% (99 mmol/mol). Her outpatient regimen consists of NPH insulin 70/30, 30 units at breakfast and 20 units before dinner. The primary team requests a consultation for inpatient diabetes management. The patient is scheduled to have surgical debridement the next morning. The team is planning to place the patient on nothing-by-mouth status after midnight.

Which of the following is the most appropriate management plan for this patient during her hospital stay?

A. Continue NPH 70/30 at the current dosage
B. Continue NPH 70/30 but decrease the dosage
C. Discontinue NPH 70/30 and initiate correction scale insulin
D. Discontinue NPH 70/30 and initiate metformin and as-needed correctional scale insulin
E. Switch to a basal-correction regimen and initiate prandial insulin when full diet is ordered

99 A 27-year-old woman presents for follow-up of primary hypothyroidism due to Hashimoto thyroiditis. Hypothyroidism was diagnosed 4 years ago and levothyroxine was initiated at that time. Although the patient's serum TSH values normalized after starting levothyroxine, she reported persistent cold intolerance, fatigue, and poor concentration. Her regimen was subsequently transitioned to combination therapy with levothyroxine, 100 mcg daily, and liothyronine, 5 mcg twice daily. After starting this new regimen, her symptoms resolved, and she has remained on this same treatment. Her only other medication is a prenatal vitamin, which she takes with her evening meal daily. In the past, she took an oral contraceptive pill, but she stopped this 2 months ago because of her desire to conceive. Her last menstrual period was 3 days ago.

On physical examination, her height is 66 in (167.6 cm) and weight is 160 lb (72.6 kg) (BMI = 25.8 kg/m^2). Her blood pressure is 112/65 mm Hg, and pulse rate is 62 beats/min supine. The thyroid gland is normal to palpation without nodules. Reflexes are 2+ and symmetric throughout.

Laboratory test results:

TSH = 0.8 mIU/L (0.5-5.0 mIU/L)
Urine pregnancy test, negative

Which of the following is the best next step in this patient's management?

A. Continue liothyronine, continue levothyroxine
B. Continue liothyronine, increase levothyroxine
C. Continue liothyronine, decrease levothyroxine
D. Discontinue liothyronine, continue levothyroxine
E. Disontinue liothyronine, increase levothyroxine

100 A 24-year-old man presents for management of hypocalcemia and hypoparathyroidism. He initially came to medical attention at age 6 months with severe hypocalcemia and seizures. He did not have dysmorphic features, findings on cardiac evaluation were normal, and hearing was normal. Since that time, he has taken calcium and calcitriol, and he describes paresthesia and muscle cramps if he misses doses. CT documents asymptomatic basal ganglia calcifications. His brother also presented with hypocalcemia in infancy, and his father was later incidentally found to have hypocalcemia in adulthood. Kidney ultrasonography demonstrates normal size and shape with moderate to severe nephrocalcinosis.

On physical examination, he has a positive Chvostek sign, but findings are otherwise normal, including normal stature.

Current medications are calcium carbonate, 600 mg calcium, 1 tablet 2 times daily at meals; cholecalciferol, 1000 units daily; calcitriol, 0.25 mcg twice daily; magnesium oxide, 800 mg twice daily; and hydrochlorothiazide, 25 mg daily.

Laboratory test results:

Calcium = 7.2 mg/dL (8.2-10.2 mg/dL) (SI: 1.8 mmol/L [2.1-2.6 mmol/L])
Albumin = 4.6 g/dL (3.5-5.0 g/dL) (SI: 46 g/L [35-50 g/L])
Creatinine = 0.98 mg/dL (0.7-1.3 mg/dL) (SI: 86.6 μmol/L [61.9-114.9 μmol/L])
Alkaline phosphatase = 77 U/L (50-120 U/L) (SI: 1.29 μkat/L [0.84-2.00 μkat/L])
Intact PTH = 6.3 pg/mL (10-65 pg/mL) (SI: 6.3 ng/L [10-65 ng/L])
25-Hydroxyvitamin D = 36 ng/mL (30-80 ng/mL [optimal]) (SI: 89.9 nmol/L [74.9-199.7 nmol/L])
Phosphate = 4.7 mg/dL (2.3-4.7 mg/dL) (SI: 1.5 mmol/L [0.7-1.5 mmol/L])
Magnesium = 1.6 mg/dL (1.5-2.3 mg/dL) (SI: 0.66 mmol/L [0.6-0.9 mmol/L])
Urinary calcium-to-creatinine ratio = 0.32 mg/mg (<0.22 mg/mg) (SI: 0.88 mmol/mmol [<0.61 mmol/mmol])

Which of the following is the best management approach for this patient's hypocalcemia?

A. Continue current therapy
B. Decrease the hydrochlorothiazide dosage
C. Increase the calcitriol dosage
D. Increase the calcium dosage
E. Start sevelamer

101 A 63-year-old woman with type 2 diabetes mellitus presents to the emergency department with the symptoms of blurred vision in her right eye that began yesterday evening and subsequently progressed to complete vision loss when she woke this morning. She has no eye pain. She reports otherwise feeling well and has no polyuria or polydipsia. She has a 10-year-history of type 2 diabetes complicated by peripheral neuropathy. She takes metformin, 1000 mg twice daily; canagliflozin, 100 mg daily; semaglutide, 0.5 mg weekly; and insulin glargine, 20 units once daily. Her last hemoglobin A_{1c} measurement was 8.4% (68 mmol/mol). She has a 30 pack-year history of cigarette smoking, and a history of hypertension treated with lisinopril/hydrochlorothiazide and hyperlipidemia treated with atorvastatin. An urgent ophthalmology consultation identifies retinal vein occlusion as the etiology of her vision loss.

On physical examination, her blood pressure is 162/78 mm Hg and pulse rate is 88 beats/min. Her height is 68 in (173 cm), and weight is 194 lb (88 kg) (BMI = 29.5 kg/m^2).

Laboratory test result:

Hemoglobin A_{1c} = 8.4% (4.0%-5.6%) (68 mmol/mol [20-38 mmol/mol])

Which of the following medications most likely contributed to this patient's vision issue?

A. Atorvastatin
B. Canagliflozin
C. Insulin glargine
D. Metformin
E. Semaglutide

102 A 46-year-old woman presents to discuss how to improve her metabolic health. Type 2 diabetes mellitus was recently diagnosed, and her primary care provider advised her to lose weight. She has hypertension and hyperlipidemia. She has met with a dietician in the past but has not consistently implemented the dietary strategies discussed, as her children are picky eaters. She also states that she does not have enough time to exercise every day. She cites her preference to eat foods that align with her cultural identity and that food cost can be a barrier to eating well.

On physical examination, her blood pressure is 148/88 mm Hg and pulse rate is 92 beats/min. Her height is 65.7 in (167 cm), and weight is 224 lb (102 kg) (BMI = 36.2 kg/m^2). She has an obese abdomen with no stigmata of hypercortisolism.

Her current medications are atorvastatin, 20 mg daily; metformin, 1000 mg twice daily; hydrochlorothiazide, 25 mg daily; and a combined oral contraceptive pill.

Laboratory test results:

Hemoglobin A_{1c} = 6.9% (4.0%-5.6%) (52 mmol/mol [20-38 mmol/mol])
Total cholesterol = 250 mg/dL (<200 mg/dL) (SI: 6.48 mmol/L [<5.18 mmol/L])
LDL cholesterol = 110 mg/dL (<100 mg/dL) (SI: 2.85 mmol/L [<2.59 mmol/L])
HDL cholesterol = 35 mg/dL (>60 mg/dL) (SI: 0.91 mmol/L [>1.55 mmol/L])
Triglycerides = 320 mg/dL (<150 mg/dL) (SI: 3.62 mmol/L [<1.70 mmol/L])

Which of the following strategies is most likely to help this patient achieve her goal of better metabolic health?

A. Advise a plant-based, Mediterranean-style dietary pattern
B. Recommend 150 minutes of physical activity of any type each week
C. See a dietician to discuss how to incorporate foods with lower simple carbohydrates and less salt
D. Start sitagliptin
E. Stop the combined oral contraceptive pill

103 A 23-year-old man with no notable medical history has been experiencing polydipsia and polyuria for the last 10 months. He reports waking every 1 to 2 hours at night to urinate and drink water. He recently developed a feeling of fullness and ringing in the right ear. Review of systems is notable for fatigue and decreased libido.

On physical examination, there is dullness of the eardrum to external light (absent light reflex), bulging of the right ear canal, and few small lymph nodes in the inguinal region. His temperature is 98.2°F (36.8°C), blood pressure is 126/82 mm Hg, and pulse rate is 71 beats/min. His height is 72 in (182.9 cm), and weight is 220.5 lb (100 kg) (BMI = 29.9 kg/m^2). He has noncentripetal fat distribution. Evaluation by an otolaryngologist identifies an ear canal lesion.

Laboratory test results:

- Serum sodium = 141 mEq/L (136-142 mEq/L) (SI: 141 mmol/L [136-142 mmol/L])
- Calcium = 10.2 mg/dL (8.2-10.2 mg/dL) (SI: 2.6 mmol/L [2.1-2.6 mmol/L])
- Albumin = 4.2 g/dL (3.5-5.0 g/dL) (SI: 42 g/L [35-50 g/L])
- Creatinine = 1.2 mg/dL (0.7-1.3 mg/dL) (SI: 106.1 µmol/L [61.9-114.9 µmol/L])
- TSH = 1.17 mIU/L (0.5-0.5 mIU/L)
- Free T_4 = 0.7 ng/dL (0.8-1.8 ng/dL) (SI: 9.0 pmol/L [10.30-23.17 pmol/L])
- Testosterone = <10 ng/dL (300-900 ng/dL) (SI: <0.3 nmol/L [10.4-31.2 nmol/L])
- LH = 1.0 mIU/mL (1.0-9.0 mIU/mL) (SI: 1.0 IU/L [1.0-9.0 IU/L])
- FSH = 1.6 mIU/mL (1.0-13.0 mIU/mL) (SI: 1.6 IU/L [1.0-13.0 IU/L])
- Prolactin = 17 ng/mL (4-23 ng/mL) (SI: 0.74 nmol/L [0.17-1.00 nmol/L])
- Cortisol (8 AM) = 19 µg/dL (5-25 µg/dL) (SI: 524.2 nmol/L [137.9-689.7 nmol/L])
- ACTH = 12 pg/mL (10-60 pg/mL) (SI: 2.6 pmol/L [2.2-13.2 pmol/L])
- Serum osmolality = 287 mOsm/kg (275-295 mOsm/kg) (SI: 287 mmol/kg [275-295 mmol/kg])
- Urine osmolality = 87 mOsm/kg (150-1150 mOsm/kg) (SI: 87 mmol/kg [150-1150 mmol/kg])
- Complete blood cell count, normal
- C-reactive protein, normal
- ACE, normal
- hCG, normal
- α-Fetoprotein, normal
- Urinalysis, low specific gravity

MRI of the pituitary gland and PET-CT are shown (*see images*).

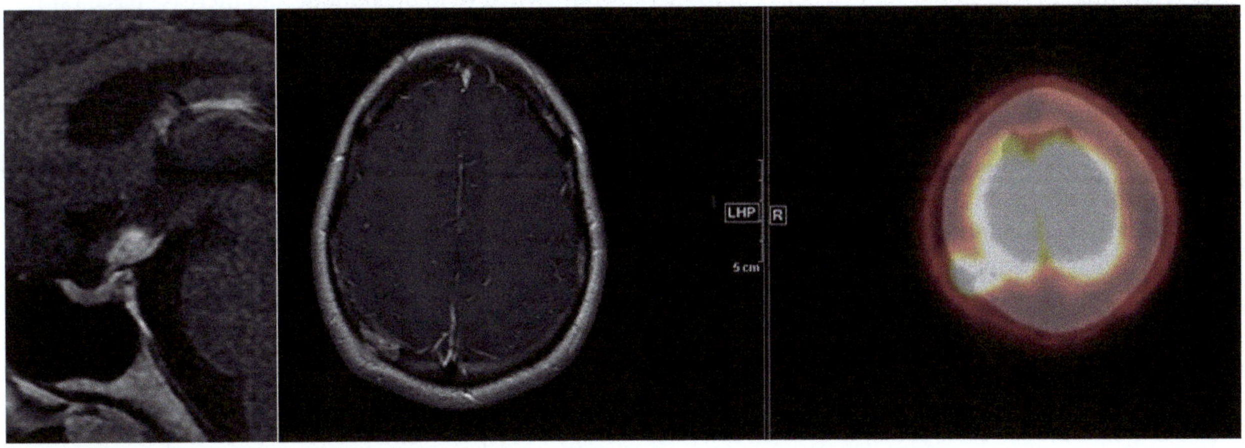

Which of the following is the best next step in this patient's management?

A. Biopsy of the ear canal lesion
B. Cerebral spinal fluid analysis (cytology, flow cytometry, immunohistochemistry for ACE, human chorionic hCG, α-fetoprotein, and lactate dehydrogenase)
C. Prednisone, 60 mg daily, and MRI imaging in 3 months
D. Reduction of fluid intake and repeated urine osmolality measurement
E. Transsphenoidal biopsy of the hypothalamic lesion

104 A 31-year-old woman with a history of type 1 diabetes mellitus presents for initial evaluation and management. One year ago, she started using a hybrid closed-loop insulin pump. Her current hemoglobin A_{1c} value is 7.2% (55 mmol/mol). Continuous glucose monitoring download shows the following values:

Average glucose concentration = 160 mg/dL (SI: 8.9 mmol/L)
Time in range (70-180 mg/dL [SI: 3.9-10.0 mmol/L]) = 67%
Time above range (>180 mg/dL [SI: >10.0 mmol/L]) = 23%
Time above range (>250 mg/dL [SI: >13.9 mmol/L]) = 9.5%
Time below range (<70 mg/dL [SI: <3.9 mmol/L]) = 0.5%
Time below range (<54 mg/dL [SI: <3.0 mmol/L]) = 0%
Coefficient of variation = 30.1%

Nocturnal and fasting glucose values are mostly between 110 and 130 mg/dL (6.1-7.2 mmol/L), and 2-hour postprandial glucose values for all meals are mostly between 160 and 190 mg/dL (8.9-10.5 mmol/L).

Auto mode is used 96% of the time. Basal rates, insulin-to-carbohydrate ratio, and insulin sensitivity factor ratio are shown (*see table*).

Start time	Basal rate (manual mode)	Insulin-to-carbohydrate ratio	Insulin sensitivity factor
Midnight	0.75 units/h	1:13	1:50 mg/dL (1:2.8 mmol/L)
6 AM	0.85 units/h	1:13	1:50 mg/dL (1:2.8 mmol/L)
9 AM	1.0 units/h	1:13	1:50 mg/dL (1:2.8 mmol/L)
2 PM	1.15 units/h	1:13	1:50 mg/dL (1:2.8 mmol/L)

Last week, she learned that she is pregnant. She would like to achieve excellent glycemic control.

Which of the following is the most appropriate management plan for this patient?

A. Continue hybrid closed-loop insulin pump therapy but switch to manual mode and increase basal rate settings throughout the day to achieve tighter control
B. Continue hybrid closed-loop insulin pump therapy but switch to manual mode, increase nocturnal basal rate, and change the insulin-to-carbohydrate ratio to increase prandial insulin coverage
C. Continue hybrid closed-loop insulin pump therapy on auto mode and change correction factor settings to increase insulin delivered through correction boluses
D. Continue hybrid closed-loop insulin pump therapy on auto mode and decrease the insulin-to-carbohydrate ratio to increase prandial insulin coverage
E. Discontinue hybrid closed-loop insulin pump therapy and initiate a basal-bolus multiple daily injection regimen at 10% higher insulin dosing

105 A 48-year-old woman (G3P1) seeks evaluation of menopausal symptoms. Her medical history is notable for osteopenia, Graves disease, and estrogen receptor– and progesterone receptor–positive breast cancer, status post bilateral mastectomy at age 47 years followed by adjuvant endocrine therapy with anastrozole after surgical menopause. She reports severe vasomotor symptoms that interrupt her workday and lead to frequent nighttime awakenings to change pajamas and even sheets at times. She describes low libido, vaginal dryness that has been unresponsive to vaginal moisturizers, and urinary stress incontinence. These symptoms have worsened since starting the aromatase inhibitor.

On physical examination, she appears well.

Before referral, her primary care physician ordered the following laboratory tests:

TSH = 2.1 mIU/L (0.5-5.0 mIU/L)

Free T_4 = 1.4 ng/dL (0.8-1.8 ng/dL) (SI: 18.02 pmol/L [10.30-23.17 pmol/L])

FSH = 67.8 mIU/mL (2.0-12.0 mIU/mL [follicular]) (SI: 67.8 IU/L [2.0-12.0 IU/L])

Which of the following is the best next step in managing this patient's menopausal symptoms?

A. After consultation with breast oncology, start low-dosage vaginal estrogen in the form of a 17β-estradiol vaginal ring
B. Continue use of vaginal moisturizers with recommendation to increase frequency to daily
C. Counsel on behavior modifications and avoidance of triggers given contraindications to hormone therapy use
D. Start estradiol therapy alone with a 17β-estradiol patch
E. Start menopausal hormone therapy with a transdermal continuous combined regimen of 17β-estradiol and a progestin

106

A 29-year-old man with a history of atrial fibrillation and a mechanical aortic valve due to congenital aortic stenosis has a history of recurrent nephrolithiasis in adulthood. Evaluation demonstrates hypercalcemia with an elevated PTH concentration. Review of his prior laboratory testing indicates that hypercalcemia developed 2 years ago. He undergoes sequential parathyroidectomy twice, and each time 1 enlarged parathyroid gland is removed. After each operation, he has transient improvement of calcium (into the upper normal range), but hypercalcemia returns several weeks later. He has intermittent nausea and vomiting and is treated for reflux. He has no known family history of endocrine disorders.

Current medications are omeprazole, 20 mg daily; cholecalciferol, 600 units daily; warfarin, 5 mg daily; hydrochlorothiazide, 25 mg daily; furosemide, 40 mg daily; amiodarone, 200 mg daily; and carvedilol, 25 mg daily.

On physical examination, his height is 70 in (177.8 cm) and weight is 160 lb (72.6 kg) (BMI = 23.0 kg/m^2). Findings on examination of the head, eyes, ears, nose, and throat are normal. A surgical scar is visible on his neck, and he has no thyromegaly or palpable masses. Lungs are clear to auscultation, and pulse rate is 72 beats/min with a regular rhythm. There is a systolic murmur and mechanical click. His abdomen is soft, nontender, and nondistended. There is no hepatomegaly. He has surgical scars on his chest and a subcutaneous implantable cardioverter-defibrillator. He has a lipoma on his back, and a few hemangiomas. He has normal reflexes and trace edema. There are no skeletal deformities.

Laboratory test results (6 months after most recent parathyroidectomy):

Calcium = 12.3 mg/dL (8.2-10.2 mg/dL) (SI: 3.1 mmol/L [2.1-2.6 mmol/L])

Albumin = 4.5 g/dL (3.5-5.0 g/dL) (SI: 45 g/L [35-50 g/L])

Creatinine = 1.1 mg/dL (0.7-1.3 mg/dL) (SI: 97.2 µmol/L [61.9-114.9 µmol/L])

Alkaline phosphatase = 94 U/L (50-120 U/L) (SI: 1.57 µkat/L [0.84-2.00 µkat/L])

Intact PTH = 238 pg/mL (10-65 pg/mL) (SI: 238 ng/L [10-65 ng/L])

25-Hydroxyvitamin D = 29 ng/mL (30-80 ng/mL [optimal]) (SI: 72.4 nmol/L [74.9-199.7 nmol/L])

Phosphate = 2.0 mg/dL (2.3-4.7 mg/dL) (SI: 0.6 mmol/L [0.7-1.5 mmol/L])

Urinary calcium = 368 mg/dL (100-300 mg/24 h) (SI: 9.2 mmol/d [2.5-7.5 mmol/d])

TSH = 0.15 mIU/L (0.5-5.0 mIU/L)

Hemoglobin A_{1c} = 5.2% (4.0%-5.6%) (33 mmol/mol [20-38 mmol/mol])

Which of the following is the most likely cause of this patient's recurrent hypercalcemia?

A. Amiodarone-induced hyperthyroidism
B. Hydrochlorothiazide
C. Pathogenic variant in the gene encoding menin
D. Pathogenic variant in the gene encoding the calcium-sensing receptor
E. Pathogenic variant in the gene encoding the sodium-phosphate cotransporter

107 A 58-year-old man is prescribed transdermal testosterone replacement after resection of a nonfunctioning macroadenoma. Other pituitary axes are intact. Prior to testosterone replacement, he reported low libido, low energy, and fatigue. Eight months after starting testosterone treatment, his libido has markedly improved, but he is still fatigued and has low energy. His medical history is relevant for obesity, type 2 diabetes mellitus, hypertension, and hyperlipidemia. Medications include an SGLT-2 inhibitor, metformin, an angiotensin-receptor blocker, and a statin. He has been on these medications for 2 years, without any recent changes. He has smoked 10 cigarettes daily since his teenage years, and he consumes 1 to 2 standard drinks 2 days per week.

On physical examination, his blood pressure is 139/86 mm Hg without a postural drop and pulse rate is 84 beats/min and regular. His height is 71 in (180.3 cm) and weight is 269 lb (122 kg) (BMI = 37.5 kg/m^2). While examination is limited by body habitus, findings on cardiac examination are normal and lungs are clear to auscultation. There are no palpable abdominal masses.

Serial laboratory testing demonstrates the following:

Measurement	Baseline (prior to testosterone replacement)	3 Months after commencing testosterone replacement	6 Months after commencing testosterone replacement	8 Months after commencing testosterone replacement
Serum testosterone	105 ng/dL (SI: 3.6 nmol/L)	420 ng/dL (SI: 14.6 nmol/L)	380 ng/dL (SI: 3.2 nmol/L)	430 ng/dL (SI: 14.9 nmol/L)
Hematocrit	42% (SI: 0.41)	48% (SI: 0.48)	52% (SI: 0.52)	56% (SI: 0.55)

Reference ranges: testosterone, 300-900 ng/dL (SI: 10.4-31.2 nmol/L); hematocrit, 41%-51% (SI: 0.41-0.51).

Which of the following is the best investigation to perform next?

A. CT of the abdomen and pelvis
B. *JAK2* genetic testing
C. Polysomnography
D. Red blood cell mass measurement by ^{51}Cr labeling
E. Six-minute walk test with pulse oximetry

108 A 62-year-old man with hypertension and impaired fasting glucose presents for discussion of optimal cardiovascular prevention strategies. Hypertension is well controlled on amlodipine, 5 mg daily, and he takes no other medications. His mother had a stroke at age 70 years, and his father died of lung cancer at age 76 years. The patient had normal findings on stress testing 2 years ago, and he remains active playing golf 3 days a week in the summer and regularly exercising on a treadmill 30 minutes daily. He avoids refined sugars and tries to follow a Mediterranean diet. He occasionally has a glass of wine at dinner and has never smoked cigarettes.

On physical examination, his blood pressure is 130/80 mm Hg and pulse rate is 76 beats/min. His height is 69 in (175.3 cm), and weight is 197 lb (89.4 kg) (BMI = 29 kg/m^2). He has no tendon xanthomas or corneal arcus or clouding.

Laboratory test results:

Fasting plasma glucose = 110 mg/dL (70-99 mg/dL) (SI: 6.1 mmol/L [3.9-5.5 mmol/L])
Hemoglobin A_{1c} = 6.2% (4.0%-5.6%) (44 mmol/mol [20-38 mmol/mol])
Serum creatinine = 1.1 mg/dL (0.7-1.3 mg/dL) (SI: 97.2 μmol/L [61.9-114.9 μmol/L])
ALT = 34 U/L (10-40 U/L) (SI: 0.57 μkat/L [0.17-0.67 μkat/L])
AST = 30 U/L (20-48 U/L) (SI: 0.50 μkat/L [0.33-0.80 μkat/L])
TSH = 1.6 mIU/L (0.5-5.0 mIU/L)
Total cholesterol = 265 mg/dL (<200 mg/dL) (SI: 6.86 mmol/L [<5.18 mmol/L])
Triglycerides = 151 mg/dL (<150 mg/dL) (SI: 1.71 mmol/L [<1.70 mmol/L])
HDL cholesterol = 95 mg/dL (>60 mg/dL) (SI: 2.46 mmol/L [>1.55 mmol/L])
LDL cholesterol = 145 mg/dL (<100 mg/dL) (SI: 3.76 mmol/L [<2.59 mmol/L])

In addition to dietary advice to help with weight loss, which of the following is the best recommendation now?

A. Abstain from drinking alcohol
B. Order genetic testing for cholesteryl ester transfer protein deficiency
C. Start fenofibrate
D. Start metformin
E. Start moderate-intensity statin therapy

109 A 48-year-old woman palpated a right thyroid nodule in her neck 1 month ago. She has had 1 year of difficulty sleeping, anxiety, and palpitations and a 2- to 3-month history of more frequent bowel movements. She has no dysphagia, difficulty breathing, voice changes, or anterior neck pain. There is no history of head or neck ionizing radiation exposure or family history of thyroid malignancy.

On physical examination, her blood pressure is 122/74 mm Hg and pulse rate is 85 beats/min. Her height is 67 in (170.2 cm), and weight is 140 lb (63.5 kg) (BMI = 21.9 kg/m^2). There is a 4-cm nodule replacing the right thyroid lobe. There is no cervical lymphadenopathy. She has a fine tremor of the upper extremities. The rest of the examination findings are normal.

Neck ultrasonography documents a 4.5 × 2.9 × 3.0-cm nodule in the right thyroid lobe and a 2.7 × 1.6 × 1.7-cm nodule in the left thyroid lobe (*see images*). There are no suspicious lymph nodes.

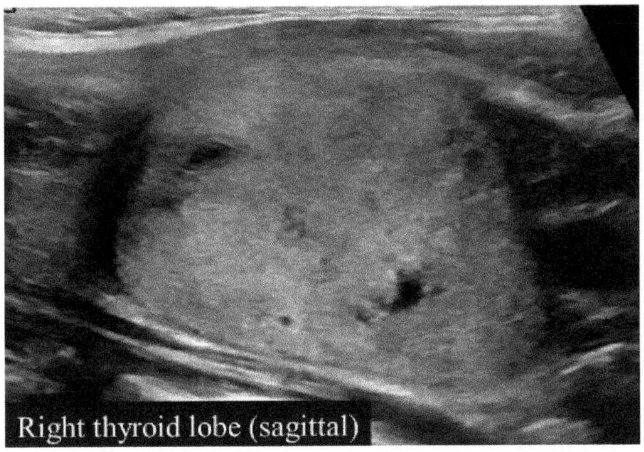

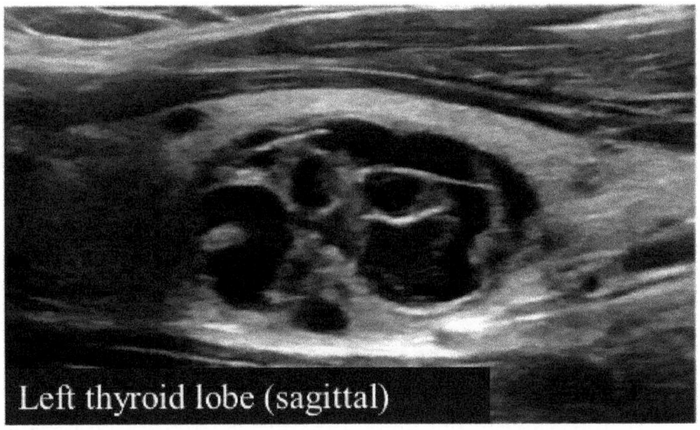

Laboratory test results:

TSH = 0.01 mIU/L (0.5-5.0 mIU/L)
Free T_4 = 1.56 ng/dL (0.8-1.8 ng/dL) (SI: 20.18 pmol/L [10.30-23.17 pmol/L])
Total T_3 = 172 ng/dL (70-200 ng/dL) (SI: 2.65 nmol/L [1.08-3.08 nmol/L])

Thyroid uptake and scan is performed (*see image*). Uptake at 6 hours is 12.5% (normal, 7%-20%).

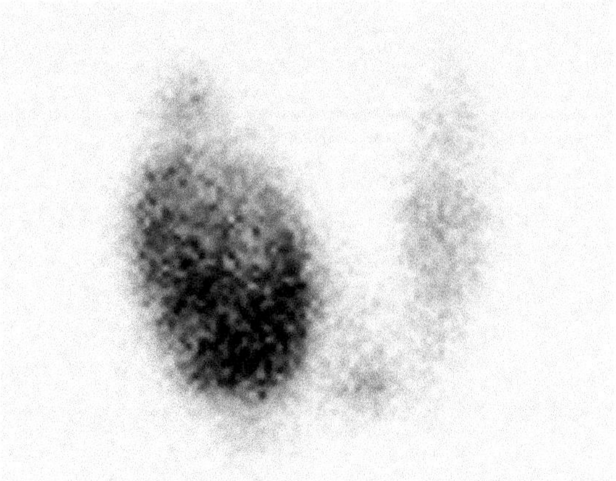

Which of the following is the most appropriate management to recommend next?

A. Referral for right thyroid lobectomy
B. TRAb measurement
C. Ultrasound-guided FNA of left thyroid nodule
D. Ultrasound-guided FNA of right and left thyroid nodules
E. Ultrasound-guided FNA of right thyroid nodule

110 A 76-year-old man is hospitalized for a total hip replacement. He has a known history of type 2 diabetes mellitus controlled with lifestyle intervention. His preoperative hemoglobin A_{1c} value was 7.3% (56 mmol/mol). His blood glucose values range from 95 mg/dL (5.3 mmol/L) (fasting) to 220 mg/dL (12.2 mmol/L) (postprandial). He requires 25 units of correctional regular insulin on postoperative day 1, and 14 units of correction insulin over the past 24 hours (postoperative day 2) with 1 episode of symptomatic nocturnal hypoglycemia (blood glucose = 62 mg/dL [3.4 mmol/L]) after 5 units of regular insulin are administered to correct a blood glucose concentration of 212 mg/dL (11.8 mmol/L) at bedtime. His wound is healing well, and he plans to start ambulating tomorrow.

His weight is 172 lb (78 kg) (BMI = 25.2 kg/m^2).

He is currently on a 60-g carbohydrate-consistent diet and eats all of his food without nausea or vomiting. His laboratory data show normal kidney function.

Which of the following is the best management plan?

A. Continue regular insulin correction scale with a bedtime snack
B. Start glipizide
C. Start insulin glargine, 10 units at bedtime, and schedule 3 units of insulin aspart before each meal
D. Start insulin glargine, 14 units at bedtime, and low-dose insulin aspart correction
E. Start sitagliptin and low-dose insulin aspart correction

111 A 52-year-old woman is referred for hypertension and hypokalemia. She also has type 2 diabetes mellitus, which is well controlled with metformin, 1000 mg twice daily, and lifestyle measures. She has a 10-year history of hypertension treated with lisinopril and hydrochlorothiazide. Since the COVID-19 pandemic, she has been working from home, and she reports that she has been more sedentary and more stressed due to numerous virtual meetings. At her recent visit with her primary care physician, her blood pressure was 190/100 mm Hg and pulse rate was 79 beats/min.

Laboratory test result:

Serum potassium = 3.0 mEq/L (3.5-5.0 mEq/L) (SI: 3.0 mmol/L [3.5-5.0 mmol/L])

Her current medications are lisinopril, 40 mg daily; labetalol 100 mg twice daily; amlodipine, 10 mg daily; potassium chloride, 10 mEq twice daily; 1 baby aspirin daily; and rosuvastatin, 20 mg daily.

At today's visit, her blood pressure is 182/98 mm Hg and pulse rate is 76 beats/min. Her height is 65.7 in (167 cm), and weight is 220 lb (99.8 kg) (BMI = 35.8 kg/m^2).

Findings on cardiovascular and respiratory examinations are unremarkable. She has uniformly distributed excess adiposity. There is no plethora, striae, or bruises. Her muscle strength is normal. She has no edema.

Laboratory test results:

Serum potassium = 3.6 mEq/L (3.5-5.0 mEq/L) (SI: 3.6 mmol/L [3.5-5.0 mmol/L])
Serum sodium = 140 mEq/L (136-142 mEq/L) (SI: 140 mmol/L [136-142 mmol/L])
Serum creatinine = 1.2 mg/dL (0.6-1.1 mg/dL) (SI: 106 µmol/L [53.0-97.2 µmol/L])
Serum cortisol = 13 µg/dL (5-25 µg/dL) (SI: 358.6 nmol/L [137.9-689.7 nmol/L])
ACTH = 23 pg/mL (10-60 pg/mL) (SI: 5.1 pmol/L [2.2-13.2 pmol/L])
Serum aldosterone = <4 ng/dL (4-21 ng/dL) (SI: <111.0 pmol/L [111.0-582.5 pmol/L])
Plasma renin activity = 0.1 ng/mL per h (0.6-4.3 ng/mL per h)

Which of the following is the best next step in this patient's management?

A. Initiate spironolactone
B. Measure 24-hour urinary cortisol and cortisone
C. Perform a 1-mg overnight dexamethasone-suppression test
D. Perform a salt-loading confirmatory test
E. Review diet and over-the-counter supplements

112 A 42-year-old woman is referred for difficulty with treatment of hypothyroidism. Initial laboratory testing ordered by her primary care physician during an evaluation for weight gain revealed an elevated serum TSH concentration of 9.6 mIU/L and a free T_4 concentration of 1.2 ng/mL (SI: 15.44 pmol/L). Her physician prescribed levothyroxine, 50 mcg daily, but subsequent TSH measurements were still elevated. Despite further levothyroxine dosage adjustment (as high as 100 mcg daily), her serum TSH did not decrease. She describes taking levothyroxine every day, on an empty stomach. She takes no over-the-counter supplements, and her only other medication is lisinopril for hypertension. Her mother has hypothyroidism treated with levothyroxine.

On physical examination, her blood pressure is 120/66 mm Hg and pulse rate is 88 beats/min. Her thyroid gland is not palpable. There is no hand tremor, and patellar reflexes are normal.

Laboratory test results:

Basic metabolic panel, normal
25-Hydroxyvitamin D = 32 ng/dL (30-80 ng/dL [optimal]) (SI: 79.9 nmol/L [74.9-199.7 nmol/L])
TSH = 8.8 mIU/L (0.5-5.0 mIU/L)
Free T_4 = 1.7 ng/dL (0.8-1.8 ng/dL) (SI: 21.88 pmol/L [10.30-23.17 pmol/L])

Which of the following is the most likely explanation for this patient's abnormal thyroid test results?

A. Heterophilic antibody interference with the TSH assay
B. Macro TSH
C. Malabsorption syndrome
D. Resistance to thyroid hormone
E. TSH-secreting pituitary adenoma

113 A 26-year-old man with no notable medical history sustains a closed head injury and brief loss of consciousness in a motor vehicle crash. Head CT without contrast in the emergency department does not identify abnormalities. After 3 months, he has headaches, fatigue, low libido, weight gain, and difficulty with focus and concentration. Medications include acetaminophen/oxycodone, 325/2.5 mg, which he takes as needed approximately twice daily.

On physical examination, his blood pressure is 130/88 mm Hg and pulse rate is 88 beats/min. His height is 71 in (180.3 cm), and weight is 230 lb (104.3 kg) (BMI = 32.1 kg/m^2). Fat distribution is noncentripetal.

Laboratory test results:

Chemistry panel, normal
TSH = 2.2 mIU/L (0.5-0.5 mIU/L)
Free T_4 = 1.5 ng/dL (0.8-1.8 ng/dL) (SI: 19.3 pmol/L [10.30-23.17 pmol/L])
Testosterone = 301 ng/dL (300-900 ng/dL) (SI: 10.4 nmol/L [10.4-31.2 nmol/L])
Cortisol (4 PM) = 3 µg/dL (2-14 µg/dL) (SI: 82.8 nmol/L [55.2-386.2 nmol/L])
IGF-1 = 130 ng/mL (117-321 ng/mL) (SI: 17.0 nmol/L [15.3-42.1 nmol/L])

The score on the adult GH deficiency questionnaire is 15 (range, 0-21).

Which of the following is the best next step in this patient's management?

A. Advise against GH replacement because his IGF-1 concentration is normal
B. Evaluate for adrenal insufficiency
C. Perform a 6-month trial of GH replacement
D. Start hydrocortisone replacement
E. Start testosterone replacement

114 A 32-year-old woman with maturity-onset diabetes of the young (MODY) due to a *GCK* pathogenic variant presents for preconception counseling. She and her partner are considering having a child, and she would like to discuss management of blood glucose before and during pregnancy. *GCK*-related MODY was diagnosed 5 years ago. Her blood glucose concentrations have always been in the range of 100 to 140 mg/dL (5.6-7.8 mmol/L). Three months ago, her hemoglobin A_{1c} value was 6.4% (46 mmol/mol).

She has never been treated with a glucose-lowering agent and has no diabetes-related complications.

Which of the following is the best recommendation for managing this patient's blood glucose peripartum?

A. Perform amniocentesis in the second trimester and start insulin if the fetus does not have the *GCK* pathogenic variant
B. Perform fetal ultrasonography starting week 26 of pregnancy and treat with insulin if macrosomia is observed
C. Start a sulfonylurea when pregnancy has been confirmed
D. Start insulin now (preconception)
E. Start insulin when pregnancy has been confirmed

115 A 31-year-old Black woman presents for recently diagnosed papillary thyroid cancer. She initially came to medical attention due to a palpable right thyroid nodule that was associated with anterior neck pressure and globus sensation. Neck ultrasonography confirmed the presence of a 3.9-cm right thyroid nodule, and ultrasound-guided FNA demonstrated cytopathology findings consistent with papillary thyroid carcinoma (Bethesda VI).

On physical examination, her blood pressure is 110/62 mm Hg and pulse rate is 80 beats/min. Her height is 64 in (162.6 cm), and weight is 122 lb (55 kg) (BMI = 20.9 kg/m^2). There is a firm nodule in the right thyroid lobe measuring approximately 4 cm. There is no palpable cervical lymphadenopathy. The rest of the examination findings are normal.

Laboratory test result:

TSH = 3.0 mIU/L (0.5-5.0 mIU/L)

Regarding this patient's thyroid cancer–related outcomes, her race is associated with an increased likelihood of which of the following?

A. Being operated on by a low-volume thyroid surgeon
B. Excessive worry about thyroid cancer recurrence
C. Receiving an early cancer diagnosis
D. Receiving treatment at an academic medical center
E. Treatment with radioactive iodine

116 A 72-year-old man is referred for management of type 2 diabetes mellitus complicated by peripheral neuropathy. He has had type 2 diabetes for 20 years, and his treatment was transitioned to a basal-bolus regimen approximately 8 years ago. His comorbidities include coronary artery disease status post coronary artery stenting 8 years ago, class 3 obesity, obstructive sleep apnea, hypertension, hyperlipidemia, and stage 3 chronic kidney disease with microalbuminuria. His peripheral neuropathy is well controlled with gabapentin. He has no chest pain or shortness of breath. Current medications are atorvastatin, 80 mg daily; gabapentin, 100 mg 3 times daily; lisinopril, 40 mg daily; metoprolol extended release, 25 mg daily; empagliflozin, 10 mg daily; and furosemide, 20 mg twice daily.

On physical examination, his blood pressure is 126/74 mm Hg and pulse rate is 56 beats/min. His height is 64 in (162.6 cm), and weight is 220 lb (99.8 kg) (BMI = 37.8 kg/m^2). His heart has a regular rhythm with bradycardia, and lungs are clear to auscultation bilaterally. There is no abdominal tenderness. He has +1 pitting edema in his lower extremities bilaterally.

Laboratory test results:

Hemoglobin A_{1c} = 8.4% (4.0%-5.6%) (68 mmol/mol [20-38 mmol/mol])
Estimated glomerular filtration rate = 48 mL/min per 1.73 m^2 (>60 mL/min per 1.73 m^2)
Triglycerides = 120 mg/dL (<150 mg/dL [optimal]) (SI: 1.36 mmol/L [<1.70 mmol/L])
LDL cholesterol = 48 mg/dL (<70 mg/dL [optimal]) (SI: 1.24 mmol/L [<1.81 mmol/L])
Potassium = 4.5 mEq/L (3.5-5.0 mEq/L) (SI: 4.5 mmol/L [3.5-5.0 mmol/L])

Which of the following is the best next step in this patient's management?

A. Add finerenone
B. Double the dosage of furosemide
C. Double the dosage of lisinopril
D. Switch to bumetanide
E. Switch to rosuvastatin

117 A 54-year-old man is referred to endocrinology for evaluation of osteoporosis. Type 1 diabetes mellitus was diagnosed at age 19 years. He is prescribed a basal-bolus insulin regimen and has had varying glycemic control. His most recent hemoglobin A_{1c} value is 8.2% (66 mmol/mol). He also has a history of depression, hypertension, and gastroesophageal reflux disease. He consumes 2 to 3 beers daily.

Current medications:

Insulin glargine, 22 units once daily
Insulin lispro, 2 to 10 units with meals
Hydrochlorothiazide, 25 mg daily
Metoprolol extended release, 50 mg daily
Sertraline, 50 mg daily
Omeprazole, 20 mg daily

Two weeks ago, he fell while walking his dog and experienced a left femoral neck fracture. He was hospitalized and underwent placement of an intramedullary pin with fixation of the femoral neck. After discharge, he was seen by his primary care physician, who then ordered DXA.

DXA results:

Lumbar spine (L1-4) T-score = −2.8
Right femoral neck T-score = −3.1
Right total neck T-score = −2.8

Which of the following is the largest contributor to this patient's osteoporosis and elevated fracture risk?

A. Alcohol consumption
B. Proton-pump inhibitor
C. Selective serotonin reuptake inhibitor
D. Thiazide diuretic
E. Type 1 diabetes mellitus

118 A 22-year-old medical student is referred for low testosterone, which was measured when he presented to his primary care provider with low libido and fatigue. He describes undergoing normal puberty. He has never attempted paternity. He has a history of chronic constipation that has been evaluated by a gastroenterologist, without a clear diagnosis. Findings on colonoscopy performed 2 years ago were reportedly normal. He states that he has lactose and fructose intolerance. Although his gastroenterologist found no evidence of celiac disease, he follows a gluten-free diet. He has always been a picky eater. He has a history of depression previously treated with a selective serotonin reuptake inhibitor. Recently, he has been experiencing increasing anxiety and difficulty coping with his studies and has been referred to a psychologist. He runs regularly (about 7.5 miles 3 to 4 times weekly), but he has stopped because of a tibial stress fracture.

On physical examination, his height is 70 in (177.8 cm) and weight is 122 lb (52.2 kg) (BMI = 17.4 kg/m^2). Blood pressure is 100/60 mm Hg lying down and 92/62 mm Hg standing, and pulse rate is 48 beats/min and regular. Muscle bulk and body hair are normal. Findings on genital examination are normal, and testes are 20 mL bilaterally.

Laboratory test results (sample drawn at 8 AM while fasting):

Total testosterone = 100 ng/dL (300-900 ng/dL) (SI: 3.5 nmol/L [10.4-31.2 nmol/L]) (repeated measurement 2 weeks later = 120 ng/dL [SI: 4.2 nmol/L])
SHBG = 9.4 µg/mL (1.1-6.7 µg/mL) (SI: 84 nmol/L [10-60 nmol/L])
LH = 3.2 mIU/mL (1.0-9.0 mIU/mL) (SI: 3.2 IU/L [1.0-9.0 IU/L])
FSH = 4.5 IU/L (1.0-13.0 mIU/mL) (SI: 4.5 IU/L [1.0-13.0 IU/L])
Hemoglobin = 12.4 g/dL (13.8-17.2 g/dL) (SI: 124 g/L [138-172 g/L])
TSH = 1.2 mIU/L (0.5-5.0 mIU/L)
Free T_4 = 0.95 ng/dL (0.8-1.8 ng/dL) (SI: 12.2 pmol/L [10.30-23.17 pmol/L])
Free T_3 = 2.3 pg/mL (2.3-4.2 pg/mL) (SI: 3.5 pmol/L [3.53-6.45 pmol/L])
Serum cortisol = 33 µg/dL (5-25 µg/dL) (SI: 910.4 nmol/L [137.9-689.7 nmol/L])
Prolactin = 20 ng/mL (4-23 ng/mL) (SI: 0.87 nmol/L [0.17-1.00 nmol/L])

MRI shows a 2-mm pituitary microadenoma.

Which of the following is the best step to address this patient's hypogonadism?

A. Measure macroprolactin
B. Refer to an eating disorder clinic
C. Start a dopamine agonist
D. Start clomiphene
E. Start topical testosterone gel at 50% of replacement dosage

119

A healthy 40-year-old man is seen for further evaluation of hypertriglyceridemia. He has no symptoms of cardiovascular disease and has never had pancreatitis. He currently takes no medications and eats a regular diet. He describes himself as a social drinker, consuming alcohol only at parties. He works as a software engineer and does not do any regular leisure time physical activity except walking his dog. His father also has high triglycerides and takes statin therapy and fish oil, but he has no known cardiovascular disease.

On physical examination, his blood pressure is 124/76 mm Hg and pulse rate is 72 beats/min. His height is 73 in (185.4 cm), and weight is 214 lb (97.1 kg) (BMI = 28.2 kg/m^2) He has no eruptive or palmar xanthomas.

Laboratory test results (sample drawn while fasting):

Total cholesterol = 210 mg/dL (<200 mg/dL) (SI: 5.44 mmol/L [<5.18 mmol/L])
Triglycerides = 634 mg/dL (<150 mg/dL) (SI: 7.16 mmol/L [<1.70 mmol/L])
HDL cholesterol = 44 mg/dL (>60 mg/dL) (SI: 1.14 mmol/L [>1.55 mmol/L])
Apolipoprotein B = 82 mg/dL (50-110 mg/dL) (SI: 0.82 g/L [0.5-1.1 g/L])
Plasma glucose = 86 mg/dL (70-99 mg/dL) (SI: 4.8 mmol/L [3.9-5.5 mmol/L])
TSH = 1.2 mIU/L (0.5-5.0 mIU/L)

Which of the following is the best next step in this patient's management?

A. A moderate-intensity statin
B. A moderate-intensity statin and omega-3 fatty acids
C. Fenofibrate
D. Lifestyle counseling
E. Omega-3 fatty acids

120 A 55-year-old man with type 2 diabetes mellitus is seen for routine follow-up. He reports feeling well. Diabetes was diagnosed at age 45 years on routine blood testing (hemoglobin A_{1c} = 8.2% [66 mmol/mol]). At that time, his BMI was 34.0 kg/m². He undertook lifestyle modifications and is now treated with metformin, 1000 mg twice daily, and semaglutide, 0.5 mg weekly, which has been his regimen for the last 2 years. During treatment, his hemoglobin A_{1c} level has ranged from 6.8% to 7.2% (51-55 mmol/mol). His medical history is notable for hypertension. There is no history of other cardiovascular disease. His only other medications are amlodipine, 10 mg daily, and rosuvastatin, 10 mg daily. He does not smoke cigarettes, and he drinks 3 to 4 alcoholic beverages per week.

On physical examination, his blood pressure is 130/78 mm Hg and pulse rate is 90 beats/min. His BMI is 31.0 kg/m². There is no acanthosis.

Laboratory test results:

Hemoglobin A_{1c} = 7.0% (4.0%-5.6%) (53 mmol/mol [20-38 mmol/mol])
Serum urea nitrogen = 22 mg/dL (8-23 mg/dL) (SI: 7.9 mmol/L [2.9-8.2 mmol/L])
Creatinine = 1.2 mg/dL (0.7-1.3 mg/dL) (SI: 106.1 µmol/L [61.9-114.9 µmol/L])
Urinary albumin-to-creatinine ratio = 28 mg/g creat (<30 mg/g creat)
ALT = 40 U/L (10-40 U/L) (SI: 0.67 µkat/L [0.17-0.67 µkat/L])
AST = 30 U/L (20-48 U/L) (SI: 0.50 µkat/L [0.33-0.80 µkat/L])
Total bilirubin = 0.5 mg/dL (0.3-1.2 mg/dL) (SI: 8.6 µmol/L [5.1-20.5 µmol/L])
Total cholesterol = 190 mg/dL (<200 mg/dL [optimal]) (SI: 4.92 mmol/L [<5.18 mmol/L])
Triglycerides = 175 mg/dL (<150 mg/dL [optimal]) (SI: 1.98 mmol/L [<1.70 mmol/L])
HDL cholesterol = 40 mg/dL (>60 mg/dL [optimal]) (SI: 1.04 mmol/L [>1.55 mmol/L])
LDL cholesterol = 115 mg/dL (<100 mg/dL [optimal]) (SI: 2.98 mmol/L [<2.59 mmol/L])

Which of the following is the most important next step?

A. Administer the Montreal Cognitive Assessment
B. Check complete blood cell count and calculate Fibrosis-4 score
C. Determine coronary artery calcium score
D. Measure lipoprotein(a)
E. Perform abdominal ultrasonography

ANSWERS

ENDOCRINE SELF-ASSESSMENT PROGRAM 2024

Part II

1 ANSWER: C) Preoperative serum TSH concentration

This patient developed compressive symptoms (anterior neck pressure, choking) in the context of a slowly enlarging left thyroid nodule with benign FNA cytology on 2 separate occasions. The risk of malignancy in this context is extremely low (<1%); however, the patient elected to undergo a left lobectomy for relief of compressive symptoms. Final surgical pathology was benign in this case. There is a reduced risk of surgical complications (recurrent laryngeal nerve injury, hematoma, and postoperative hypoparathyroidism) when thyroid lobectomy is performed instead of total thyroidectomy. Another argument in favor of thyroid lobectomy is a lower likelihood of postoperative hypothyroidism requiring thyroid hormone replacement. In cases of papillary thyroid carcinoma, thyroid lobectomy is also a recommended surgical option for tumors smaller than 4 cm if they are confined to the thyroid gland.

The likelihood of developing postoperative hypothyroidism following thyroid lobectomy is estimated to be 20% to 50%. Without immediate initiation of thyroid hormone replacement, up to two-thirds of patients with subclinical hypothyroidism identified early in the postoperative period recover normal thyroid function if simply observed. The strongest predictor of postoperative hypothyroidism and failure of subsequent recovery to euthyroidism is the preoperative TSH concentration (Answer C). Higher normal preoperative serum TSH concentrations above 1.7 to 2.5 mIU/L have been identified as a significant risk factor for subsequent postoperative hypothyroidism. Other risk factors include positive TPO antibodies, presence of thyroiditis, older age, smaller volume of the contralateral thyroid lobe, and the presence of malignancy on final pathology (likely secondary to more stringent TSH goals in this setting).

The presence of positive TPO antibodies (Answer E) has been identified as a predictor in many but not all studies. A recently published study with long-term follow-up (15 years) demonstrated no significant difference in the number of patients who required postoperative thyroid hormone replacement when those with Hashimoto thyroiditis were excluded from the analysis. This study also demonstrated that nearly half of patients eventually required thyroid hormone replacement following lobectomy for benign disease, with almost 25% not needing treatment until 2 or more years after surgery. The only predictor of late hypothyroidism in another study was a TSH concentration of 3.1 mIU/L or higher at 1 year postoperatively. Therefore, it is prudent that patients continue to be monitored for the development of postoperative hypothyroidism for at least 2 to 3 years after surgery.

Isthmus-sparing surgery (Answer A), male sex (Answer B), and technical expertise of the surgeon (Answer D) have not been shown to be significant predictors of postoperative thyroid hormone status. Access to a high-volume thyroid surgeon (variably defined as those performing more than 25 or 50 thyroid operations per year) is associated with a lower risk of other surgical complications, including risk of ipsilateral recurrent laryngeal nerve injury.

Educational Objective

Identify risk factors for postoperative hypothyroidism after thyroid lobectomy.

Reference(s)

Barranco H, Fazendin J, Lindeman B, Chen H, Ramonell KM. Thyroid hormone replacement following lobectomy: long-term institutional analysis 15 years after surgery. *Surgery.* 2022:S0039-6060. PMID: 36202649

Cao Z, Liu R, Wu M, Xu X, Liu Z. Risk factors for thyroid hormone replacement therapy after hemithyroidectomy and development of a predictive nomogram. *Endocrine.* 2022;76(1):85-94. PMID: 35067900

Park S, Jeon MJ, Song E, et al. Clinical features of early and late postoperative hypothyroidism after lobectomy. *J Clin Endocrinol Metab.* 102(4):1317-1324. PMID 28324106

Verloop H, Louwerens M, Schoones JW, Kievit J, Smit JWA, Dekkers OM. Risk of hypothyroidism following hemithyroidectomy: systematic review and meta-analysis of prognostic studies. *J Clin Endocrinol Metab.* 2012;97(7):2243-2255. PMID: 22511795

2 ANSWER: D) Perform diagnostic continuous glucose monitoring

Managing diabetes mellitus in patients older than 65 years can be challenging. Older patients with diabetes may or may not develop microvascular or macrovascular complications, depending on their life expectancy. Older patients are also more vulnerable to hypoglycemia than younger individuals. Hypoglycemia can lead to neuroglycopenic manifestations such as dizziness or confusion, which may lead to traumatic falls. Hypoglycemia is also associated with adverse cardiovascular events and increased mortality among patients with diabetes mellitus. Older patients with diabetes, especially those who have established cardiovascular disease, such as the patient in this vignette, may be more vulnerable to hypoglycemia than those who do not have underlying cardiovascular disease.

GLP-1 receptor agonists are effective weight-loss medications that can significantly decrease glucose concentrations. This patient has achieved a hemoglobin A_{1c} level of 7.5% (58 mmol/mol). However, glycemic control in this tight range can lead to hypoglycemia, and this should be suspected, especially among patients who have a long history of diabetes. Although he currently recognizes symptoms of hypoglycemia at night, prolonged history of diabetes can lead to hypoglycemia unawareness.

Assessing for nocturnal hypoglycemia is the best next step in this patient's care. Checking blood glucose before meals and at bedtime (Answer E) would not reveal nocturnal hypoglycemia before meals, as these episodes occur overnight. Diagnostic continuous glucose monitoring devices (Answer D) that check glucose values every 1 to 5 minutes can identify hypoglycemia in the overnight hours. Continuous glucose monitoring provides comprehensive information in the form of graphs and diagrams, which can not only identify the presence or absence of hypoglycemia but can also reveal the severity and duration of these events. Appropriate changes can be made to the treatment regimen after reviewing the detailed reports.

Continuing the current diabetes regimen (Answer A) is not appropriate for this elderly patient, who has multiple comorbidities and is suspected to have clinical hypoglycemia severe enough to wake him at night.

Similarly, stopping semaglutide (Answer B) would not be the best next step. GLP-1 receptor agonists do not usually cause hypoglycemia.

Basal insulin and sulfonylureas are more likely to lead to hypoglycemia. Adding a GLP-1 receptor agonist may necessitate reduction of insulin or sulfonylureas dosages, as achieving tight glucose control can lead to hypoglycemia. In addition to their important weight-loss properties, GLP-1 receptor agonists have significant cardioprotective effects and, therefore, semaglutide should be continued in this patient.

One of the major limitations of relying on hemoglobin A_{1c}, fructosamine (Answer C), or any other glycemic markers is that they provide information about average glycemic control. Thus, patients who have significant hyperglycemia and hypoglycemia may have a desired ("on target") hemoglobin A_{1c} value, although their glycemic control is at least suboptimal. Measuring fructosamine would, therefore, only reveal an average estimate of this patient's glycemic control and would not identify the hypoglycemia, which is necessary to make safe adjustments to his diabetes regimen.

Educational Objective

Recommend continuous glucose monitoring to identify hypoglycemia.

Reference(s)

Lee AK, Warren B, Lee CJ, et al. The association of severe hypoglycemia with incident cardiovascular events and mortality in adults with type 2 diabetes. *Diabetes Care.* 2018;41(1):104-111. PMID: 29127240

Bergenstal RM, Ahmann AJ, Bailey T, et al. Recommendations for standardizing glucose reporting and analysis to optimize clinical decision making in diabetes: the ambulatory glucose profile. *J Diabetes Sci Technol.* 2013;7(2):562-578. PMID: 23567014

Danne T, Nimri R, Battelino T, et al. International consensus on use of continuous glucose monitoring. *Diabetes Care.* 2017;40(12):1631-1640. PMID: 29162583

3 ANSWER: E) SHBG measurement

Although sexual symptoms, especially low libido, have a syndromic association with low serum testosterone (referred to as late-onset hypogonadism), even these relatively specific sexual symptoms have a high prevalence in middle-aged and older men with normal serum testosterone concentrations. In this patient, total testosterone was unexpectedly above the upper limit of the reference range. This was confirmed using validated liquid chromatography–tandem mass spectrometry, indicating that the elevated serum testosterone was not a spurious result. Endocrine Society guidelines recommend measuring fasting morning total testosterone concentrations using an accurate and reliable assay as the initial diagnostic test to confirm a clinical suspicion of androgen deficiency. Total testosterone is largely protein bound, about 60% with high affinity to SHBG and 40% with low affinity to albumin (the latter is therefore considered bioavailable). Only 2.0% to 4.0% of circulating testosterone is unbound or free. Therefore, in the presence of conditions that alter SHBG concentrations, in the context of a normally functioning hypothalamic-pituitary-gonadal axis, total testosterone concentrations change in parallel to changes in SHBG to maintain adequate tissue androgenization (ie, total testosterone increases if SHBG increases and decreases if SHBG decreases). If there is a discrepancy between the clinical picture and the total testosterone value, abnormalities in SHBG concentrations should be considered, especially in the appropriate clinical context (Answer E). The most common scenario is reduced

SHBG leading to low total testosterone (with normal bioavailable/free testosterone) in the context of obesity/insulin resistance (ie, pseudohypogonadism). In this patient, SHBG was elevated (13.4 µg/mL [1.1-6.7 µg/mL] [SI: 119 nmol/L (10-60 nmol/L)]). Given the clinical presentation (clinical and biochemical features consistent with alcoholic hepatitis), the most likely cause of his elevated SHBG value is high alcohol consumption. Other potential causes of elevated SHBG, such as thyrotoxicosis, HIV infection, a hyperestrogenic state, or the use of anticonvulsant agents, have been excluded or are not supported by the clinical history. While increased SHBG concentrations are common in men with liver cirrhosis, chronic consumption of high amounts of alcohol can increase SHBG (and cortisol-binding globulin), even in the absence of liver cirrhosis. Longitudinal studies have reported that alcohol abstinence for at least 3 months is necessary to normalize SHBG concentrations.

In situations where abnormalities of SHBG are suspected, the Endocrine Society guidelines recommend measuring free testosterone using either equilibrium dialysis or estimating its concentration with an accurate formula. While equilibrium dialysis is considered the gold standard for measuring free testosterone, in practice, free testosterone is usually determined with calculations that use total testosterone, SHBG, and albumin concentrations (eg, the Vermeulen formula). Of note, direct analogue-based free testosterone immunoassays should not be used because they are inaccurate. In contrast to reference ranges for total testosterone, harmonized reference ranges for free testosterone have not been established, so reference ranges may vary considerably depending on the specific equilibrium dialysis method or the algorithm used to calculate free testosterone. This patient's calculated free testosterone was normal, consistent with the lack of specific clinical features of androgen deficiency on physical examination. The elevated total testosterone indicates that his hypothalamic-pituitary-gonadal axis is functioning normally and compensating for the elevated SHBG.

Androgen insensitivity syndromes can present with increased serum testosterone (and occasionally high or high-normal SHBG) and nonsuppressed (or more typically frankly elevated) LH concentrations. However, the absence of clinical features of androgen deficiency and his normal reproductive history with prior paternity are not consistent with this diagnosis. Therefore, genetic testing of the gene encoding the androgen receptor (Answer B) is not indicated.

Functioning pituitary gonadotroph adenomas secreting biologically active gonadotropins can present with elevated total testosterone and nonsuppressed or frankly elevated gonadotropins (often FSH is elevated, leading to testicular enlargement). Functioning pituitary gonadotroph adenomas are extremely rare, and SHBG would not be expected to be elevated. Therefore, pituitary-directed MRI (Answer D) is not indicated.

Hemochromatosis can present with evidence of liver disease and (usually central) hypogonadism. However, the hepatitis is most likely due to alcohol excess and he is not hypogonadal, so iron studies (Answer C) are not the best next step.

Similar to total testosterone, serum cortisol (measured as total cortisol) is largely protein-bound (80% to 90% to cortisol-binding globulin). Like SHBG, serum cortisol-binding globulin is increased in active hepatitis, and this patient's increased serum total cortisol is simply a consequence of the increased cortisol-binding globulin, indicating a functioning hypothalamic-pituitary-adrenal axis. Given that there is no clinical suspicion of Cushing syndrome, a 1-mg dexamethasone-suppression test (Answer A) is not indicated. Of note, although not evident in this case, alcoholism can be associated with pseudo-Cushing syndrome, which is another reason to hold off evaluation of the hypothalamic-pituitary-adrenal axis in the context of excessive alcohol use.

This patient gradually stopped drinking alcohol. After 4 months of abstinence, SHBG, total testosterone, and cortisol concentrations normalized. His libido improved, and he reported satisfactory erectile function occasionally requiring the use of a phosphodiesterase-5 inhibitor.

Educational Objective

Recommend determination of free testosterone when SHBG abnormalities are present and identify excessive alcohol intake as a cause of elevated SHBG (and secondarily total testosterone), even in the absence of cirrhosis.

References

Bhasin S, Brito JP, Cunningham GR, et al. Testosterone therapy in men with hypogonadism: an Endocrine Society clinical practice guideline. *J Clin Endocrinol Metab.* 2018;103(5):1715-1744. PMID: 29562364

Iturriaga H, Lioi X, Valladares L. Sex hormone-binding globulin in non-cirrhotic alcoholic patients during early withdrawal and after longer abstinence. *Alcohol Alcohol.* 1999;34(6):903-909. PMID: 10659727

Orbach O, Schussler GC. Increased serum cortisol binding in chronic active hepatitis. *Am J Med.* 1989;86(1):39-42. PMID: 2910094

4 **ANSWER: A) Perform MRI again in 12 months**

The decision whether to recommend active surveillance or early adjuvant therapy following primary surgery for a clinically nonsecretory (nonfunctioning) pituitary adenoma (NFPA) should be made by a specialist multidisciplinary team (ideally in a pituitary tumor center of excellence), and informed by postoperative endocrine and ophthalmic assessments, histopathological findings of the resected tumor, follow-up imaging (performed 3 to 6 months after surgery), and an understanding of the patient's treatment preference(s).

In the absence of pathologic hormone secretion, the main goals of pituitary surgery for NFPAs are:

- Protection, stabilization, and rescue of vision
- Preservation and recovery of pituitary function

These goals may be achieved without complete tumor resection, and more "aggressive surgery" can result in less favorable outcomes, including injury to key neurovascular structures within the cavernous sinus or damage to the remaining normal gland with widespread pituitary dysfunction, including arginine vasopressin deficiency (central diabetes insipidus).

The demonstration of possible, or even likely, residual tumor on early postoperative imaging should not therefore be considered an immediate indication for adjuvant therapy, especially if the visual pathways have been adequately decompressed, as in this case. Surveillance is a reasonable—indeed preferred—option, especially in the early phase after surgery when histology has not identified any concerning features (including Ki-67 index <3%). This approach also acknowledges the potential limitations of standard clinical MRI in the discrimination of residual tumor from postoperative remodeling, as not all apparent remnants turn out to be tumor.

In this case, excellent surgical decompression has been achieved, with a good ophthalmic outcome and preservation of normal pituitary function. Therefore, even though it is not possible to exclude residual tumor within the sella on the initial postoperative MRI, it is reasonable to wait and see whether appearances change with time. Twelve months is an appropriate interval to the next surveillance scan (Answer A), assuming the patient does not report any new vision symptoms in the intervening period and ophthalmology findings are unchanged.

A second transsphenoidal surgery (Answer C) by a highly skilled pituitary surgeon may be considered for patients with an NFPA, especially when there is evidence of tumor regrowth. Additional debulking can protect vision and facilitate more effective tumor control in response to subsequent radiotherapy. However, in this case, further surgery is not currently indicated given the clinical, laboratory, and radiologic findings.

Routine use of postoperative radiotherapy (Answer B) to mitigate regrowth of NFPAs is no longer supported. However, in patients with significant tumor remnants that are enlarging and not amenable to further surgery, radiotherapy can arrest growth or induce tumor shrinkage. Conventional fractionated radiotherapy (eg, 45-55 Gy, delivered in 25 to 30 fractions, using image-guided, intensity-modulated techniques) achieves high control rates at 10 and 20 years (75%-90%) but carries a risk of hypopituitarism (~50% at 10 years) and second tumors (~1%-2%) and may predispose to premature cerebrovascular disease, although the latter is debated. Stereotactic radiosurgery has been reported to achieve control rates of up to 95% at 5 years. However, larger tumors, suprasellar extension, and lower radiation doses have all been linked to suboptimal control, while hypopituitarism, vision disturbance, and cranial neuropathies can complicate treatment.

Several retrospective studies have reported tumor stabilization or even shrinkage in patients with residual or recurrent NFPAs treated with dopamine agonists (most commonly cabergoline) (Answer D) following primary surgery. Timing of treatment initiation (early [preventive, ie, when residual tumor is suspected on postoperative MRI] vs delayed [remedial, ie, upon detection of regrowth during follow-up]) may influence effectiveness. However, routine adoption of such an approach must be balanced against the potential risks of long-term dopamine agonist therapy, and further prospective multicenter studies will be required to establish the effectiveness and safety of this approach. In this case, the mildly elevated serum prolactin level is likely due to disruption to normal inhibitory dopaminergic tone following surgery. Additionally, histopathology demonstrated a tumor of SF-1 lineage with only focal FSH staining.

Evidence for the routine use of first-generation somatostatin receptor ligands (octreotide, lanreotide) (Answer E) in the management of residual or recurrent NFPAs is currently lacking. Although tumor stabilization has been reported in some small-scale studies, there is little evidence of tumor shrinkage. Similarly, there is a paucity of data to support combined treatment with dopamine agonists and somatostatin receptor ligands or with second-generation somatostatin receptor ligand therapy (eg, pasireotide).

Educational Objective

Appropriately recommend active surveillance after primary surgery for a nonsecretory pituitary adenoma and explain the benefits and limitations of possible adjuvant therapies.

Reference(s)

Raverot G, Burman P, McCormack A, et al; European Society of Endocrinology. European Society of Endocrinology Clinical Practice Guidelines for the management of aggressive pituitary tumours and carcinomas. *Eur J Endocrinol.* 2018;178(1):G1-G24. PMID: 29046323

Esposito D, Olsson DS, Ragnarsson O, Buchfelder M, Skoglund T, Johannsson G. Non-functioning pituitary adenomas: indications for pituitary surgery and post-surgical management. *Pituitary.* 2019;22(4):422-434. PMID: 31011999

Yavropoulou MP, Tsoli M, Barkas K, Kaltsas G, Grossman A. The natural history and treatment of non-functioning pituitary adenomas (non-functioning PitNETs). *Endocr Relat Cancer.* 2020;27(10):R375-R390. PMID: 32674070

5 ANSWER: A) Alendronate

Prescription medication cost is a major barrier to many patients with limited resources who require treatment for diseases such as osteoporosis. According to the prescription cost website Good Rx at the time of this writing, the following lists the generic (if available) lowest retail price for a 1-year course of the medications:

Alendronate	$29.96
Denosumab	$1509.00 + administration costs
Ibandronate	$79.96
Risedronate	$203.40
Zoledronic acid	$120.43 + administration costs

Administration costs of twice-yearly denosumab and once-yearly zoledronic acid vary widely across the United States and depend on the geographic location and the type of facility where the medication is administered, such as a private physician's office or a hospital-based infusion center. Irrespective of the treatment location, administration costs for denosumab and zoledronic acid are often at least in the hundreds-of-dollars range. Of the 5 medications listed, alendronate (Answer A) is the least expensive and the most reasonable option for this patient. Denosumab (Answer B), ibandronate (Answer C), risedronate (Answer D), and zoledronic acid (Answer E) are reasonable options to treat osteoporosis, but the cost of these agents is significantly more and they almost certainly represent unaffordable options for this particular patient. Despite the lower cost of alendronate, denosumab is marginally superior to bisphosphonates in reducing fracture risk and should be considered in patients with a moderate to high risk of fragility fractures.

Educational Objective

Recommend the best options for osteoporosis medications when cost is a concern.

Reference(s)

Nayak S, Roberts MS, Greenspan SL. Impact of generic alendronate cost on the cost-effectiveness of osteoporosis screening and treatment. *PLoS One.* 2012;7(3):e32879. PMID: 22427903

Kanis JA, Adams J, Borgström F, et al. The cost-effectiveness of alendronate in the management of osteoporosis. *Bone.* 2008;42(1):4-15. PMID: 18156107

Pedersen AB, Heide-Jørgensen U, et al. Comparison of risk of osteoporotic fracture in denosumab vs alendronate treatment within 3 years of initiation. *JAMA Netw Open.* 2019;2(4):e192416. PMID: 31002319

6 ANSWER: D) Switch insulin lispro to a GLP-1 receptor agonist

Many patients find basal-bolus regimens overwhelming and burdensome. In addition, because of the risk of hypoglycemia associated with multiple daily insulin injections, achieving glycemic targets can be challenging. Patients are often discouraged by the weight gain that can accompany insulin therapy. In the past, most patients with suboptimally controlled type 2 diabetes were relegated to complex and burdensome regimens to control glycemia. With the advent of GLP-1 receptor agonist therapy, the need to initiate prandial insulin can now be delayed or negated in some patients. Recently, it has been shown that patients with type 2 diabetes requiring basal-bolus insulin, after insulin optimization, can be transitioned from a basal-bolus regimen to a once-weekly GLP-1 receptor agonist in combination with basal insulin. Rosenstock et al demonstrated that prandial insulin can be substituted with once-weekly GLP-1 receptor agonist therapy in 54% of patients, substantially reducing the number of prandial insulin injections. In this treat-to-target study, basal plus prandial insulin was optimized over 4 weeks before participants were randomly assigned (1:1) to albiglutide plus optimized basal insulin glargine and lispro (dosage reduced by 50% at randomization. Subsequently, lispro injections were fully discontinued 4 weeks later) (n = 402) or continued with optimized lispro plus optimized glargine (n = 412). Key eligibility criteria at screening were age 18 to 75 years, hemoglobin A_{1c} ≥7.0% and ≤9.5% (≥53 and ≤80 mmol/mol), fasting C-peptide ≥0.8 ng/mL (≥0.26 nmol/L), BMI ≤40.0 kg/m^2, and current use of a basal plus prandial insulin regimen (3 or more injections per day and ≤140 units daily) for ≥3 months. Baseline hemoglobin A_{1c} (mean ± SD), after lead-in insulin optimization was 7.7% ± 0.6% (60 mmol/mol ± 7 mmol/mol) and 7.7% ± 0.6% (60 mmol/mol ± 7 mmol/mol), in the albiglutide + glargine and insulin lispro + insulin glargine groups, respectively. The baseline daily mean prandial insulin dose was 38.7 ± 19.0 units and 41.3 ± 21.6 units, in the albiglutide + glargine and insulin lispro + insulin glargine groups, respectively.

Glycemic control is also reported to improve with GLP-1 receptor agonists, with the added benefits of weight loss and less hypoglycemia. Replacing prandial insulin with once-weekly GLP-1 receptor agonist therapy (Answer D) can simplify regimens of multiple daily insulin injections and achieve better outcomes in patients with type 2 diabetes. Accordingly, this approach should be considered in patients with type 2 diabetes receiving basal-bolus therapy, particularly those frustrated with the burden of management that accompanies multiple daily insulin injections, as well as those experiencing weight gain and/or frequent hypoglycemia.

Increasing this patient's insulin lispro dosage (Answer B) would not reduce her burden of management, and it would likely only potentiate further weight gain.

Adding a sulfonylurea (Answer A) is unlikely to provide much benefit in a patient taking basal-bolus insulin and may also result in further weight gain.

There is no indication to change her basal insulin from insulin glargine to insulin degludec (Answer C), nor would such a switch reduce the management burden associated with a basal-bolus insulin regimen.

Insulin lispro-aabc is a mealtime insulin that works more quickly than insulin lispro. The insulin lispro-aabc formulation contains a microdose of treprostinil to enhance insulin lispro absorption by local vasodilation, and sodium citrate is added to further enhance the absorption from the site of subcutaneous injection. While changing this patient's bolus insulin to insulin lispro-aabc (Answer E) may help improve postprandial glucose control, it would not reduce her management burden or her frustration with weight gain associated with her regimen of multiple daily insulin injections.

Educational Objective

Determine when replacement of prandial insulin with a GLP-1 receptor agonist may be appropriate for patients with type 2 diabetes mellitus on a basal-bolus regimen.

Reference(s)

Rosenstock J, Nino A, Soffer J, et al. Impact of weekly glucagon-like peptide 1 receptor agonist, albiglutide, on glycemic control and on reducing prandial insulin use in type 2 diabetes inadequately controlled on multiple insulin therapy: a randomized trial. *Diabetes Care.* 2020;43(10):2509-2518. PMID: 32694215

7 ANSWER: B) Place an etonogestrel implant

This transgender man is seeking gender-affirming hormone therapy with testosterone for masculinization. Transgender men who seek a binary gender identity and presentation often desire facial and body hair, deepening of the voice, increased strength, change in body fat distribution, and cessation of menses. It is important to counsel transgender men about the varying effects of testosterone on the body, and also about the potential risks. On testosterone therapy, the serum testosterone target is the mid-normal range for cisgender men of the same age (250-750 ng/dL [8.7-26.0 nmol/L]). Although most transgender men on physiologic dosages of testosterone therapy experience estradiol suppression and cessation of menses by 6 months of continuous treatment, in some cases, this does not occur and other treatment modalities must be considered.

In general, gender-affirming therapy is associated with decreased gender dysphoria in both transgender men and women. In this patient, the continuation of menses has led to persistent gender dysphoria and suicidal ideation. Therefore, a change must be made in his therapeutic plan. In addition, it is important to note that this transgender man engages in sexual behavior with a partner who produces sperm (where sperm can meet egg); this puts him at risk for pregnancy, and he does not presently desire pregnancy. Transgender men on testosterone therapy should be counseled that if they become pregnant, they should not take testosterone because it is a category X medication that may cause fetal harm. Therefore, appropriate contraception should be addressed as well.

The only answer option that will prevent conception, lead to cessation of menses, and not require increasing the testosterone dosage is an etonogestrel implant (Answer B). The etonogestrel implant is a progestin contraceptive placed subdermally in the inner upper arm for long-acting, reversible contraception. This patient does not have a history of or current breast cancer or active liver disease and would be a good candidate. One might also consider a levonorgestrel intrauterine device to induce amenorrhea, but this would require a speculum examination and may lead to worsening of gender dysphoria.

Switching to subcutaneous formulations of testosterone gender-affirming hormone therapy (Answer E) would not be expected to alleviate menses without increasing the testosterone dosage (Answer A), which he has already tried but cannot tolerate due to the associated onset of dizziness, both at rest and with movement.

Combined oral contraceptive pills (Answer C), when taken continuously, could be considered as an approach to stop menstrual bleeding. However, taking estrogen may induce dysphoria and be incongruent with gender-affirming goals. The use of exogenous estrogen may also counteract the desired masculinizing effects of testosterone therapy.

Salpingectomy (Answer D) is surgical removal of one or both fallopian tubes. In this situation, the patient could still pursue egg retrieval and in vitro fertilization to carry a pregnancy in the future. However, this approach would not help the patient achieve the goal of menses cessation. Salpingectomy is akin to tubal ligation, which also does not affect the menstrual cycle given that intact ovaries and uterus remain.

Educational Objective

Treat vaginal bleeding in transgender men.

Reference(s)

Hembree WC, Cohen-Kettenis PT, Gooren L, et al. Endocrine treatment of gender-dysphoric/gender-incongruent persons: an Endocrine Society clinical practice guideline. *J Clin Endocrinol Metab.* 2017;102(11):3869-3903. PMID: 28945902

Center of Excellence for Transgender Health, Department of Family and Community Medicine, University of California, San Francisco. *Guidelines for the Primary and Gender-Affirming Care of Transgender and Gender Nonbinary People.* 2nd ed. Deutsch MB, ed. June 2016. Available at: www.transhealth.ucsf.edu/guidelines.

Irwig MS. Testosterone therapy for transgender men. *Lancet Diabetes Endocrinol.* 2017;5(4):301-311. PMID: 27084565

Schwartz AR, Russell K, Gray BA. Approaches to vaginal bleeding and contraceptive counseling in transgender and gender nonbinary patients. *Obstet Gynecol.* 2019;134(1):81-90. PMID: 31188325

8 ANSWER: A) Adenomas

Adrenal incidentalomas are a common finding on cross-sectional imaging studies of the abdomen (estimated to occur in 4% to 7% of adults older than 40 years). A systematic approach to assessment is important and must address 2 key questions:

1. Could this be a primary (eg, adrenocortical carcinoma) or secondary (eg, metastasis) malignant tumor?
2. Is the lesion functioning?

With modern imaging techniques (unenhanced ± triple-phase CT; chemical shift MRI), most adrenal incidentalomas are readily classified as benign in nature. Unenhanced CT and chemical shift MRI provide an assessment of lipid content within the adrenal mass. In a homogeneous lesion, a Hounsfield unit value less than 10 on noncontrast CT or clear signal drop-out on opposed phase images during chemical shift MRI identifies a lipid-rich lesion and confidently excludes malignancy.

In this patient, both adrenal lesions are less than 4 cm in diameter and both demonstrate a clear drop in signal intensity on the out-of-phase MR sequences when compared with in-phase signal intensity (*see images, arrows*). These findings strongly suggest that both adrenal nodules are likely to be adenomas (solitary unilateral adenomas are the most common type of adrenal incidentaloma, but bilateral adenomas are found in a subgroup of patients). It is likely that unenhanced CT would also have confirmed the diagnosis without needing to proceed to a triple-phase washout study. In the absence of clinical or biochemical evidence to suggest endocrine hyperfunction, the most likely diagnosis is bilateral nonsecretory adrenal adenomas (Answer A).

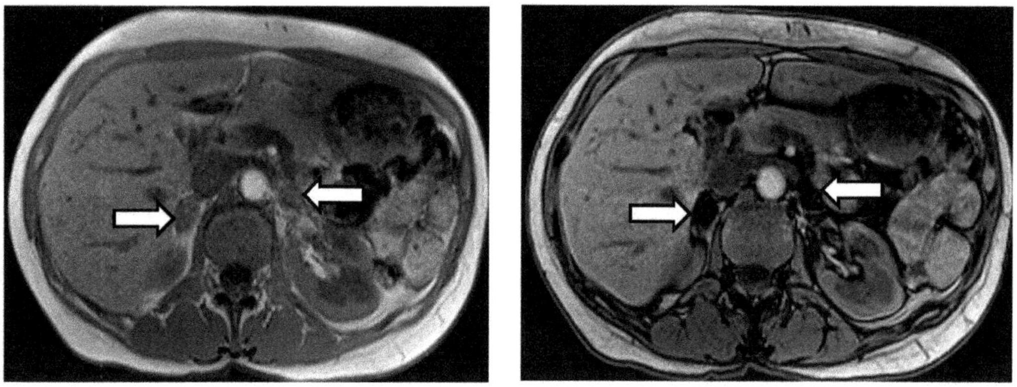

Adrenal hemorrhage (Answer B) can result from a variety of traumatic and nontraumatic causes. Risk factors for adrenal hemorrhage include anticoagulation, disseminated intravascular coagulation, sepsis (including meningococcemia, Waterhouse-Friderichsen syndrome), primary antiphospholipid syndrome, or an underlying adrenal tumor. On CT, adrenal hematomas characteristically appear round or oval and are often accompanied by stranding of periadrenal fat. The attenuation value of an adrenal hematoma depends on its age, with high attenuation in the acute/subacute phase but reduced attenuation (and size) over time. Some resolve completely, while others remain visible as a nonenhancing mass with a hypoattenuating center, with or without calcification(s). The radiologic findings in this case show no significant change in size over a 2-month interval and are not typical of adrenal hemorrhage. In addition, although the demonstration of well-preserved adrenocortical function (with normal values of early-morning cortisol and plasma renin) does not exclude bilateral adrenal hemorrhage or infiltration, it is not suggestive of significant bilateral adrenal insults.

Adrenal metastases (Answer C) are estimated to account for 8% to 9% of all adrenal incidentalomas, and bilateral adrenal involvement may be observed, especially in some malignancies such as renal cell carcinoma. However, the radiologic appearance in this vignette is not consistent with metastases, and it is likely that a whole-body trauma CT would have identified a primary site in most patients with bilateral metastases.

Adrenal myelolipomas (Answer D), which can be bilateral, typically contain macroscopic fat, which means that they are readily diagnosed on both CT and MRI. The amount of fat varies, ranging from only a few small regions in an otherwise largely soft-tissue density mass (~10%), to lesions containing roughly equal proportions of fat and soft tissue (~50%), to those that are almost completely composed of fatty tissue (~40%). Because of this heterogeneity, density estimation with Hounsfield units is typically not performed and indeed is often considered unnecessary given the distinctive radiologic appearance. The imaging findings here are not typical of adrenal myelolipomas.

Plasma free metanephrines or 24-hour urinary fractionated metanephrines are often measured to exclude pheochromocytoma (Answer E) in patients with adrenal incidentalomas . However, recent data suggest that if the imaging findings effectively exclude pheochromocytoma (eg, homogeneous mass with unenhanced CT density <10 Hounsfield units or clear signal drop-out on chemical shift MRI), then this assessment is not necessary unless there are other clinical indicators for biochemical screening. In this patient, the finding of bilateral adrenal abnormalities, which could not be characterized as adenomas on initial contrast-enhanced CT, coupled with the mildly elevated blood pressure, triggered measurement of plasma metanephrines. However, this approach caused significant confusion due to the confounding effects of the medications that the patient was taking. An initial short period off venlafaxine resulted in a lowering, but not complete normalization, of plasma normetanephrine. As lamotrigine has also been implicated in causing false-positive normetanephrine values, both agents were withdrawn for 7 days, following which plasma normetanephrine fully normalized. Plasma metanephrine levels were normal throughout. If the patient had subsequently been found to have bilateral pheochromocytomas, then genetic screening for an inherited cause (eg, multiple endocrine neoplasia type 2 or von Hippel-Lindau syndrome) would have been indicated.

Educational Objective

Identify typical radiologic appearances of adrenal adenomas on chemical shift MRI and determine when measurement of metanephrines may confound the diagnostic pathway.

Reference(s)

Fassnacht M, Arlt W, Bancos I, et al. Management of adrenal incidentalomas: European Society of Endocrinology clinical practice guideline in collaboration with the European Network for the Study of Adrenal Tumors. *Eur J Endocrinol.* 2016;175(2):G1-G34. PMID: 27390021

Bancos I, Prete A. Approach to the patient with adrenal incidentaloma. *J Clin Endocrinol Metab.* 2021;106(11):3331-3353. PMID: 34260734

9 ANSWER: D) Switch to a hybrid closed-loop insulin pump system

A hybrid closed-loop system (HCLS) automatically adjusts basal insulin rates based on sensor glucose concentrations. Adjustments depend on the algorithm used, which is unique to each HCLS. In addition, certain algorithms include microboluses that are automatically administered in the setting of hyperglycemia to improve time-in-range (TIR). Prandial insulin boluses, however, are manually administered by users. HCLSs are associated with a 9% to 16% increase in TIR and a reduction in hypoglycemia. Its predictive glucose system can alert users of impending hypoglycemia while simultaneously suspending basal insulin delivery. This patient's TIR is below the recommended 70% and time-below-range is above the recommended 4%. His fear of hypoglycemia is most likely prohibiting him from achieving satisfactory glucose concentrations during exercise (basketball). He would purposefully allow hyperglycemia before basketball by eating a snack without insulin coverage, as can be seen by his continuous glucose monitor tracing. Switching to an HCLS (Answer D) is the best option to improve his TIR, reduce hypoglycemia, and reduce glycemic variability. The newer HCLS systems have the ability to target a higher glucose concentration ("exercise mode"), which was designed specifically to prevent exercise-induced hypoglycemia and hyperglycemia. This feature would be beneficial for this patient who specifically aims for a higher glucose concentration before exercise (in this case, severe hyperglycemia due to his fear of hypoglycemia with exercise).

Changing the carbohydrate ratio to 1 unit for every 10 g carbohydrates (Answer A) or changing the correction factor to 1 unit of insulin aspart for every 40 mg/dL (2.2 mmol/L) over a blood glucose concentration of 180 mg/dL (>10.0 mmol/L) at night (Answer B) would reduce time-above-range but would not improve time-below-range or his intentional hyperglycemia during exercise.

Switching to insulin degludec (Answer C) may reduce overnight hypoglycemia; however, his continuous glucose tracing is more suggestive of aggressive overcorrection of high blood glucose due to short-acting insulin use rather than basal insulin.

Although smart insulin pens (Answer E) can calculate and log insulin doses administered, the patient does not exhibit issues to related to insulin dose calculations, so they would not likely help his glycemic control.

Educational Objective

Explain the benefit of closed-loop systems in improving time-in-range in patients with type 1 diabetes mellitus.

Reference(s)

Phillip M, Nimri R, Bergenstal RM, et al. Consensus recommendations for the use of automated insulin delivery (AID) technologies in clinical practice. *Endocr Rev.* 2023;44(2):254-280. PMID: 36066457

American Diabetes Association Professional Practice Committee. 7. Diabetes technology: standards of medical care in diabetes-2022. *Diabetes Care.* 2022;45(Suppl 1):S97-S112. PMID: 34964871

10 ANSWER: D) Reduce the calcitriol dosage

Patients with hypoparathyroidism require treatment to prevent hypocalcemia, usually with active vitamin D (calcitriol) plus calcium, although a PTH receptor agonist may also be used. Treatment must be balanced against the risk of hypercalciuria, which can result in nephrocalcinosis. This patient's condition is currently complicated by pregnancy, which has additional influences on mineral metabolism. During the course of a normal pregnancy, PTH decreases during the first and second trimesters and then rises again in the third trimester, while PTHrP produced by the breast and placenta begins increasing in the first trimester. Calcitriol concentrations (1,25-dihydroxyvitamin D) increase 2- to 3-fold, enhancing intestinal calcium absorption and bone resorption. These adaptations increase calcium availability to the developing fetus, but the net effect also increases urinary calcium excretion.

Some women with hypoparathyroidism demonstrate fewer hypocalcemic symptoms and require lower treatment dosages. Especially late in pregnancy, maternal hypercalcemia and hypercalciuria can occur unless the calcitriol dosage is reduced. Calcitriol dosage requirements are also expected to decrease during lactation. However, treatment must be individualized during pregnancy based on frequent laboratory assessments, as some women with hypoparathyroidism instead require intensified therapy to avoid worsening hypocalcemia. Maternal hypocalcemia can lead to fetal hyperparathyroidism and fetal demise.

Treatment of hypoparathyroidism usually targets a low-normal serum calcium concentration. This pregnant patient's urinary calcium-to-creatinine ratio is elevated, and her albumin-adjusted calcium concentration is 10.1 mg/dL (2.5 mmol/L) (high-normal). Thus, the appropriate adjustment is to reduce the calcitriol dosage (Answer D). Although decreasing her calcium dosage is an alternative approach to addressing this patient's mild hypercalcemia and hypercalciuria, the presence of a borderline-high phosphate value supports a decrease in calcitriol dosage instead, which will also reduce intestinal phosphate absorption. Calcium citrate may be better absorbed than calcium carbonate. However, increasing the calcium dosage or increasing its absorption by changing formulation (Answer C) would not address her high serum calcium and hypercalciuria.

Thiazide diuretics (Answer B) can be used to decrease urinary calcium excretion in patients with hypoparathyroidism; however, they should be discontinued during pregnancy (pregnancy category C).

Reducing the levothyroxine dosage (Answer E) in the setting of a slightly low TSH concentration would not improve the calcium balance, and this patient's TSH concentration is within the range of reasonable third-trimester values.

PTH receptor agonists (Answer A) have not been thoroughly evaluated as treatment during pregnancy and are classified as pregnancy category C medications.

Educational Objective

Explain how pregnancy influences the management of hypoparathyroidism.

Reference(s)

Kovacs CS. Maternal mineral and bone metabolism during pregnancy, lactation, and post-weaning recovery. *Physiol Rev.* 2016;96(2):449-547. PMID: 26887676

Khan AA, Clarke B, Rejnmark L, Brandi ML. Management of endocrine disease: hypoparathyroidism in pregnancy: review and evidence-based recommendations for management. *Eur J Endocrinol.* 2019;180(2):R37-R44. PMID: 30444723

Khan AA, Koch CA, Van Uum S, et al. Standards of care for hypoparathyroidism in adults: a Canadian and International Consensus. *Eur J Endocrinol.* 2019;180(3):P1-P22. PMID: 30540559

11 ANSWER: D) Refer to an otolaryngologist

Graves orbitopathy is an orbital inflammatory condition that not only causes patient stress because of disfigurement but also vision loss when it is severe. Orbitopathy occurs in approximately 40% of patients with Graves disease. The thyrotropin receptor (TSHR), which is expressed in the thyroid, adipocytes, and orbital fibroblasts, was thought to be the main autoantigen in the pathogenesis of Graves disease. However, recent data indicate that the IGF-1 receptor is overexpressed by orbital fibroblasts and B and T cells in Graves disease and Graves orbitopathy, and these cells have a central role in the pathogenesis of this condition. TSHR forms a functional complex with the IGF-1 receptor. Stimulation of the TSHR and IGF-1 receptor complex by thyroid-stimulating immunoglobulins causes hyaluronic acid accumulation and cytokine expression, resulting in inflammation, edema, and expansion of extraocular muscle and adipose tissue. The management of Graves orbitopathy can sometimes be challenging and depends on severity of the Clinical Activity Score.

In moderate to severe Graves orbitopathy, treatment options include steroid therapy (glucocorticoids) combined with orbital radiation therapy, which can improve symptoms of lid swelling or proptosis but are insufficient for diplopia. Intravenous steroids are usually preferred, but if they are not available, oral prednisone may be prescribed. Surgery on extraocular muscles is recommended in the inactive phase and can relieve diplopia or strabismus. In the setting of severe sight-threatening disease, the recommended therapy is intravenous steroids followed by orbital decompression surgery in unresponsive cases.

In 2021, teprotumumab, a fully human monoclonal antibody, was approved for the treatment of active Graves orbitopathy. Teprotumumab attenuates signaling initiated at either receptor (TSHR or IGF-1 receptor), thereby blocking pathologic immune responses in active Graves orbitopathy. Douglas et al reported that this novel medication has beneficial effects on proptosis and diplopia, reduces the Clinical Activity Score, and improves the quality of life. Severe adverse effects are rare, and thus teprotumumab could be considered as an alternative to surgical treatment in Graves orbitopathy. The most common adverse effects from combined data of phase 2 and phase 3 trials evaluated by Kahaly et al include muscle spasms (18%), hyperglycemia (8%), and hearing loss (10%). Other adverse effects are nausea, hair loss, diarrhea, fatigue, taste changes, headache, dry skin, and changes in menstruation. Subsequent publications have reported that the incidence of hearing symptoms, such as subjective hearing loss, hypoacusis, autophony, and tinnitus, could be as high as 81.5%. Otologic symptoms occur after an average of 3.6 infusions. The IGF-1 receptor has been implicated in homeostatic regulation of the inner ear and may have a role in maintaining sensorineural auditory function. Sensorineural hearing loss results from damaged hair cells in the inner ear. Patulous eustachian tube dysfunction has also been observed, a disorder in which the channel between the middle ear and back of the nose and throat remains open. In the normal state, the eustachian tubes remain closed but open occasionally to regulate air pressure around the ear drum.

Prescribers should be sensitive to hearing issues. Performing baseline audiography with patulous eustachian tube testing before the initiation of teprotumumab is recommended, and testing should be repeated during the treatment course in case of new otologic symptoms. There is no consensus as to whether teprotumumab should be continued or discontinued when hearing issues arise. Hearing loss and patulous eustachian tube symptoms from teprotumumab often, but not always, improve after stopping therapy. Some patients experience permanent hearing loss from this medication. If patients continue teprotumumab, hearing loss will most likely worsen. Similar to the decision faced by patients taking other known ototoxic drugs, if there is not a good alternative treatment option, patients may choose to live with hearing loss for the sake of improving their primary disease. Thus, patients should be counseled about this risk and engaged in shared decision-making.

The patient in this vignette has severe Graves orbitopathy and is treated with teprotumumab. After a couple of treatment cycles, he is experiencing hearing loss and tinnitus. He should be referred to an otolaryngologist for evaluation and audiography (Answer D).

His eye symptoms have improved, although he has some mild persistent diplopia. He does not require eye surgery given symptom improvement, so referral to an oculoplastic surgeon (Answer C) is not necessary.

Brain MRI (Answer B) is not indicated because his hearing issues are related to teprotumumab.

His serum TSH concentration is within an acceptable range, and he does not need a higher levothyroxine dosage (Answer A).

Selenium (Answer E) has been suggested in the management of mild Graves orbitopathy because selenium decreases inflammation. The European Group on Graves Orbitopathy recommends a 6-month course of selenium (100 mg twice daily) for patients with mild Graves orbitopathy of short duration. There is no evidence of a beneficial adjuvant effect of selenium in patients with moderate-to-severe and active Graves orbitopathy. It seems that selenium supplementation would not be effective in selenium-replete areas such as the United States. Because this patient has severe Graves orbitopathy, initiating selenium is not the best option.

Educational Objective

Identify the adverse effects of teprotumumab in a patient with Graves orbitopathy.

Reference(s)

Douglas RS, Kahaly GJ, Patel A, et al. Teprotumumab for the treatment of active thyroid eye disease. *N Engl J Med.* 2020;382(4):341-352. PMID: 31971679

Kahaly GJ, Douglas RS, Holt RJ, Sile S, Smith TJ. Teprotumumab for patients with active thyroid eye disease: a pooled data analysis, subgroup analyses, and off-treatment follow-up results from two randomised, double-masked, placebo-controlled, multicentre trials. *Lancet Diabetes Endocrinol.* 2021;9(6):360-372. PMID: 33865501

Bartalena L, Kahaly GJ, Baldeschi L, et al. The 2021 European Group on Graves' orbitopathy (EUGOGO) clinical practice guidelines for the medical management of Graves' orbitopathy. *Eur J Endocrinol.* 2021;185(4):G43-G67. PMID: 34297684

Chow A, Silkiss RZ. Teprotumumab-associated chronic hearing loss screening and proposed treatments. *BMJ Case Rep.* 2022;15(4):e248335. PMID: 35418378

Sears CM, Azad AD, Amarikwa L, et al. Hearing dysfunction after treatment with teprotumumab for thyroid eye disease. *Am J Ophthalmol.* 2022;240:1-13. PMID 35227694

12

ANSWER: A) Discontinue methadone

This patient presents with the Whipple triad, meaning she has neuroglycopenic symptoms of hypoglycemia concurrent with a plasma glucose concentration less than 55 mg/dL (<3.1 mmol/L) and resolution of symptoms after her glucose concentration normalizes. The results of the supervised fast suggest endogenous hyperinsulinism due to elevated insulin and C-peptide concentrations and a low plasma glucose concentration. This pattern is suggestive of insulinoma or ingestion of sulfonylureas, but the latter was ruled out. Therefore, it was reasonable perform localization studies. Endoscopic ultrasonography did not demonstrate a pancreatic mass. Cross-sectional imaging was deferred because of chronic kidney disease. In this setting, it would be reasonable to pursue a selective arterial calcium-stimulation test for localization, but this was not presented as an answer choice. However, alternative diagnoses should be considered before ordering a more invasive diagnostic test.

Of the medications mentioned in this vignette, only methadone is known to be a potential cause of hypoglycemia, and it should be discontinued (Answer A). Several case reports and 2 retrospective studies suggest that methadone should be considered as a cause of hypoglycemia, particularly in individuals with chronic kidney disease and during rapid dosage escalation. Moryl et al conducted a review of 59 patients who were treated for cancer-related pain and found that 11 developed documented hypoglycemia. In these 11 patients, the methadone dosage had been doubled within 2 days of the hypoglycemic episode. Flory et al reported on a retrospective observational cohort of 641 patients with cancer-related pain treated with at least 1 dose of opioid analgesics. Of the opioids described, only methadone was associated with hypoglycemia. This relationship was dose-responsive; a dosage of 80 mg daily had an odds ratio of 3.1 for development of hypoglycemia. In the case presented by Kanbour et al, supervised fasts were repeated over 13 days after discontinuation of methadone. The authors documented that in conjunction with declining methadone levels (from 610 to 99 mg/dL), concentrations of insulin and C-peptide also decreased.

Six months after remaining off methadone, the patient in this vignette had normal fasting glucose levels and no further symptomatic episodes. The mechanism of methadone-induced hypoglycemia is not well elucidated. Data from experiments in animals suggest that methadone can stimulate opioid receptors in pancreatic islets and may increase glucose-stimulated insulin secretion. Intrathecal methadone is associated with reduced hepatic glycogen stores. Whether there is an indirect effect on pancreatic islets through methadone action in the central nervous system is not known.

Thiazides (Answer B) are associated with hyperglycemia. Prescription of acarbose (Answer C) or diazoxide (Answer D) and consumption of small, frequent meals (Answer E) would not address the likely cause of this patient's hypoglycemia, which in this case is modifiable.

Educational Objective

Identify methadone as a cause of hypoglycemia in persons with chronic kidney disease.

Reference(s)

Moryl N, Pope J, Obbens E. Hypoglycemia during rapid methadone dose escalation. *J Opioid Manag.* 2013;9(1):29-34. PMID: 23709301

Flory JH, Wiesenthal AC, Thaler HT, Koranteng L, Moryl N. Methadone use and the risk of hypoglycemia for inpatients with cancer pain. *J Pain Symptom Manage.* 2016;51(1):79-87. PMID: 26342726

Kanbour S, Balaji A, Chae K, Mathioudakis N. Insulinoma mimic: methadone-induced hypoglycaemia. *BMJ Case Rep.* 2022;15(7):e245890. PMID: 35882435

Cryer PE, Axelrod L, Grossman AB, et al; Endocrine Society. Evaluation and management of adult hypoglycemic disorders: an Endocrine Society clinical practice guideline. *J Clin Endocrinol Metab.* 2009;94(3):709-728. PMID: 19088155

13 ANSWER: A) Measure IGF-1, cortisol, TSH, and free T_4

Diagnosis and management of hyperprolactinemia in patients taking antipsychotic medications can be challenging. Risperidone is an atypical antipsychotic agent that increases prolactin levels in up to 65% patients because of dopaminergic blockade at the tuberoinfundibular tract. Many other antipsychotic medications (phenothiazines, butyrophenones) have a dopamine receptor 2 (DR2) antagonist effect resulting in severe or moderate hyperprolactinemia. In contrast, aripiprazole has unique pharmacology, with DR2 partial agonist and antagonist properties. Most patients taking aripiprazole experience a decrease in prolactin levels from baseline.

This patient developed breast enlargement and low libido after initiating risperidone. However, he also has a pituitary macroadenoma, which could be contributing to hyperprolactinemia because of infundibular compression (stalk effect). Endocrine Society guidelines recommend stopping the medication potentially responsible for hyperprolactinemia for 3 days and repeating prolactin measurement; however, this is not an option offered here.

Switching risperidone to aripiprazole (Answer C) is incorrect because aripiprazole could decrease his prolactin concentration and confound the differential diagnosis of hyperprolactinemia. Also, he previously tried aripiprazole, and his psychiatric condition could worsen if his medication regimen is altered.

Transsphenoidal surgery (Answer B) is incorrect because he has a pituitary adenoma that is not causing mass effect symptoms and does not contact the optic chiasm. Further biochemical evaluation for hyperpituitarism and hypopituitarism is warranted. Elective transsphenoidal surgery could be considered depending on symptoms and future imaging changes.

Starting cabergoline (Answer D) is incorrect because the adenoma is unlikely to be a prolactinoma, which is expected to be associated with a more pronounced prolactin elevation. The prolactin concentration is usually greater than 200 ng/mL (>8.7 nmol/L) in patients with macroprolactinomas. In this case, the degree of prolactin elevation is consistent with stalk effect and/or being medication-induced. Also, cabergoline could exacerbate psychiatric disease. Cabergoline binds to type 3 dopamine receptors in the mesolimbic tracts, which can reduce the effectiveness of antipsychotic agents. Based on a recent retrospective study, starting a low dosage of cabergoline in patients with macroprolactinomas and optic chiasmopathy may improve vision and reduce tumor size; however, this patient does not likely have a prolactinoma and the suggested cabergoline dosage is not low.

Testosterone replacement (Answer E) is incorrect because the diagnosis of hypogonadism has not been clearly demonstrated. Blood was drawn in the afternoon and the testosterone concentration was only minimally below the reference range. This patient also has obesity and elevated fasting glucose. Lifestyle interventions and weight loss could improve his testosterone level. If hypogonadism persists, testosterone replacement would be indicated after a complete evaluation of pituitary function.

Given that this patient has a pituitary macroadenoma that could cause ACTH and TSH deficiencies and that acromegaly screening with IGF-1 measurement is recommended for all patients with pituitary adenomas, the best next step is to measure IGF-1, cortisol, TSH, and free T_4 (Answer A).

Educational Objective

Describe the effects of antipsychotic agents on prolactin concentrations and guide the management of pituitary adenomas.

Reference(s)

Tasaki M, Yasui-Furukori N, Yokoyama S, Shinozaki M T, Sugarawa N, Shimoda K. Hypoprolactinemia and hyperprolactinemia in male schizophrenia patients treated with aripiprazole and risperidone and their relationships with testosterone levels. *Neuropharmacol Rep.* 2021;41(3):379-384. PMID: 34189861

Allard L, Albarel F, Bertherat J, et al. Efficacy and safety of dopamine agonists in patients treated with antipsychotics and presenting a macroprolactinoma. *Eur J Endocrinol.* 2020;183(2):221-231. PMID: 32583656

Melmed S, Casanueva FF, Hoffman AR, et al; Endocrine Society. Diagnosis and treatment of hyperprolactinemia: an Endocrine Society clinical practice guideline. *J Clin Endocrinol Metab.* 2011;96(2):273-288. PMID: 21296991

Huang W, Molitch ME. Management of nonfunctioning pituitary adenomas (NFAs): observation. *Pituitary.* 2018;21(2):162-167. PMID: 29280025

14 ANSWER: C) Change to levothyroxine oral solution

When a person's serum TSH concentration measures outside the desired range, the levothyroxine dosage may need to be adjusted. However, it is first important to determine whether the medication is being administered consistently and correctly. Patients should be counseled on the importance of regular daily administration but also that it is safe to take skipped tablets the next day in cases of missed doses. With the goal of optimizing absorption, levothyroxine is preferably taken on an empty stomach 30 to 60 minutes prior to food and coffee consumption and several hours prior to the administration of known interfering substances, such as calcium carbonate and ferrous sulfate. Absorption of levothyroxine occurs in the jejunum and ileum, with up to 75% to 80% of the administered dose absorbed in the fasting state vs 59% to 68% with food consumption. However, bedtime administration (administration a few hours after final food consumption) is a viable alternative, although absorption is modestly lower when compared with morning administration 1 hour before breakfast.

The patient described in this vignette is administering levothyroxine optimally (ie, in the fasting state 1 hour before breakfast). He also does not take any vitamins or supplements that may be interfering with absorption. Therefore, changing levothyroxine administration time to bedtime (Answer A) would not be expected to improve absorption and lower his serum TSH.

An acidic gastric environment is needed to promote levothyroxine absorption. Levothyroxine requirements have been demonstrated to increase proportionately to rising gastric pH. The patient described in this vignette is prescribed proton-pump inhibitor therapy twice daily for Barrett esophagus. This is the most likely explanation for the elevated serum TSH concentrations that are observed. Discontinuation of omeprazole (Answer D) would not be indicated in this clinical scenario; however, substituting an H2-blocker could be considered with alternative indications for acid-reducing therapy (eg, gastroesophageal reflux disease without esophagitis).

Treatment with an oral levothyroxine solution has been associated with lower serum TSH levels compared with levothyroxine tablets administered at the same daily dose (mean TSH 1.7 vs 5.4 mIU/L) in a prospective observational cohort study of 24 patients treated with proton-pump inhibitor therapy. Changing to levothyroxine oral solution (Answer C) would be an appropriate management strategy in the current clinical scenario. Another liquid levothyroxine preparation is composed of levothyroxine dissolved in glycerol that is enclosed in a gelatin capsule. The dissolution of the gelatin capsule also appears to be relatively unchanged by gastric pH. Liquid preparations may also be better absorbed with tube feeds or in the context of malabsorptive disorders. In contrast, changing to a branded levothyroxine tablet (Answer B) without up-titration of the prescribed dosage would offer little advantage over a generic formulation when the suspected driver of inadequate treatment is impaired absorption secondary to increased gastric pH.

Carbamazepine, phenytoin, and phenobarbital are all anticonvulsant drugs that have been shown to increase the metabolism of T_4 and T_3 leading to hypothyroidism in patients who were previously euthyroid on the same levothyroxine dosage. However, levetiracetam is not known to affect the metabolism of thyroid hormone. Therefore, substituting another anticonvulsant drug for levetiracetam (Answer E) would not be recommended.

Educational Objective

Explain the effect of proton-pump inhibitor therapy on the absorption of levothyroxine.

Reference(s)

Jonklaas J. Optimal thyroid hormone replacement. *Endocr Rev.* 2022;43(2):366-404. PMID: 34543420

Virili C, Bruno G, Santaguida MG, et al. Levothyroxine treatment and gastric juice pH in humans: the proof of concept. *Endocrine.* 2022;77(1):102-111. PMID: 35477833

Vita R, Saraceno G, Trimarchi F, Benvenga S. Switching levothyroxine from the tablet to the oral solution formulation corrects the impaired absorption of levothyroxine induced by proton-pump inhibitors. *J Clin Endocrinol Metab.* 2014;99(12):4481-4486. PMID: 25259910

15 ANSWER: C) Start moderate-intensity statin therapy

Estimation of 10-year ASCVD risk is an essential part of deciding which patients require statin therapy for primary prevention. Many risk engines are available that incorporate both traditional and nontraditional risk factors to help estimate risk. The Pooled Cohort equations introduced in the 2018 multisociety guidelines are widely used, with a recommendation to start statin therapy for primary prevention in those without diabetes or severe hypercholesterolemia (LDL cholesterol ≥190 mg/dL [>4.92 mmol/L]) if the estimated 10-year risk is greater than 7.5%. Reclassification of estimated risk is possible using other nontraditional risk markers, including coronary artery calcium (CAC) scoring. In patients at borderline risk (5.0%-7.4%), the presence or absence of CAC helps to reclassify them as being at high or low risk, respectively. CAC's greatest utility is considered to be its ability to identify those at low risk when the score is zero, with the implication that these individuals have a very low risk of ASCVD events in the next 10 years. Repeating CAC in 5 years in such patients is reasonable. A recent meta-analysis confirmed the slight increase in discrimination index when using CAC scoring with traditional risk factors, although it is not yet recommended by the US Preventive Services Taskforce for risk estimation in the general population.

This patient is indeed at borderline risk with a predicted 10-year ASCVD risk of 5.2%, and his CAC score is zero. However, it is important to recognize the limitations of this approach in patients at high risk such as those who smoke cigarettes, have diabetes mellitus, or have a strong family history of premature ASCVD. Given this patient's family history of premature ASCVD, he most likely has familial combined hyperlipidemia with a very atherogenic lipid profile and would benefit from early initiation of statin therapy. In some young patients with genetic dyslipidemia and soft atherosclerotic plaques, coronary CT may fail to detect subclinical atherosclerosis due to absence of calcium deposition in these lesions. The negative predictive value of a CAC score of zero is more reliable in older patients than in younger patients. It has been estimated from various longitudinal studies that one-third to one-fourth of myocardial infarctions occur in individuals with a CAC score of zero. The optimal approach to ASCVD risk reduction in individuals who most likely have genetic dyslipidemia and a strong family history of premature ASCVD is early initiation of statin therapy (Answer C) in combination with heart-healthy lifestyles. Obtaining a CAC score is not necessary to decide whether statin therapy should be prescribed in this situation. Similarly, repeating coronary CT (Answer A) or a lipid panel (Answer B) would not be adequate or appropriate.

There is no benefit to repeating CAC scoring after statin initiation (Answer D). Statin therapy is known to be associated with an increased CAC score despite plaque regression and ASCVD risk reduction.

The benefit of combination lipid-lowering therapy with statins and omega-3 fatty acids (Answer E) in this patient population has not been established.

Educational Objective

List appropriate indications for obtaining coronary artery calcium scoring to help reclassify risk for atherosclerotic cardiovascular disease.

Reference(s)

Grundy SM, Stone NJ, Bailey AL, et al. 2018 AHA/ACC/AACVPR/AAPA/ABC/ACPM/ADA/AGS/APhA/ASPC/NLA/PCNA guideline on the management of blood cholesterol: a report of the American College of Cardiology/American Heart Association Task Force on Clinical Practice Guidelines. *J Am Coll Cardiol.* 2019;73(24):e285-e350. PMID: 30423393

US Preventive Services Task Force, Curry SJ, Krist AH, et al. Risk assessment for cardiovascular disease with nontraditional risk factors: US Preventive Services Task Force recommendation statement. *JAMA.* 2018;320(3):272-280. PMID: 29998297

Hussain A, Ballantyne CM, Nambi V. Zero coronary artery calcium score: desirable, but enough? *Circulation.* 2020;142(10):917-919. PMID: 32897743

Bell KJL, White S, Hassan O, et al. Evaluation of the incremental value of a coronary artery calcium score beyond traditional cardiovascular risk assessment: a systematic review and meta-analysis. *JAMA Intern Med.* 2022;182(6):634-642. PMID: 35467692

Puri R, Nicholls SJ, Shao M, et al. Impact of statins on serial coronary calcification during atheroma progression and regression. *J Am Coll Cardiol.* 2015;65(13):1273-1282. PMID: 25835438

16 ANSWER: E) Bisphosphonates: decrease/decrease; teriparatide: increase/increase; romosozumab: increase/decrease

Osteoporosis medication classes have different mechanisms of action. Understanding those differences is important, especially when assessing medication adherence and effectiveness and determining when to consider medication "holidays."

The bisphosphonates approved to treat osteoporosis in the United States have a nitrogen within a sidechain of the structure that makes them more potent than bisphosphonates without a nitrogen. The nitrogen-containing bisphosphonates inhibit farnesyl-pyrophosphate synthase, an enzyme involved in cholesterol synthesis and in the prenylation of signaling proteins such as small GTPases. These signaling molecules are essential for osteoclast survival, and a block in production leads to apoptosis of these cells. Given the strong affinity of bisphosphonates for mineralized tissues such as bone, these medications primarily target the osteoclast. When an osteoclast adheres to a bone surface containing bisphosphonate, the osteoclast dissolves the hydroxyapatite and protein matrix. This action releases the bisphosphonate, which is biologically active and can be taken up by active osteoclasts, leading to apoptosis and decreased bone resorption. Since the activity of osteoclasts and osteoblasts are tightly coupled, osteoblast-dependent bone formation also decreases with bisphosphonate treatment.

Teriparatide is the first 34 amino acids of PTH, and it functions like PTH. Since teriparatide is administered as a once-daily subcutaneous injection and has a short circulating half-life, the pulsatile nature of teriparatide results in an anabolic effect on the skeleton leading to increased bone formation. Although bone resorption also increases because of the coupling of osteoblasts and osteoclasts, the net effect is more bone formation than resorption, leading to increased bone mineral density and decreased fracture risk.

Romosozumab is a humanized monoclonal antibody that targets the protein sclerostin, an inhibitor of osteoblast Wnt signaling. Blocking the inhibitor leads to an increase in osteoblast Wnt signaling and an increase in the number of osteoblasts and bone formation in the initial 6 months of treatment. For reasons that are not quite understood, romosozumab results in an uncoupling of osteoclast action from that of osteoblasts, leading to a concomitant decrease in bone resorption.

Answer is E is the only option that describes the effects of (1) bisphosphonates to decrease both bone formation and resorption, (2) teriparatide to increase both bone formation and resorption, and (3) romosozumab to increase bone formation and decrease bone resorption within the first 6 months after treatment initiation. Answers A, B, C and D describe inaccurate effects on osteoblast and/or osteoclast biology for one or more of these osteoporosis therapies.

No consensus exists regarding when and how to use bone turnover makers. The best-validated approaches to using bone turnover markers include ensuring adherence to oral bisphosphonates, reassuring patients of the effectiveness of osteoporosis medications after initiation, and determining when bisphosphonate "holidays" end.

Educational Objective

Explain how different osteoporosis medications change bone turnover markers.

Reference(s)

Dunford JE, Kwaasi AA, Rogers MJ, et al. Structure-activity relationships among the nitrogen containing bisphosphonates in clinical use and other analogues: time-dependent inhibition of human farnesyl pyrophosphate synthase. *J Med Chem.* 2008;51(7):2187-95. PMID: 18327899

Black DM, Schwartz AV, Ensrud KE, et al; FLEX Research Group. Effects of continuing or stopping alendronate after 5 years of treatment: the Fracture Intervention Trial Long-term Extension (FLEX): a randomized trial. *JAMA.* 2006;296(24):2927-2938. PMID: 17190893

Leder BZ, Tsai JN, Uihlein AV, et al. Denosumab and teriparatide transitions in postmenopausal osteoporosis (the DATA-Switch study): extension of a randomised controlled trial. *Lancet.* 2015;386(9999):1147-1155. PMID: 26144908

Cosman F, Crittenden DB, Adachi JD, et al. Romosozumab treatment in postmenopausal women with osteoporosis. *N Engl J Med.* 2016;375(16):1532-1543. PMID: 27641143

Saag KG, Petersen J, Brandi ML, et al. Romosozumab or alendronate for fracture prevention in women with osteoporosis. *N Engl J Med.* 2017;377(15):1417-1427. PMID: 28892457

17 ANSWER: E) Hemoglobin A_{1c} is inaccurate, so glucose management indicator/time-in-range should be used to guide therapy

While hemoglobin A_{1c} has been the primary outcome measure in many large-scale diabetes trials, its use is limited in certain populations. The most common scenarios that lead to an inaccurate hemoglobin A_{1c} measurement are altered red cell turnover (eg, anemia due to vitamin B_{12} or folate deficiency or hemolysis, or treatment of anemia with iron, vitamin B_{12}, folate, or erythropoietin), hemoglobin variants (dependent on the manufacturer's assay), recent blood transfusion, and advanced chronic kidney disease. The measured hemoglobin A_{1c} should be compared with measured glucose concentrations (either via continuous glucose monitoring or mean fingerstick glucose value). If there is discrepancy between them, further investigation into the underlying cause is warranted. In this case, the patient has stage 5 chronic kidney disease, which can lead to falsely low hemoglobin A_{1c} concentrations via altered red cell turnover. The glucose management indicator is calculated from the regression line–derived formula of mean glucose concentrations on the x-axis and hemoglobin A_{1c} concentrations on the y-axis. The glucose management indicator can therefore serve as a surrogate for hemoglobin A_{1c}. Because hemoglobin A_{1c} is inaccurate in this case, the glucose management indicator/time-in-range should be used to guide therapy (Answer E).

The accuracy of continuous glucose monitoring in patients with advanced chronic kidney disease is reasonably accurate (mean absolute relative difference = 13.8% in one study) and can be relied on for clinical management. Although the hemoglobin A_{1c} level is inaccurate in this patient, the glucose management indicator is accurate (thus, Answer A is incorrect).

Similarly, given that hemoglobin A_{1c} is inaccurate in this patient, relying on this measurement to assess her treatment goals is wrong (Answers B, C, and D).

Educational Objective

Explain the utility of the glucose management indicator when hemoglobin A_{1c} is inaccurate.

Reference(s)

American Diabetes Association Professional Practice Committee. 6. Glycemic targets: *standards of medical care in diabetes-2022. Diabetes Care.* 2022;45(Suppl 1):S83-S96. PMID: 34964868

Bergenstal RM, Beck RW, Close KL, et al. Glucose management indicator (GMI): a new term for estimating A1C from continuous glucose monitoring. *Diabetes Care.* 2018;41(11):2275-2280. PMID: 30224348

Villard O, Breton MD, Rao S, et al. Accuracy of a factory-calibrated continuous glucose monitor in individuals with diabetes on hemodialysis. *Diabetes Care.* 2022;45(7):1666-1669. PMID: 35485908

18 ANSWER: D) Perform parathyroidectomy with multigland resection

X-linked hypophosphatemia (XLH) due to pathogenic variants in the *PHEX* gene has a prevalence of 1 in 20,000 to 1 in 25,000. Deficiency of PHEX activity causes lifelong renal phosphate wasting and hypophosphatemia due to elevated circulating FGF-23. Phosphate is freely filtered at the glomerulus and FGF-23 downregulates the surface expression of sodium phosphate cotransporters (NPT2a and NPT2c) in the renal proximal tubule, which decreases phosphate reabsorption. In addition, FGF-23 downregulates renal vitamin D 1α-hydroxylase and upregulates 24-hydroxylase, together resulting in serum levels of 1,25-dihydroxyvitamin D that are typically low or low-normal. When FGF-23 concentrations are chronically elevated as in XLH, these effects cause rickets, skeletal deformities, and growth impairment in growing children. Adults with XLH manifest hypophosphatemic osteomalacia, insufficiency fractures, bone pain, joint and muscle stiffness, enthesopathy, and osteoarthritis. Dental abscesses are also common at all ages, often leading to tooth loss. In adults with XLH, the goal of medical treatment is to improve osteomalacia and associated symptoms, such as bone pain, fractures, muscle weakness, and impaired mobility.

Conventional therapy for XLH uses active forms of vitamin D (calcitriol, alfacalcidol, etc) plus phosphate salts, which must be administered multiple times daily. Conventional therapy generally does not normalize fasting serum phosphate but can improve osteomalacia. Complications of conventional therapy include gastrointestinal symptoms (due to administration of phosphate salts), nephrocalcinosis (due to the effects of both active vitamin D and phosphate salts), and hyperparathyroidism (due to the effect of phosphate salts to reduce serum calcium and thereby stimulate PTH production). Nephrocalcinosis occurs in 50% or more of individuals treated with conventional therapy. Secondary hyperparathyroidism is sometimes present before initiating therapy, when it is thought to be due to the effect of high FGF-23 to limit production of 1,25-dihydroxyvitamin D. Secondary hyperparathyroidism may then be improved by administering active vitamin D. However, administering phosphate salts has the opposite effect of increasing PTH as detailed above. Thus, secondary hyperparathyroidism is also a complication of conventional therapy with phosphate salts, occurring in more than 80% of persons with XLH at some point during their treatment. Over time, multigland hyperplasia develops and approximately 25% to 30% of adults with XLH progress to hypercalcemic (or "tertiary") hyperparathyroidism, as seen in this patient. She has a symptomatic insufficiency fracture, which is a clear indication for medical therapy in a patient with XLH. However, the complication of hypercalcemic hyperparathyroidism must be addressed to effectively reduce cortical bone resorption that occurs with PTH excess. This patient has been treated with very imbalanced dosages of conventional therapy, with a lower dosage of calcitriol and a higher dosage of phosphate salts, likely contributing to the development of hypercalcemic hyperparathyroidism.

For this patient, the best next step in management is to address hyperparathyroidism. Given longstanding treatment with phosphate salts, this patient almost certainly has multigland involvement and will require multigland resection (3 and one-half glands) (Answer D) with the goal of normalizing calcium and PTH.

During monitoring of patients with XLH, it is important to adjust medical therapy dosages to normalize PTH, but this becomes more complicated when the patient is hypercalcemic. Increasing the calcitriol dosage (Answer B) may lower PTH, but it would not correct and would likely worsen hypercalcemia in this patient. Decreasing the calcitriol dosage may lower calcium to some extent, but tertiary hyperparathyroidism and resultant hypercalcemia would persist. She is taking the lowest calcitriol dosage available in capsules, and patients should not stop taking active vitamin D while continuing phosphate salts, as this would be undermine the treatment of osteomalacia in the setting of XLH and could also worsen secondary hyperparathyroidism, which can coexist in patients who have developed parathyroid autonomy. Similarly, increasing the phosphate dosage (Answer C) is likely to worsen hyperparathyroidism. If calcitriol is stopped, then the phosphate salts should also be stopped. Starting magnesium treatment (Answer E) in a patient with a low-normal magnesium concentration is not expected to significantly alter hypercalcemic hyperparathyroidism.

Burosumab (Answer A) is a monoclonal antibody to FGF-23 that was approved by the US FDA in 2018. By blocking FGF-23, burosumab increases renal phosphate reabsorption and activation of vitamin D. Burosumab can normalize serum phosphate and improve osteomalacia and rickets in XLH, as well as heal insufficiency fractures. Risks of burosumab include hyperphosphatemia (overcorrection, indicating a need to decrease the dosage), injection-site reactions, and restless legs syndrome. There may still be a risk of nephrocalcinosis with burosumab. Burosumab can decrease PTH in the setting of secondary hyperparathyroidism, but there is no evidence that it corrects hypercalcemic hyperparathyroidism. Thus, while switching to burosumab may be useful regarding her insufficiency fracture, it would not effectively address her hypercalcemia.

Educational Objective

Manage complications related to treatment of X-linked hypophosphatemia.

Reference(s)

Haffner D, Emma F, Eastwood DM, et al. Clinical practice recommendations for the diagnosis and management of X-linked hypophosphataemia. *Nat Rev Nephrol.* 2019;15(7):435-455. PMID: 31068690

Portale AA, Carpenter TO, Brandi ML, et al. Continued beneficial effects of burosumab in adults with X-linked hypophosphatemia: results from a 24-week treatment continuation period after a 24-week double-blind placebo-controlled period. *Calcif Tissue Int.* 2019;105(3):271-284. PMID: 31165191

Ackah SA, Imel EA. Approach to hypophosphatemic rickets. *J Clin Endocrinol Metab.* 2023;108(1):209-220. PMID: 35981346

DeLacey S, Liu Z, Broyles A, et al. Hyperparathyroidism and parathyroidectomy in X-linked hypophosphatemia patients. *Bone.* 2019;127:386-392. PMID: 31276850

19 ANSWER: C) Mammography

Physicians should engage in organ-based preventive screening for all individuals, regardless of gender identification. Specifically, understanding which existing internal and external organs each patient has allows for appropriate cancer screening as recommended by the American Cancer Society, Centers for Disease Control, and US Preventive Services Task Force. Currently, there are no evidence-based screening guidelines specific for transgender and gender-diverse individuals given the insufficient evidence to determine whether transgender people are at increased or decreased overall cancer risk or organ-specific cancer risk. Therefore, if an individual has a particular body part or organ and otherwise meets criteria for screening based on age, risk factors, etc, then screening should be ordered, independent of gender-affirming hormone use.

Given that this transgender man has chest tissue and has not had a mastectomy, he should be advised to undergo standard mammography screening (Answer C), which is recommended for individuals with breast tissue who are older than 50 years and are at average risk for breast cancer.

This patient has no indication for *BRCA* genetic testing (Answer A) based on the provided history.

Clinical breast examination (Answer B) during the office visit has been reported to be gender-affirming for transgender women, and yet it is no longer recommended for the detection of breast cancer for screening purposes. In transgender men, clinical breast examination may increase gender dysphoria.

This patient reports that he is comfortable with his appearance and has not expressed a desire for masculinizing chest reconstruction (Answer D).

Finally, based on history and organ inventory, this transgender man no longer has a cervix given total hysterectomy, and referral for a Papanicolaou test (Answer E) is not needed.

Educational Objective

Guide cancer screening for transgender men.

Reference(s)

Center of Excellence for Transgender Health, Department of Family and Community Medicine, University of California, San Francisco. *Guidelines for the Primary and Gender-Affirming Care of Transgender and Gender Nonbinary People.* 2nd edition. Deutsch MB, ed. June 2016. Available at: www.transhealth.ucsf.edu/guidelines.

Coleman E, Radix AE, Bouman WP, et al. Standards of care for the health of transgender and gender diverse people, version 8. *Int J Transgend Health.* 2022;23(Suppl 1):S1-S259. PMID: 36238954

Salibian AA, Axelrod DM, Smith JA, Fischer BA, Agarwal C, Bluebond-Langner R. Oncologic considerations for safe gender-affirming mastectomy: preoperative imaging, pathologic evaluation, counseling, and long-term screening. *Plast Reconstr Surg.* 2021;147(2):213e-221e. PMID: 33565823

Wierckx K, Elaut E, Declercq E, et al. Prevalence of cardiovascular disease and cancer during cross-sex hormone therapy in a large cohort of trans persons: a case-control study. *Eur J Endocrinol.* 2013;169(4):471-478. PMID: 23904280

Wierckx K, Mueller S, Weyers S, et al. Long-term evaluation of cross-sex hormone treatment in transsexual persons. *J Sex Med.* 2012;9(10):2641-2651. PMID: 22906135

20

ANSWER: C) Recommend no further workup or follow-up

As in this patient, adrenal nodules can be found incidentally on cross-sectional imaging performed for a variety of reasons. Hormonal testing for primary aldosteronism, autonomous hypercortisolism, and pheochromocytoma is commonly performed in patients with adrenal incidentalomas. Testing for primary aldosteronism can be skipped in patients without hypertension, and testing for pheochromocytoma is superfluous in patients with lipid-rich adenomas, as these are always of cortical origin. Most adrenal incidentalomas are hormonally inactive. Mild autonomous hypercortisolism is the most common hormonal abnormality in patients with adrenal incidentalomas. The most sensitive test for mild autonomous cortisol excess is a 1-mg dexamethasone-suppression test, but many things can lead to false-positive results. Examples include failure to follow the test instructions, medications that accelerate the metabolism of dexamethasone by inducing CYP3A4 (eg, barbiturates, phenytoin, rifampin, and carbamazepine), malabsorption, and elevated cortisol-binding globulins. Serum cortisol assays measure total cortisol (free and bound to proteins), while salivary and urinary cortisol assays measure free cortisol. Estrogens, whether endogenous (during pregnancy) or exogenous (eg, in women taking oral contraceptive pills), induce the synthesis of cortisol-binding globulins, and hence total cortisol, while free cortisol remains normal.

In patients who might not be willing or able to undergo a 1-mg dexamethasone-suppression test, alternative tests for hypercortisolism can be performed, including measurement of midnight salivary cortisol and 24-hour urinary cortisol excretion. Midnight salivary cortisol can be elevated in patients with disrupted circadian rhythm (shift work, recent travel across time zones, etc), acute illness, severe depression, alcoholism, or when there is contamination with blood. Blood contamination of salivary samples is not uncommon in patients with gum disease (as suggested in the patient presented), mouth ulcers, or hemoptysis. This patient had no specific signs of cortisol excess, and her result from 1-mg dexamethasone testing was normal. Therefore, further testing for hypercortisolism, such as 24-hour urinary cortisol (Answer A), is not indicated. However, when hypercortisolism is suspected clinically and 2 tests have discrepant results, additional testing should be conducted.

Adrenalectomy (Answer B) is the treatment of choice for malignant and hyperfunctioning adrenal nodules. This patient has a nonfunctioning, lipid-rich adrenal cortical adenoma, and surgery is not recommended.

Mifepristone (Answer D) is a glucocorticoid receptor and progesterone receptor antagonist, and osilodrostat (Answer E) is an inhibitor of 11β-hydroxylase (CYP11B1), an enzyme required for cortisol synthesis. Mifepristone and osilodrostat are medical treatment options for Cushing syndrome. Medical treatment for hypercortisolism is reserved for patients who cannot be cured by surgery. The patient in this vignette has a nonfunctioning, benign adrenal incidentaloma, and she does not require treatment (surgical or medical).

In patients with adrenal nodules smaller than 4 cm with clear imaging features of benign adrenal adenomas, the European Society of Endocrinology and the American Association of Endocrine Surgeons practice guidelines recommend against follow-up imaging, as the risk of malignant transformation is extremely low. Similarly, follow-up for hormonal hypersecretion is not recommended for nonfunctional adenomas, unless clinical changes suggest hormonal excess is occurring. Thus, no further workup or follow-up is recommended (Answer C).

Educational Objective

Identify caveats of testing for hypercortisolism in patients with adrenal incidentalomas.

Reference(s)

Sherlock M, Scarsbrook A, Abbas A, et al. Adrenal incidentaloma. *Endocr Rev.* 2020;41(6):775-820. PMID: 32266384

Elhassan YS, Alahdab F, Prete A, et al, Natural history of adrenal incidentalomas with and without mild autonomous cortisol excess: a systematic review and meta-analysis, *Ann Intern Med.* 2019;171(2):107-116. PMID: 31234202

Fassnacht M, Arlt W, Bancos I, et al. Management of adrenal incidentalomas: European Society of Endocrinology Clinical Practice Guideline in collaboration with the European Network for the Study of Adrenal Tumors. *Eur J Endocrinol.* 2016;175(2):G1-G34. PMID: 27390021

Castro M, Elias PC, Quidute AR, Halah FP, Moreira AC. Out-patient screening for Cushing's syndrome: the sensitivity of the combination of circadian rhythm and overnight dexamethasone suppression salivary cortisol tests. *J Clin Endocrinol Metab.* 1999;84(3):878-882. PMID: 10084565

21 ANSWER: A) Hydrocortisone, 100 mg intravenously, followed by levothyroxine, 300 mcg intravenously

The patient described in this vignette is presenting with myxedema coma, more aptly referred to as decompensated hypothyroidism. Although presentation with coma constitutes one of the most severe clinical manifestations of this condition, it is not required for the diagnosis. Myxedema coma is a life-threatening form of hypothyroidism that previously was associated with mortality rates of 60% to 70% (now 20% to 25% due to advances in intensive supportive care). Manifestations of myxedema coma reflect multisystem decompensation and include decreased mental status (eg, somnolence, as seen in this patient); hypothermia; bradycardia (present); cardiovascular dysfunction (pericardial and pleural effusions and QT prolongation in this patient); and metabolic disturbances, which may include hyponatremia, hypoglycemia, hypoxemia, hypercarbia (present), and decreased glomerular filtration rate (present). Precipitating events can be infection or significant medical events (eg, myocardial event), cold exposure, trauma, or surgery, among others. In patients with a known diagnosis of hypothyroidism, a history of recent thyroid hormone discontinuation is often encountered.

Although the diagnosis of myxedema coma is largely made on clinical grounds, a diagnostic scoring system, such as that proposed by Popoveniuc and colleagues in 2014, can be supportive. The myxedema coma score is determined based on the combination of thermoregulatory, central nervous system, gastrointestinal, cardiovascular, and metabolic disturbances in the presence or absence of a precipitating event. A score of 60 or higher is considered diagnostic, while a score below 25 makes myxedema unlikely. Scores between 25 and 60 may suggest myxedema but are indeterminate. The score calculated for this patient is 95 (0 thermoregulatory + 10 CNS + 0 GI + 55 CV + 20 metabolic + 10 precipitating event).

Management of myxedema coma includes supportive measures to address hypothermia, hypoventilation, hypovolemia, and electrolyte imbalances, evaluation for precipitating causes (eg, infection) with empiric broad-spectrum antibiotic coverage if sepsis is suspected, and rapid repletion of the thyroid hormone deficit. There are no randomized controlled trials comparing different thyroid hormone replacement strategies for myxedema. Treatment with intravenous levothyroxine alone or in combination with intravenous liothyronine is recommended. The 2014 guidelines of the American Thyroid Association for the treatment of hypothyroidism advise a loading dose of 200 to 400 mcg of levothyroxine, with lower doses for older patients or those with a history of coronary artery disease or dysrhythmia, followed by a daily replacement dose of 1.6 mcg/kg body weight, reduced to 75% for the intravenous route of administration. Concurrent administration of intravenous liothyronine should prompt lower levothyroxine loading doses (200 to 300 mcg). The intention of using relatively large loading doses in patients with severe hypothyroidism is to hasten the saturation of thyroid-binding proteins and ensure that the free/bioavailable thyroid hormone is more quickly normalized. When intravenous liothyronine is administered, the American Thyroid Association guidelines suggest a loading dose of 5 to 20 mcg, followed by a maintenance dose of 2.5 to 10 mcg every 8 hours. If levothyroxine monotherapy is selected initially, liothyronine can be added if there is no significant clinical improvement within 1 to 2 days.

Empiric stress-dose glucocorticoids should be given intravenously for the initial management of myxedema coma before the administration of thyroid hormone. Treatment of hypothyroidism may accelerate cortisol metabolism and could precipitate adrenal crisis in at risk individuals, including those with undiagnosed autoimmune adrenal disease and hypothalamic-pituitary disease. Furthermore, abnormal cortisol responses to stress have been observed in the context of severe hypothyroidism and are thought to be mediated by blunted

ACTH secretion. Therefore, administering hydrocortisone, 100 mg intravenously, followed by levothyroxine, 300 mcg intravenously (Answer A), is an appropriate initial management approach for this patient with myxedema coma. Alternatively, intravenous loading doses of hydrocortisone, levothyroxine, and liothyronine could be recommended, although this is not among the listed answer choices.

Levothyroxine, 125 mcg intravenously (Answer C); levothyroxine, 175 mcg orally (Answer D); and levothyroxine, 200 mcg intravenously, and liothyronine, 10 mcg intravenously (Answer E) are incorrect in that they do not include glucocorticoid therapy. Administering hydrocortisone, 100 mg intravenously, followed by liothyronine, 75 mcg intravenously (Answer B) is incorrect. Although not a common treatment strategy, liothyronine monotherapy in dosages up to 25 to 50 mcg daily has been used successfully. However, higher dosages of liothyronine (≥75 mcg daily) are associated with an increased risk of adverse outcomes.

Educational Objective

Recommend initial therapy for severe hypothyroidism/myxedema coma.

Reference(s)

Jonklaas J, Bianco AC, Bauer AJ, et al; American Thyroid Association Task Force on Thyroid Hormone Replacement. Guidelines for the treatment of hypothyroidism: prepared by the American Thyroid Association task force on thyroid hormone replacement. *Thyroid.* 2014;24(12):1670-1751. PMID: 25266247

McDermott MT. Hypothyroidism. *Ann Intern Med.* 2020;173(1):ITC1-ITC6. PMID: 32628881

Popoveniuc G, Chandra T, Sud A, et al. A diagnostic scoring system for myxedema coma. *Endocr Pract.* 2014;20(8):808-817. PMID: 24518183

Rodriguez I, Fluiters E, Perez-Mendez LF, Luna R, Paramo C, Garcia-Mayor RV. Factors associated with mortality of patients with myxoedema coma: prospective study in 11 cases treated in a single institution. *J Endocrinol.* 2004;180(2), 347-350. PMID: 14765987

22 **ANSWER: C) Stop cabergoline and refer for pituitary surgery**

Dopamine agonists (eg, cabergoline, bromocriptine, quinagolide) are generally well-tolerated, and they achieve good laboratory and radiologic control in most patients with prolactinomas. Accordingly, dopamine agonists are normally recommended as first-line therapy. The most commonly encountered adverse effects are nausea and dizziness (especially postural) during the initial phase of treatment, but fortunately these symptoms often subside with continued use. However, other adverse effects may be more troublesome and can prevent effective management. These include drowsiness/somnolence, headache, dyspepsia/gastritis, constipation, edema, and altered mood. Less commonly, digital vasospasm, exacerbation of angina, or overt psychosis occur in predisposed individuals.

In recent years, concerns have also been raised regarding 2 specific and potentially serious adverse effects of dopamine agonist therapy:

(1) Fibrotic reactions: Cabergoline and bromocriptine (both of which are ergot-derivatives) have been associated with cardiac, pulmonary, and retroperitoneal fibrotic reactions. Although most commonly observed in clinical contexts where higher dosages are used (eg, cabergoline therapy in Parkinson disease), reports have also emerged of fibrotic disorders in patients treated with lower dosages for endocrine conditions, especially if required long-term. Accordingly, surveillance measures such as clinical examination and periodic echocardiography are recommended for patients with prolactinomas who are treated with dopamine agonists, and surveillance should be tailored according to dosage and duration of treatment.

(2) Impulse control disorders (ICDs): Treatment with dopamine agonists has been linked to the development of ICDs, including pathologic gambling, binge eating, and hypersexuality. Patients and their trusted contacts or caregivers should be informed about the risk of ICDs, and any history of psychiatric illness should be discussed before starting dopamine agonist therapy. Ergot- and non–ergot-derived (eg, quinagolide) dopamine agonists do not differ in their propensity to cause ICDs, so switching between drugs will not avoid these adverse effects.

There are several reasons why continuing dopamine agonist therapy in this patient is not advisable. Most importantly, her partner clearly describes behavior that is not consistent with her normal character and which is strongly suggestive of an ICD, most likely related to an increased cabergoline dosage in light of ongoing hyperprolactinemia and secondary amenorrhea. Therefore, while reducing the cabergoline dosage (Answer A) might alleviate the impulse control manifestations if these were not present when taking a lower dosage, symptoms could persist and discontinuation is generally preferred. If continued treatment is being considered, then formal psychiatric advice should be sought. In addition, even if a trial of a reduced cabergoline dosage is determined to be acceptable from a psychiatry perspective, it is not the most appropriate option here because the patient has persistent hyperprolactinemia and secondary amenorrhea while taking a higher dosage. Similarly, bromocriptine (Answer D), which is less potent than cabergoline, would be unlikely to achieve prolactin normalization and would present a similar risk of provoking an ICD.

For patients with microprolactinomas who are intolerant of dopamine agonist therapy and who are not troubled by galactorrhea, hormone therapy (with combined estrogen and progesterone) (Answer E) may suffice, and this is generally considered a safe alternative, provided that serum prolactin levels and radiologic appearances remain stable. A small number of microprolactinomas demonstrate increased growth in response to exogenous estrogen. In this case, hormone therapy is not an appropriate choice because primary infertility is a key concern for this patient. In addition, some clinicians might consider the apparent refractoriness of the tumor to reasonable dosages of cabergoline as a cautionary note for estrogen therapy.

Recognizing that an important subgroup of patients with prolactinomas are unable to tolerate dosages of dopamine agonists sufficient to control hyperprolactinemia and ameliorate symptoms, there has been a recent resurgence in interest in the potential role of transsphenoidal surgery in the management of microprolactinomas. Several groups have reported the effectiveness and safety of prolactinoma surgery. Not surprisingly, most studies have documented higher remission rates for microprolactinomas compared with macroprolactinomas, and adenomas that are enclosed within the gland may have a more favorable outcome than adenomas located at the lateral margins. These findings have been endorsed in several systematic reviews and meta-analyses, which have reported transsphenoidal surgery to deliver superior clinical outcomes compared with those of dopamine agonist therapy, along with superior cost-effectiveness. However, the absence of randomized controlled trials remains a significant limitation. Accepting this, recent guidelines acknowledge that surgery can be considered as a first-line treatment option for microprolactinomas when complete resection is deemed possible following specialist neurosurgical evaluation. In this vignette, the finding of a clearly visible lesion on MRI, contained within the gland and without cavernous sinus extension, indicates that pituitary surgery (Answer C) in the hands of an experienced neurosurgeon offers a high probability of remission, without compromising remaining pituitary function, which is an important consideration for a patient desiring future fertility.

Pituitary radiotherapy (Answer B) may also achieve good control and permit future fertility. However, even when delivered as a single fraction (eg, stereotactic radiosurgery), it is likely to be associated with a delay in achieving biochemical control (months to years), and it also carries a risk of secondary pituitary dysfunction. Radiation therapy is therefore usually reserved for patients who show poor response to or are intolerant of dopamine agonist therapy, have nonresectable residual tumor after surgery, or are not a candidate for curative surgery.

Educational Objective

Diagnose impulse-control disorder as an important, potentially serious adverse effect of dopamine agonist therapy and explain management options for patients with prolactinomas who develop dopamine agonist intolerance.

Reference(s)

Hamidianjahromi A, Tritos N. Impulse control disorders in hyperprolactinemic patients on dopamine agonist therapy. *Rev Endocr Metab Disord.* 2022;23(5):1089-1099. PMID: 36125673

De Sousa SMC, Baranoff J, Rushworth RL, Butler J, et al. Impulse control disorders in dopamine agonist-treated hyperprolactinemia: prevalence and risk factors. *J Clin Endocrinol Metab,* 2020;105(3):dgz076. PMID: 31580439

Zamanipoor Najafabadi AH, Zandbergen IM, de Vries F, et al. Surgery as a viable alternative first-line treatment for prolactinoma patients. A systematic review and meta-analysis. *J Clin Endocrinol Metab.* 2020;105(3):e32-e41. PMID: 31665485

23 ANSWER: C) Proceed to adrenal vein sampling

The initial laboratory results are strongly suggestive of primary aldosteronism (PA) with unprovoked hypokalemia and a raised aldosterone-to-renin ratio in the context of hypertension. When plasma renin is suppressed and the aldosterone concentration is greater than 20 ng/dL (>550 pmol/L) in a patient with a history of hypokalemia, confirmatory testing (eg, saline infusion, oral salt loading, fludrocortisone suppression, or captopril challenge) is not required. Although we do not know the absolute values of the original aldosterone and renin measurements, the latest laboratory findings show continued suppression of plasma renin activity despite treatment with eplerenone, and most clinicians experienced in the management of PA would not consider further confirmatory testing (Answer B) to be required in this patient.

CT has shown an approximately 1-cm mass in the body of the right adrenal gland, which is likely to be the culprit lesion. The left adrenal gland appears normal on imaging. However, given the relatively high prevalence of adrenal incidentalomas in the general population (4% to 7% in adults older than 40 years), further investigation is required to ensure the patient does not have bilateral PA or unilateral PA that is localized to the side opposite of the anatomical lesion. In most centers, once surgery is being contemplated, adrenal vein sampling (AVS) (Answer C), performed by an experienced radiologist, is recommended to make the distinction between unilateral and bilateral adrenal disease. Although traditional teaching has recommended that AVS should not be performed until the patient's regimen has been changed to nonconfounding medications (eg, discontinuing mineralocorticoid receptor antagonist therapy) (Answer E), several groups have now shown that AVS can be reliably performed even on mineralocorticoid receptor antagonist therapy, provided that plasma renin remains suppressed. Hence, this patient can now proceed to AVS as the next step in management.

The patient's current treatment regimen could be improved, specifically an increase in the eplerenone dosage (Answer A). This would likely further reduce her blood pressure and spare the need for ongoing supplemental potassium. However, a reasonable case can be made for delaying this until AVS has been performed, assuming it can be done in a timely manner. Her blood pressure and serum potassium are satisfactory in the short-term, and increasing the eplerenone dosage risks de-suppression of plasma renin, which could then confound the interpretation of AVS through masking of unilateral disease. In the longer term, however, de-suppression of plasma renin is considered an important criterion for assessing the adequacy of mineralocorticoid receptor blockade.

Recently, molecular imaging with the PET radiotracer ^{11}C-metomidate (MTO) has been shown to be a noninferior alternative to AVS for lateralization in PA and may even confer additional benefits through its ability to go beyond lateralization and precisely localize the causative aldosterone-producing adenoma or nodule in unilateral PA.

In limited circumstances, it is reasonable to proceed directly to surgery (Answer D), but this is only advised if the patient meets all of the following criteria:

1. Age <35 years
2. Spontaneous hypokalemia
3. Marked aldosterone excess
4. Unilateral adrenal lesion(s) with radiologic features of a cortical adenoma on adrenal CT

However, this is not the case here, as the patient exceeds the age threshold.

Educational Objective

Determine when additional testing to establish diagnosis and/or determine lateralization is indicated in the evaluation of primary aldosteronism.

Reference(s)

Funder JW, Carey RM, Mantero F, et al. The management of primary aldosteronism: case detection, diagnosis, and treatment: an Endocrine Society clinical practice guideline. *J Clin Endocrinol Metab.* 2016;101(5):1889-1916. PMID: 26934393

Haase M, Riester A, Kropil P, et al. Outcome of adrenal vein sampling performed during concurrent mineralocorticoid receptor antagonist therapy. *J Clin Endocrinol Metab.* 2014;99(12):4397-4402. PMID: 25222758

Wu X, Senanayake R, Goodchild E, et al. [^{11}C]-metomidate PET-CT versus adrenal vein sampling for diagnosing surgically curable primary aldosteronism: a prospective, within-patient trial. *Nat Med.* 2023;29(1):190-202. PMID: 36646800

24 ANSWER: B) Cardiovascular disease and peripheral neuropathy

Prediabetes, which is defined by a hemoglobin A_{1c} value of 5.7% to 6.4% (39-47 mmol/mol) per the American Diabetes Association, is an independent risk factor for cardiovascular disease. The increased risk of cardiovascular disease in persons with prediabetes compared with the risk in those with normoglycemia has been well established in multiple studies. The risk differs depending on the definition of abnormal glycemia used (eg, impaired fasting glucose vs impaired glucose tolerance vs prediabetes defined by hemoglobin A_{1c}). Schlesinger et al conducted an umbrella review of 95 meta-analyses investigating the associated risk of complications with prediabetes. The authors subgrouped prediabetes based on various definitions used by the American Diabetes Association, World Health Organization, and the International Diabetes Federation. Impaired glucose tolerance, as defined by the 2-hour plasma glucose value during a 75-g oral glucose tolerance test, was associated with the highest risk for all complications (all-cause mortality, cardiovascular mortality, cardiovascular events, cerebrovascular events, total cancer, and dementia) compared with risks associated isolated impaired fasting glucose or with prediabetes as defined by hemoglobin A_{1c} (5.7%-6.4% [39-47 mmol/mol]). When prediabetes as defined by the American Diabetes Association hemoglobin A_{1c} criteria is used, risks of cognitive impairment (Answers A, C, and D), chronic kidney disease (Answer C), and retinopathy (Answers D and E) are not significant. The prevalence of peripheral neuropathy in persons with prediabetes (defined in most studies by glucose tolerance status) has been estimated as 10% or more (interquartile range, 6%-34%), with progression of hyperglycemia increasing the risk of developing peripheral neuropathy. This patient's highest risks are developing cardiovascular disease and peripheral neuropathy (Answer B).

Educational Objective

Identify the complications associated with prediabetes.

Reference(s)

Schlesinger S, Neuenschwander M, Barbaresko J, et al. Prediabetes and risk of mortality, diabetes-related complications and comorbidities: umbrella review of meta-analyses of prospective studies. *Diabetologia.* 2022;65(2):275-285. PMID: 34718834

Lee CC, Perkins BA, Kayaniyil S, et al. Peripheral neuropathy and nerve dysfunction in individuals at high risk for type 2 diabetes: the PROMISE Cohort. *Diabetes Care.* 2015;38(5):793-800. PMID: 25665810

Perreault L, Pan Q, Schroeder EB, et al; Diabetes Prevention Program Research Group. Regression from prediabetes to normal glucose regulation and prevalence of microvascular disease in the Diabetes Prevention Program Outcomes Study (DPPOS). *Diabetes Care.* 2019;42(9):1809-1815. PMID: 31320445

Kirthi V, Perumbalath A, Brown E, et al. Prevalance of peripheral neuropathy in pre-diabetes: a systematic review. *BMJ Open Diabetes Res Care.* 2021;9(1):e002040. PMID: 34006607

Schlesinger S, Neuenschwander M, Barbaresko J, et al. Prediabetes and risk of mortality, diabetes-related complications and comorbidities: umbreall review of meta-analyses of prospective studies. *Diabetologia.* 2022;65(2):275-285. PMID: 34718834

25 ANSWER: E) Serum total testosterone

The combination of mild normochromic normocytic anemia and vasomotor symptoms is most suggestive of hypogonadism. Therefore, measuring this patient's serum total testosterone (Answer E) is the best next step. He had a profoundly low serum testosterone concentration of 66 ng/dL (SI: 2.3 nmol/L). Further workup revealed a pituitary macroademona not abutting the optic chiasm. Unexplained anemia can be a presenting symptom of male hypogonadism. Testosterone stimulates erythropoiesis via not fully understood mechanisms that involve a direct effect on erythroid progenitor cells, regulation of iron regulatory proteins such as hepcidin, and possible stimulation of renal erythropoietin production. In a retrospective analysis of 100 older men with pituitary macroadenomas, two-thirds (67 individuals) had a low serum testosterone concentration, and 31 of these men (46%) had anemia. In the Testosterone Trials that recruited men with age-related hypogonadism, 126 of 788 had baseline anemia (baseline hemoglobin of 10.0-12.7 g/dL). Of these 126, 62 (49%) had anemia of unknown cause. After testosterone treatment over 12 months, 60% of men were no longer anemic, compared with 20% of placebo-treated men. While testosterone treatment can correct mild anemia, erythrocytosis (defined as hematocrit >54% or hemoglobin >15.5 g/dL) was the most common adverse effect of testosterone treatment (relative risk: 8.14 [95% CI, 1.87-35.40]) in a recent meta-analysis. Hot flushes are a typical feature of androgen deficiency, occurring especially if serum testosterone is markedly low and/or the decline in serum testosterone is relatively abrupt. For example, more than 70% of men commencing androgen-deprivation therapy for prostate cancer develop hot flushes.

Mechanistically, in hypogonadal men, hot flushes are not due to testosterone deficiency but rather to concomitant estradiol deficiency (because of reduced availability of testosterone, the substrate for aromatase). Of note, this patient's 6-month history of symptoms suggests that the onset of hypogonadism was relatively recent, explaining why some clinical features (reduced muscle bulk, body/sexual hair, and testicular size) were absent, as these take 12 or more months to manifest. However, constitutional symptoms (low mood, fatigue, and low libido) manifest relatively quickly over several months. In his case, these symptoms were most likely exacerbated by his hot flushes leading to sleep disturbance. Given that hot flushes due to sex steroid deficiency are neurally mediated (possibly involving dysregulation of the hypothalamic kisspeptin/neurokinin B/dynorphin [KNDy] neurons), these hot flushes are "wet," because of the concomitant neurologic control of autonomic nerve fibers of vascular smooth muscle and eccrine sweat glands.

In contrast, hot flushes mediated by circulating vasodilator substances such as kinins, prostaglandins, calcitonin, and serotonin are typically "dry" and less likely to be associated with sweating. In addition, there are no other clinical manifestations to suggest carcinoid syndrome or medullary thyroid cancer, and neither condition (unless advanced) would explain the presence of anemia. Thus, measuring 5-hydroxyindoleacetic acid (Answer A), calcitonin (Answer C), or chromogranin A (Answer D) is incorrect. Also, the serum chromogranin A concentration would most likely be high because of proton-pump inhibitor use.

Flushing is uncommon in the setting of pheochromocytoma, which typically presents with pallor due to α1 receptor–mediated vasoconstriction of cutaneous vessels. The imaging characteristics of this patient's adrenal adenoma are not suggestive of pheochromocytoma, which would have higher density. In a meta-analysis of 1217 pheochromocytomas, the overall mean unenhanced CT attenuation was 35.6 Hounsfield units (95% CI, 22.0-49.1 Hounsfield units), and a cutoff of greater than 10 Hounsfield units had 100% sensitivity for pheochromocytoma. Thus, measuring metanephrines (Answer B) is incorrect.

Educational Objective

Identify anemia and hot flushes as presenting symptoms of male hypogonadism.

References

Warren AM, Grossmann M. Haematological actions of androgens. *Best Pract Res Clin Endocrinol Metab.* 2022;36(5):101653. PMID: 35414435

Huguet I, Grossman A. Management of endocrine disease: flushing: current concepts. *Eur J Endocrinol.* 2017;177(5):R219-R229. PMID: 28982960

Gruber LM, Strajina V, Bancos I, et al. Not all adrenal incidentalomas require biochemical testing to exclude pheochromocytoma: Mayo clinic experience and a meta-analysis. *Gland Surg.* 2020;9(2):362-337. PMID: 32420260

26 ANSWER: A) *GATA3* (GATA binding protein 3)

Pathogenic variants in numerous genes have been reported to cause hypoparathyroidism. Most genetic causes are discovered by childhood, but adults are often found to have genetic etiologies of hypoparathyroidism, given the recent wider availability of genetic testing. HDR syndrome (hypoparathyroidism, sensorineural deafness, and renal disease) was first described in 1977 and is one of the most common causes of syndromic familial hypoparathyroidism. Pathogenic variants in *GATA3* (Answer A), a gene that encodes a transcription factor critical for development of the parathyroid glands, auditory sensory nerve, and kidneys, cause this autosomal dominant syndrome. Affected patients are generally diagnosed based on the presentation of hypocalcemia with a concomitant low or inappropriately normal PTH level for the degree of hypocalcemia. Most, but not all, affected patients also have some degree of chronic kidney disease, from mild vesicoureteral reflux to more serious renal aplasia. Barakat et al reported a case series of 173 patients with HDR syndrome. In those with identified *GATA3* variants, 93% had hypoparathyroidism, 96% had hearing impairment, and 72% had kidney disease. The patient in this vignette has classic features of HDR syndrome.

Pathogenic variants in *GNAS* (Answer C) are associated with important endocrine diseases, with inactivating variants resulting in the pseudohypoparathyroidism spectrum of disorders. The protein encoded by *GNAS*, the G-protein α-subunit, is required to transmit the signals from the PTH receptor. With defective PTH signaling, a syndrome of PTH resistance is created, resulting in hypocalcemia and a high serum PTH concentration. This patient has a mid-normal PTH concentration. Albright hereditary osteodystrophy, characterized by short stature and the classic shortened fourth metacarpal bone, is a disorder within pseudohypoparathyroidism type 1A that occurs when the abnormal *GNAS* variant is maternally inherited. Albright hereditary osteodystrophy is caused by PTHrP resistance in growth plate chondrocytes (PTHrP is another ligand of the PTH receptor). This patient has normal stature, normal hands, and a normal PTH concentration.

Hypercalcemia, not hypocalcemia, from primary hyperparathyroidism is typically the presenting condition in patients with pathogenic variants in the *RET* gene (Answer D) as part of multiple endocrine neoplasia type 2.

Pathogenic variants in the *GNA11* gene (Answer B) cause the rare syndrome known as autosomal dominant hypocalcemia type 2. Patients with this autosomal dominant condition have similar laboratory findings as those of the described patient, but hearing impairment and primary kidney disease are not within the spectrum of this syndrome.

DiGeorge syndrome is caused by 1.5- to 3.0-Mb microdeletions of chromosome 22q11.2. In addition to primary hypoparathyroidism, other manifestations include craniofacial abnormalities, developmental delay, immunodeficiency, and other complex conditions. The *TBX1* gene (Answer E), located within the DiGeorge syndrome deletion region, is thought to be critical in the pathogenesis of DiGeorge syndrome. Rarely, patients with pathogenic variants in *TBX1* (in the absence of chromosomal deletions) have the same phenotype as patients with chromosome 22q11.2 microdeletions. Like *GATA3, TBX1* is important for parathyroid development. However, this patient does not have an intellectual disability or craniofacial abnormalities.

Educational Objective

Diagnose hypoparathyroidism, deafness, and renal dysplasia syndrome (HDR syndrome) as a cause of hypoparathyroidism and consider genetic etiologies of hypoparathyroidism.

Reference(s)

Van Esch H, Groenen P, Nesbit MA, et al. GATA3 haplo-insufficiency causes human HDR syndrome. *Nature.* 2000;406(6794):419-422. PMID: 10935639

Barakat AJ, Raygada M, Rennert OM. Barakat syndrome revisited. *Am J Med Genet A.* 2018;176(6):1341-1348. PMID: 29663634

Mantovani G, Bastepe M, Monk D, et al. Diagnosis and management of pseudohypoparathyroidism and related disorders: first international Consensus Statement. *Nat Rev Endocrinol.* 2018;14(8):476-500. PMID: 29959430

Li D, Opas EE, Tuluc F, et al. Autosomal dominant hypoparathyroidism caused by germline mutation in GNA11: phenotypic and molecular characterization. *J Clin Endocrinol Metab.* 2014;99(9):E1774-E1783. PMID: 24823460

Haddad RA, Clines GA, Wyckoff JA. A case report of T-box 1 mutation causing phenotypic features of chromosome 22q11.2 deletion syndrome. *Clin Diabetes Endocrinol.* 2019;5:13. PMID: 31428446

27 ANSWER: D) Lipoprotein (a)

This patient not only has a personal and family history of premature coronary artery disease, but he also has progressive vascular disease despite aggressive lipid-lowering therapy. Elevated lipoprotein (a) (Answer D) can independently contribute to progressive atherosclerosis despite low levels of LDL cholesterol, and it is therefore important to measure it in this individual.

Lipoprotein (a) is an apolipoprotein B–containing lipoprotein in which apolipoprotein B is bound by disulfide linkage to another lipoprotein apo (a), which has structural similarity to plasminogen and also binds to proinflammatory and proatherogenic lipid moieties. Elevated levels of lipoprotein (a) are an independent and causal risk factor for atherosclerotic cardiovascular disease (ASCVD), thrombosis, and aortic stenosis. Lipoprotein (a) levels should be measured in individuals with a personal or family history of premature coronary artery disease, suspected familial hypercholesterolemia, or suboptimal response to traditional lipid-lowering therapy. In addition, elevated lipoprotein (a) levels can serve as a risk-enhancing factor favoring statin therapy for primary prevention in individuals with borderline or intermediate risk. However, statin therapy does not lower lipoprotein (a) levels. Modest reduction (25%-30%) has been noted with PCSK9 inhibitor therapy with some studies suggesting that it may independently contribute to risk lowering, especially in individuals with an LDL-cholesterol concentration less than 70 mg/dL (<1.81 mmol/L). The only currently approved therapy for effective lipoprotein (a) reduction is lipoprotein apheresis, which should be considered in this individual for secondary prevention. While there are no controlled studies, limited data suggest possible risk reduction with this approach. In 2020, the US FDA approved lipoprotein apheresis for individuals with established coronary artery disease or peripheral vascular disease and elevated lipoprotein (a) (>60 mg/dL [2.1 µmol/L]). Novel therapies targeting apolipoprotein (a), including an antisense oligonucleotide (pelacarsen) and siRNA, have demonstrated robust lipoprotein (a) lowering and are undergoing clinical trials.

Measurement of apolipoprotein B (Answer A) and LDL particle number (Answer C) would be more appropriate in patients with hypertriglyceridemia where there would be discordance between LDL-cholesterol concentration and LDL particle number. LDL-cholesterol concentrations alone may underestimate the atherogenic risk in such patients.

Measurement of high-sensitivity C-reactive protein (Answer B) is useful in patients at intermediate risk to help decide on initiating statin therapy. Its measurement would not be appropriate in this patient who has established ASCVD and is already on high-intensity statin therapy.

Post hoc analysis of some studies has shown that on-treatment levels of both apolipoprotein B and high-sensitivity C-reactive protein do predict risk. However, in this patient who is already on maximum dosages of a statin and PCSK9 inhibitor therapy, this additional data is unlikely to help guide therapy. Specific anti-inflammatory therapies such as colchicine and canakinumab have indeed demonstrated risk reduction without affecting lipid levels, but they are not currently recommended or routinely used in clinical practice.

Measurement of plasma phytosterol (Answer E) should be considered when sitosterolemia is suspected, a rare autosomal recessive disorder characterized by tendon xanthomas and premature ASCVD with or without elevated cholesterol levels.

Educational Objective

List the appropriate indications for measuring lipoprotein (a).

Reference(s)

Reyes-Soffer G, Ginsberg HN, Berglund L, et al; American Heart Association Council on Arteriosclerosis, Thrombosis and Vascular Biology; Council on Cardiovascular Radiology and Intervention; and Council on Peripheral Vascular Disease. Lipoprotein(a): a genetically determined, causal, and prevalent risk factor for atherosclerotic cardiovascular disease: a scientific statement from the American Heart Association. *Arterioscler Thromb Vasc Biol.* 2022;42(1):e48-e60. PMID: 34647487

Wilson DP, Jacobson TA, Jones PH, et al. Use of lipoprotein(a) in clinical practice: a biomarker whose time has come. A scientific statement from the National Lipid Association. *J Clin Lipidol.* 2019;13(3):374-392. PMID: 31147269

Szarek M, Bittner VA, Aylward P, et al; ODYSSEY OUTCOMES Investigators. Lipoprotein(a) lowering by alirocumab reduces the total burden of cardiovascular events independent of low-density lipoprotein cholesterol lowering: ODYSSEY OUTCOMES trial. *Eur Heart J.* 2020;41(44):4245-4255. PMID: 33051646

Nugent AK, Gray JV, Gorby LK, Moriarty PM. Lipoprotein apheresis: first FDA indicated treatment for elevated lipoprotein(a). *J Clin Cardiol.* 2019;1(1):16-21.

Ridker PM, Everett BM, Thuren T, et al; CANTOS Trial Group. Antiinflammatory therapy with canakinumab for atherosclerotic disease. *N Engl J Med.* 2017;377(12):1119-1131. PMID: 28845751

Ridker PM, Bhatt DL, Pradhan AD, Glynn RJ, MacFadyen JG, Nissen SE; PROMINENT, REDUCE-IT, and STRENGTH Investigators. Inflammation and cholesterol as predictors of cardiovascular events among patients receiving statin therapy: a collaborative analysis of three randomised trials. *Lancet.* 2023:S0140-6736(23)00215-5. PMID: 36893777

28 ANSWER: C) Metabolic syndrome

This woman meets the criteria for gestational diabetes mellitus based on results of oral glucose tolerance testing (100-g fasting, 1-hour, and 2-hour glucose concentrations [*see table*]). The effects of hyperglycemia on the developing fetus can be detrimental, with strict glucose control lowering the risks of neonatal congenital anomalies, prematurity, macrosomia, metabolic derangements, cardiomyopathy, and death. The long-term risks to children born to mothers with gestational diabetes include type 2 diabetes, obesity, hypertension, hyperinsulinemia, and cardiovascular disease. In the HAPO Follow-up Study, where 4832 children were followed up to age 10 to 14 years, maternal glycemia, as measured by a 75-g oral glucose tolerance test at a gestational age of 28 weeks, was positively associated with offspring glycemia and insulin resistance that was measured by the Matsuda Index. Her child's highest risk is therefore developing metabolic syndrome (Answer C).

Table. Normal Ranges for 50-g, 75-g, and 100-g Glucose Tolerance Tests in Pregnancy

Test	Fasting glucose	1-Hour glucose	2-Hour glucose	3-Hour glucose
50-g glucose	...	<130-140 mg/dL (SI: <7.2-7.8 mmol/L)	...	...
100-g glucose	<95 mg/dL (SI: <5.3 mmol/L)	<180 mg/dL (SI: <10 mmol/L)	<155 mg/dL (SI: <8.6 mmol/L)	140 mg/dL (SI: <7.8 mmol/L)
75-g glucose	< 92 mg/dL (SI: <5.1 mmol/L)	<180 mg/dL (SI: <10 mmol/L)	<155 mg/dL (SI: <8.6 mmol/L)	140 mg/dL (SI: <7.8 mmol/L)

There have been no studies showing associations between gestational diabetes mellitus and chronic kidney disease (Answer A), delayed puberty (Answer B), primary hypothyroidism (Answer D), or type 1 diabetes (Answer E)

in the offspring of women with gestational diabetes mellitus. Given that her family members with primary hypothyroidism and type 1 diabetes are not immediate, her offspring's overall risk for metabolic syndrome is higher compared with the much lower risk for either of those conditions.

Educational Objective

Describe the long-term effects of gestational diabetes on offspring.

Reference(s)

Scholtens DM, Kuang A, Lowe LP, et al; HAPO Follow-up Study Cooperative Research Group; HAPO Follow-Up Study Cooperative Research Group. Hyperglycemia and adverse pregnancy outcome follow-up study (HAPO FUS): maternal glycemia and childhood glucose metabolism. *Diabetes Care.* 2019;42(3):381-392. PMID: 30617141

Vääräsmäki M, Pouta A, Elliot P, et al. Adolescent manifestations of metabolic syndrome among children born to women with gestational diabetes in a general-population birth cohort. *Am J Epidemiol.* 2009;169(10):1209-1215. PMID: 19363101

Boney CM, Verma A, Tucker R, Vohr BR. Metabolic syndrome in childhood: association with birth weight, maternal obesity, and gestational diabetes mellitus. *Pediatrics.*2005;115(3):e290-e296. PMID: 15741354

29 ANSWER: C) Measure plasma ACTH

Primary adrenal insufficiency (Addison disease) must be promptly suspected in this young woman with type 1 diabetes and hypothyroidism. Addison disease is potentially lethal if unrecognized. Autoimmune destruction of the adrenal cortex is the most common cause of primary adrenal insufficiency in the western world, and it can occur alone or in combination with other autoimmune disorders. Autoimmune adrenal insufficiency is a feature of both polyglandular autoimmune syndrome types 1 and type 2. Polyglandular autoimmune syndrome type 1 is a rare autosomal recessive disorder caused by pathogenic variants in the autoimmune regulator (*AIRE*) gene, located on chromosome 21q22.3. Polyglandular autoimmune syndrome type 1 typically develops at a young age, and it is characterized by hypoparathyroidism, chronic mucocutaneous candidiasis, primary adrenal insufficiency, primary hypogonadism, malabsorption syndromes, and autoimmune skin manifestations (vitiligo and alopecia). Polyglandular autoimmune syndrome type 2 is more common, tends to occur later in life, and is characterized by adrenal insufficiency, autoimmune thyroid disease (typically Hashimoto thyroiditis, but sometimes Graves disease), and diabetes mellitus. Other autoimmune disorders, such as primary hypogonadism, vitiligo, and alopecia, are infrequent. Polyglandular autoimmune syndrome type 2 can be familial (autosomal recessive, autosomal dominant, and polygenic) or sporadic. In all forms, females are affected more often than males.

The young woman in this vignette has fatigue, weight loss, and hyperpigmentation ("tan" skin). Her morning cortisol concentration of 10 μg/dL (275.9 nmol/L) is much lower than expected in someone taking combined estrogen-progestin oral contraceptives. Because estrogens induce cortisol-binding globulin production, the morning cortisol concentration is commonly greater than 18 μg/dL (>497 nmol/L) in women taking estrogen preparations. In this patient, elevated ACTH (Answer C) would confirm the suspicion of primary adrenal insufficiency. High plasma renin, low plasma aldosterone, and elevated 21-hydroxylase antibodies would further support the diagnosis.

Fatigue can be caused by a variety of factors, including hypothyroidism, anemia, chronic malabsorption, and depression. This patient is appropriately treated for hypothyroidism, and her TSH is normal. Thus, increasing her levothyroxine dosage (Answer A) is not indicated. In patients with adrenal insufficiency, acceleration of cortisol metabolism induced by thyroid hormones in conjunction with a limited adrenocortical reserve can precipitate an adrenal crisis.

Measuring free T_4 (Answer B) would be indicated in a patient with suspected secondary hypopituitarism, which is not suggested in this case.

Screening for celiac disease (Answer D) and/or depression (Answer E) could be considered in a patient with fatigue and weight loss, but adrenal insufficiency testing takes priority in this case, given the patient's suggestive clinical features. This vignette emphasizes the potential for serious complications when adrenal insufficiency goes unrecognized.

Educational Objective

Suspect adrenal insufficiency based on the clinical presentation in a patient with other autoimmune disorders and order the correct diagnostic test.

Reference(s)

Eisenhofer G, Peitzsch M, Kaden D, et al. Reference intervals for plasma concentrations of adrenal steroids measured by LC-MS/MS: Impact of gender, age, oral contraceptives, body mass index and blood pressure status. *Clin Chim Acta.* 2017;470:115-124. PMID: 28479316

Hahner S, Ross RJ, Arlt W, et al. Adrenal insufficiency. *Nat Rev Dis Primers.* 2021;7(1):19. PMID: 33707469

30 **ANSWER: D) Proceed with continuous glucose monitoring evaluation**

Adjusting diabetes medications requires accurate information about glycemic control, especially in patients treated with a multiple daily injection regimen. Increasing or decreasing basal or short-acting insulin or initiating or stopping diabetes medications can lead to hypoglycemia or hyperglycemia when these decisions are based on inaccurate or inadequate information.

In this clinical case, which is not uncommon, the clinician is faced with conflicting results. The patient is reporting glucose values in an excellent range (90-140 mg/dL [5.0-7.8 mmol/L]), while his hemoglobin A_{1c} measurement (9.1% [76 mmol/mol]) suggests that he has suboptimal glycemic control. Although information about possible nonadherence to his diabetes regimen is not provided in the vignette (which is also the case in real-life situations), the clinician should always suspect nonadherence when receiving conflicting information about diabetes control. This is more significant in this clinical scenario in which the patient has a history of multiple diabetes-related complications, which should alert the clinician to possible nonadherence.

Conversely, although hemoglobin A_{1c} is an important laboratory measurement providing an estimate of glycemic control over the last 90 to 120 days, it has many limitations and can be falsely abnormal in different conditions. The medical provider can reasonably suspect that the hemoglobin A_{1c} is not accurate in this individual who has an underlying history of chronic kidney disease, a condition that can lead to false measurements.

In situations in which there is conflicting information about glycemic control, assessing another glycemic biomarker is reasonable. Although several glycemic biomarkers have been investigated, fructosamine has been used most often in clinical practice. Fructosamine is a serum protein that can be measured to evaluate glycation of proteins, predominantly albumin. Fructosamine measurement has limitations, which makes it less favorable than hemoglobin A_{1c}. The turnover of fructosamine is quicker than that of hemoglobin A_{1c} and, therefore, it can provide an estimate of glycemic control for only the last 28 days compared with the 90 to 120 days that hemoglobin A_{1c} can provide. In addition, fructosamine has not been standardized as a metric of glycemic control and there are limited studies linking fructosamine to long-term diabetes complications, compared with data available for hemoglobin A_{1c}. Also, fructosamine reflects glycated protein, and it can therefore be affected if the patient has a condition in which the protein concentrations are abnormal. As a result, fructosamine can be low in the settings of malabsorption, protein-losing enteropathy, liver cirrhosis, and, more commonly, nephrotic syndromes.

Because this patient has advanced liver cirrhosis, which affects liver synthetic function and leads to low albumin-protein levels, fructosamine may be inaccurate and another method is needed to evaluate glycemic control. Continuous glucose monitoring devices (Answer D), either as blinded (retrospective use) or as real-time continuous glucose monitoring, can provide comprehensive information on glycemic control. These systems measure glucose values every 1 to 5 minutes. Data can be downloaded and then visualized as diagrammatic reports. Among the various metrics that can be obtained in these reports is the glucose management indicator, which is an estimate of the expected hemoglobin A_{1c} value during the study period (derived from continuous glucose monitoring values documented during the observation period). One limitation of using continuous glucose monitoring for a short period, typically in the blinded-retrospective mode, is that evaluation of glycemic control is only gleaned during this observation period, typically 10 to 14 days.

Increasing the basal insulin dosage (Answer A), initiating empagliflozin (Answer B), initiating semaglutide (Answer C), or reducing the basal insulin dosage (Answer E) would be appropriate only when adequate information about glycemic control is provided. In this scenario, reported glucose and fructosamine values point to this patient having excellent glucose control, whereas the hemoglobin A_{1c} level suggests that he has uncontrolled diabetes.

Educational Objective

Describe the limitations of fructosamine in monitoring glycemic control in patients with diabetes mellitus.

Reference(s)

Howey JE, Browning MC, Fraser CG, Assay of serum fructosamine that minimizes standardization and matrix problems: use to assess components of biological variation. *Clin Chem.* 1987;33(2 Pt 1):269-272. PMID: 3802511

Selvin E, Rawlings AM, Grams M, et al. Fructosamine and glycated albumin for risk stratification and prediction of incident diabetes and microvascular complications: a prospective cohort analysis of the Atherosclerosis Risk in Communities (ARIC) study. *Lancet Diabetes Endocrinol.* 2014;2(4):279-288. PMID: 24703046

Bergenstal RM, Beck RW, Close KL, et al. Glucose management indicator (GMI): a new term for estimating A1C from continuous glucose monitoring. *Diabetes Care.* 2018;41(11):2275-2280. PMID: 30224348

31 ANSWER: B) Discontinue propylthiouracil

If possible, antithyroid medications should be avoided during the first trimester of pregnancy. If they are administered, they should be prescribed at the lowest possible dosage to maintain the maternal serum free T_4 concentration in the upper end or slightly above the trimester-specific pregnancy reference range. If a trimester-specific reference range is not available via the laboratory, the total T_4 concentration should be maintained at 1.5 times above the nonpregnant reference range. Serum TSH should be maintained below the reference range. The goal is to prevent fetal hypothyroidism because the fetal thyroid gland is very sensitive to antithyroid drugs.

Propylthiouracil is the preferred medication during the first trimester (to reduce the risk of teratogenic effects associated with methimazole during organogenesis), while methimazole is the preferred medication during the second and third trimesters. There is evidence that propylthiouracil also causes birth defects, although less severe than those associated with methimazole, which is known to cause embryopathy (*see table*).

Table. Congenital Abnormalities Associated With Antithyroid Medications

Congenital abnormalities	Methimazole	Propylthiouracil
Aplasia cutis	•	
Tracheoesophageal fistulas	•	
Patent vitellointestinal duct	•	
Choanal atresia	•	
Omphalocele	•	
Omphalomesenteric duct anomaly	•	
Preauricular sinuses abnormalities		•
Cysts and urinary tract abnormalities		•

In women on a low dosage of methimazole (5 to 10 mg daily) or propylthiouracil (100 to 200 mg daily) who become pregnant, antithyroid drugs can be discontinued if they have normal thyroid function in the early first trimester. This pregnant woman with Graves disease has T_4 and T_3 values in the mid-normal range and a low-normal TSH value. Therefore, the best answer is to discontinue propylthiouracil (Answer B). Continuing propylthiouracil or increasing the current dosage (Answers A and C) would be inappropriate. When antithyroid drugs are discontinued, TSH and free T_4 should be checked every 1 to 2 weeks to confirm euthyroidism. If clinical and biochemical euthyroidism persists during the first trimester, thyroid function may be monitored at longer intervals during the second and third trimesters.

Thyroid-stimulating immunoglobulin (Answer D) is usually monitored during the second trimester (18 to 22 weeks) and she is currently only 10 weeks pregnant. Thyroid-stimulating immunoglobulin can cross the placenta and activate the fetal thyroid gland, leading to fetal thyrotoxicosis. If elevated thyroid-stimulating immunoglobulin is detected at weeks 18 to 22 or the mother is on antithyroid drugs during the third trimester, thyroid-stimulating immunoglobulin should be measured again in the third trimester (weeks 30 to 34) to evaluate the need for neonatal monitoring and postnatal surveillance.

Thyroid ultrasonography (Answer E) is unnecessary for this patient, as there is no thyroid nodularity on physical examination and she has no compressive symptoms.

Educational Objective

Recommend the appropriate antithyroid medication dosage in a pregnant woman with Graves disease.

Reference(s)

Alexander EK, Pearce EN, Brent GA, et al. 2017 guidelines of the American Thyroid Association for the diagnosis and management of thyroid disease during pregnancy and the postpartum. *Thyroid.* 2017;27(3):315-389. PMID: 28056690

Andersen SL, Olsen J, Wu CS, Laurberg P. Birth defects after early pregnancy use of antithyroid drugs: a Danish nationwide study. *J Clin Endocrinol Metab.* 2013;98(11):4373-4381. PMID: 24151287

32 ANSWER: D) Start phentermine/topiramate, 3.75/23 mg daily

Metabolic dysfunction-associated steatotic liver disease (MASLD) (formerly termed nonalcoholic fatty liver disease [NAFLD]) is now the most prevalent chronic liver condition globally, in line with the obesity epidemic. The ultimate goal of managing MASLD is to prevent the development of cirrhosis. Weight management is a universal recommendation in the management of MASLD, with more aggressive weight management strategies strongly recommended in later stages of fibrosis. Weight loss of approximately 10% leads to regression of fibrosis and resolution of steatohepatitis in most patients.

All of the answer options listed in this vignette are reasonable in the management of MASLD. However, an appetite-suppressing agent (Answer D) for weight management is the best choice for this patient. The combination of phentermine and topiramate, when added to a lifestyle modification program, produces an average 10% weight loss from baseline. Approximately 40% of patients experience weight loss of greater than 15% on this medication. Patients who are hypertensive or tachycardic at baseline should not take phentermine/topiramate. It should also not be prescribed to women who are attempting pregnancy or who are pregnant or breastfeeding. Other appetite suppressants such as GLP-1 receptor agonists have been studied in MASLD, with semaglutide showing the best weight loss and hepatic outcomes in this patient population.

The Mediterranean-style diet (Answer B) is the dietary pattern of choice for patients with MASLD, and it improves steatosis even in the absence of weight loss. Consumption of simple carbohydrates and low-fiber foods, which increases the risk of MASLD independent of energy overconsumption, is discouraged with this dietary pattern. Although this patient could benefit from a Mediterranean-style diet, her disease stage is advanced enough that weight loss should be the top priority and this is best achieved with weight-loss modalities beyond lifestyle changes. Additionally, the patient reports that adherence to lifestyle changes is difficult. The ketogenic or very low-carbohydrate diet (Answer A) has been studied in patients with MASLD, but because long-term data on the sustainability (and risk of weight regain) of such a diet are lacking, this is not the most appropriate recommendation for this patient now.

There are good data supporting the role of bariatric surgery in patients with MASLD. Roux-en-Y gastric bypass in particular has been shown to improve several features of MASLD, including steatosis, steatohepatitis, ballooning degeneration, and fibrosis. Bariatric surgery is not recommended in patients who have decompensated cirrhosis, and as with all patients, careful patient selection is key to optimal long-term results. Although this patient could benefit from bariatric surgery, sleeve gastrectomy (Answer C) is not the best choice because she has Barrett esophagus, which is a relative contraindication to this specific type of bariatric procedure.

Pioglitazone (Answer E) or a GLP-1 receptor agonist can be considered in patients with MASLD or steatohepatitis if associated with type 2 diabetes. Pioglitazone improves hepatic insulin resistance by targeting adipose tissue behavior, and it decreases liver fat content and inflammation. Pioglitazone is associated with weight gain in a dose-dependent fashion; therefore, low-dosage pioglitazone is preferred. This patient does not have type 2 diabetes, so pioglitazone would not be the best choice, given that current guidelines most strongly support use of this medication in persons with type 2 diabetes and biopsy-proven metabolic dysfunction-associated steatohepatitis (MASH) (formerly termed nonalcoholic steatohepatitis [NASH]).

Educational Objective

List weight-loss goals and describe proven treatment modalities for advanced metabolic dysfunction-associated steatotic liver disease.

Reference(s)

Cusi K, Isaacs S, Barb D, et al. American Association of Clinical Endocrinology clinical practice guideline for the diagnosis and management of nonalcoholic fatty liver disease in primary care and endocrinology clinical settings: co-sponsored by the American Association for the Study of Liver Diseases (AASLD). *Endocr Pract.* 2022;28(5):528-562. PMID: 35569886

Garvey WT, Ryan DH, Look M, et al. Two-year sustained weight loss and metabolic benefits with controlled-release phentermine/topiramate in obese and overweight adults (SEQUEL): a randomized, placebo-controlled, phase 3 extension study. *Am J Clin Nutr.* 2012;95(2):297-308. PMID: 22158731

33 ANSWER: C) Increase the calcitriol dosage

This patient has pseudohypoparathyroidism type 1a, as evidenced by PTH resistance causing hypocalcemia, along with TSH resistance, gonadotropin resistance, brachydactyly, and subcutaneous calcifications. Hand radiographs from 3 children with pseudohypoparathyroidism are shown (*see image*), demonstrating varying degrees of metacarpal shortening. The right-most radiograph also demonstrates calcifications in the patient's thumb and first finger (calcifications were removed in adolescence due to local mass symptoms).

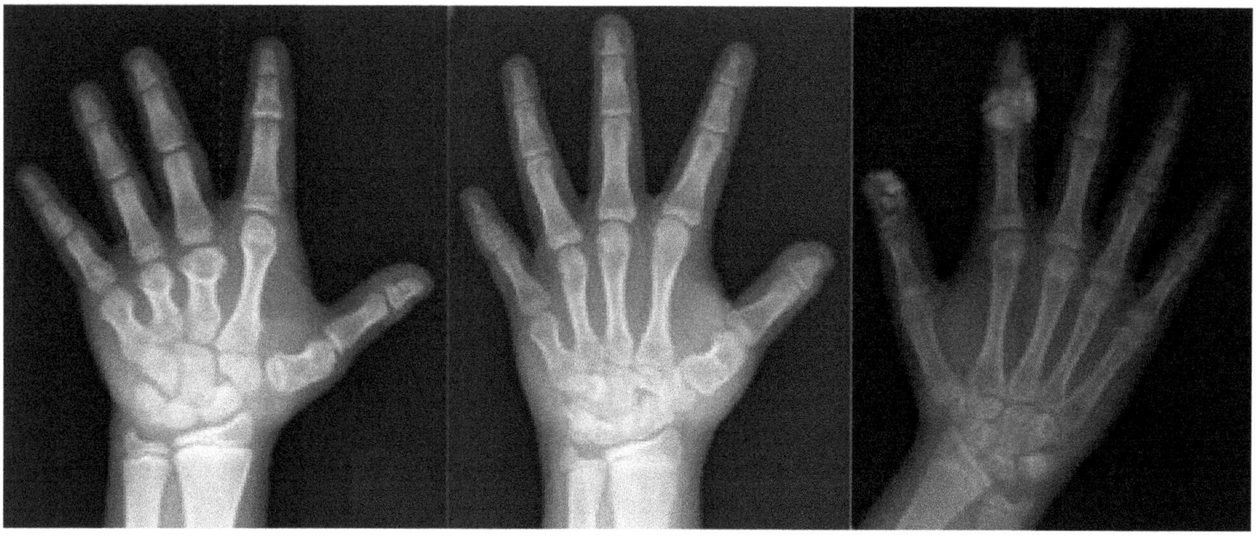

The inheritance of this disorder is affected by parental imprinting influencing tissue expression of the alleles. PTH resistance syndromes are typically caused by inactivating pathogenic variants in the *GNAS* gene that encodes $G_s\alpha$, which is involved in G-protein–coupled receptor signaling. Expression of *GNAS* is biallelic in most tissues, but only the maternal allele is expressed in the renal proximal tubule, thyroid, pituitary somatotrophs, and gonads. Thus, maternal inheritance of an inactivating *GNAS* pathogenic variant causes resistance to hormone signaling in these cells. This patient inherited the condition from her mother, who has calcifications but not PTH resistance (pseudopseudohypoparathyroidism). The proximal tubule PTH resistance manifests as hyperphosphatemia and impairments in 1,25-dihydroxyvitamin D activation, causing hypocalcemia, which is treated similarly to hypoparathyroidism. The distal renal tubule expresses both maternal and paternal alleles; thus, even with a maternal inactivating *GNAS* pathogenic variant, the distal renal tubule still expresses the normal paternal allele and is able to respond to PTH by increasing calcium reabsorption and limiting urinary calcium losses. Unlike persons with hypoparathyroidism, persons with pseudohypoparathyroidism do not appear to be at increased risk for hypercalciuria or nephrocalcinosis, likely because of this preserved PTH effect on the distal tubule. Bone resorption is still triggered by elevated PTH.

Treatment goals include maintaining a normal serum calcium concentration without hypercalciuria, normalizing PTH, and preventing elevated serum phosphate (and calcium-phosphate product). This patient has a low-normal serum calcium value and a normal serum phosphate value, which would both be within an appropriate target range for treating hypoparathyroidism. Because of the elevated PTH value in the setting of pseudohypoparathyroidism, she requires additional therapy. The best next step is to increase the calcitriol dosage (Answer C) and/or to increase the calcium dosage (not decrease [Answer B]).

A thiazide diuretic (Answer A) is often added to limit hypercalciuria in hypoparathyroidism, but that is not typically an issue in the setting of pseudohypoparathyroidism, and this patient's urinary calcium excretion is not elevated (but low), as expected given that PTH's effect on the distal renal tubule remains intact, stimulating calcium reabsorption.

This patient does not need parathyroidectomy (Answer D) because her calcium value is low-normal and the abnormality in pseudohypoparathyroidism is not at the level of PTH production and secretion (which is "appropriate"), but rather at the level of its receptor effect. Rare reports describe adults with pseudohypoparathyroidism who developed hypercalcemic tertiary hyperparathyroidism after longstanding severe PTH elevation. To prevent this development, the goal is to normalize PTH by adjusting her calcium and calcitriol dosages.

Recommending no change in her treatment regimen (Answer E) would fail to address or prevent consequences of chronically elevated PTH on skeletal metabolism.

Educational Objective

Recommend treatment targets for pseudohypoparathyroidism vs targets for hypoparathyroidism.

Reference(s)

Mantovani G, Bastepe M, Monk D, et al. Diagnosis and management of pseudohypoparathyroidism and related disorders: first international Consensus Statement. *Nat Rev Endocrinol.* 2018;14(8):476-500. PMID: 29959430

Pereda A, Elli FM, Thiele S, et al. Inactivating PTH/PTHrP signaling disorders (iPPSDs): evaluation of the new classification in a multicenter large series of 544 molecularly characterized patients. *Eur J Endocrinol.* 2021;184(2):311-320. PMID: 33270042

Imel E. Presented at Endocrine Society's Pediatric Endocrinology Board Review Course; September 24-25, 2013; New Orleans, LA.

34 **ANSWER: A) Measure IGF-1**

This patient requires screening for acromegaly with measurement of serum IGF-1 (Answer A). The clinical scenario is suggestive of a GH-secreting tumor that has not yet caused the typical changes in physical appearance or acral enlargement. Although the delay in acromegaly diagnosis has shortened over the past 2 decades in the context of improved biochemical testing and radiologic techniques, onset of clinical manifestations and/or comorbidities occurs on average 5 years before diagnosis. Carpal tunnel syndrome affects up to 24% of patients with acromegaly and has been more frequently described in women, sometimes developing many years before acromegaly is diagnosed. Studies have shown that women with acromegaly are older than men at diagnosis and undergo more medical evaluations for nonspecific symptoms such as fatigue, headaches, hyperhidrosis, and arthralgia. Compared with men, premenopausal women have lower concentrations of IGF-1 due to the estrogen effect on the GH receptor. This occurs via inhibition of Janus kinase, a signal transducer and activator of transcription signaling by GH. Findings of several studies indicate that young women have larger tumors at presentation than the tumors in men, suggesting that early diagnosis could improve the likelihood of postoperative remission.

Starting an oral contraceptive (Answer E) is incorrect because the patient is unlikely to have polycystic ovary syndrome, which usually has onset of clinical manifestations at a younger age. If her IGF-1 level is normal, further workup with ovarian ultrasonography and testosterone measurement would be necessary. At this time, while taking a combined oral contraceptive pill would resolve amenorrhea, the etiology of symptoms would remain unknown and untreated. Also, oral estrogen administration decreases IGF-1 concentrations through the mechanism described above, attenuating the typical manifestations of acromegaly while the tumor continues to enlarge. If the tumor invades the cavernous sinuses, complete surgical resection is less likely. Likewise, ovarian ultrasonography (Answer C) is incorrect because this patient is unlikely to have polycystic ovary syndrome or an ovarian tumor.

Pituitary MRI (Answer D) is indicated for women with nonphysiologic hyperprolactinemia after evaluation for drug interactions and systemic conditions that can influence prolactin levels. However, this is not the best next step in this patient's management because her prolactin concentration is only slightly elevated, possibly in context of stimulation after pelvic evaluation.

Measuring morning fasting prolactin again (Answer B) is incorrect because screening for acromegaly is still necessary even if a repeated prolactin measurement in the absence of stimulation is normal. Also, prolactin measurement does not warrant fasting early-morning blood collection.

Educational Objective

Identify signs of acromegaly before the typical physical changes occur.

Reference(s)

Ioachimescu AG. Acromegaly: achieving timely diagnosis and improving outcomes by personalized care. *Curr Opin Endocrinol Diabetes Obes.* 2021;28(4):419-426. PMID: 34101652

Vouzouneraki K, Esposito D, Mukka S, et al. Carpal tunnel syndrome in acromegaly: a nationwide study. *Eur J Endocrinol.* 2020;184(2):209-216. PMID: 33136549

Park SH, Ku CR, Moon JH, Kim EH, Kim SH, Lee EJ. Age- and sex-specific differences as predictors of surgical remission among patients with acromegaly. *J Clin Endocrinol Metab.* 2018;103(3):909-916. PMID: 29272449

Dal J, Skov BG, Andersen M, et al. Sex differences in acromegaly at diagnosis: a nationwide cohort study and meta-analysis of the literature. *Clin Endocrinol (Oxf).* 2020;94(4):625-635. PMID: 33306249

Parkinson C, Ryder WD, Trainer PJ, Sensus Acromegaly Study Group. The relationship between serum GH and serum IGF-I in acromegaly is gender-specific. *J Clin Endocrinol Metab.* 2001;86(11):5240-5244. PMID: 11701684

35 ANSWER: A) Measure gonadotropins and order semen analysis

In patients with classic congenital adrenal hyperplasia due to 21-hydroxylase deficiency, the adrenal glands produce androgens in excess. This occurs due to a combination of chronic ACTH elevation, which overstimulates the steroidogenic pathway, and defective 21-hydroxylase, with consequent diversion of steroid precursors towards the open androgen pathway (*see figure*). In addition to androstenedione and testosterone, the adrenal glands also overproduce 11-oxygenated androgens, particularly 11β-hydroxyandrostenedione and 11β-hydroxytestosterone, which are metabolized in periphery to the potent androgen 11-ketotestosterone (*see figure*). In patients with poorly controlled 21-hydroxyalse deficiency, the surplus of adrenal androgens leads to gonadotropin suppression and subsequent disruption of gonadal function. Although the serum testosterone concentration is normal in this man, it likely reflects disproportionate adrenal rather than testicular secretion. Gonadotropin measurement and semen analysis (Answer A) are valuable for assessing hypothalamic-pituitary-gonadal function. Gonadotropin suppression can be reversed with therapies that target the early-morning ACTH rise, which is the primary driver of adrenal androgen synthesis. If the patient confirms adherence to his bedtime prednisolone, intensification of therapy can be pursued by increasing the bedtime prednisolone dosage or switching to the more potent glucocorticoid dexamethasone.

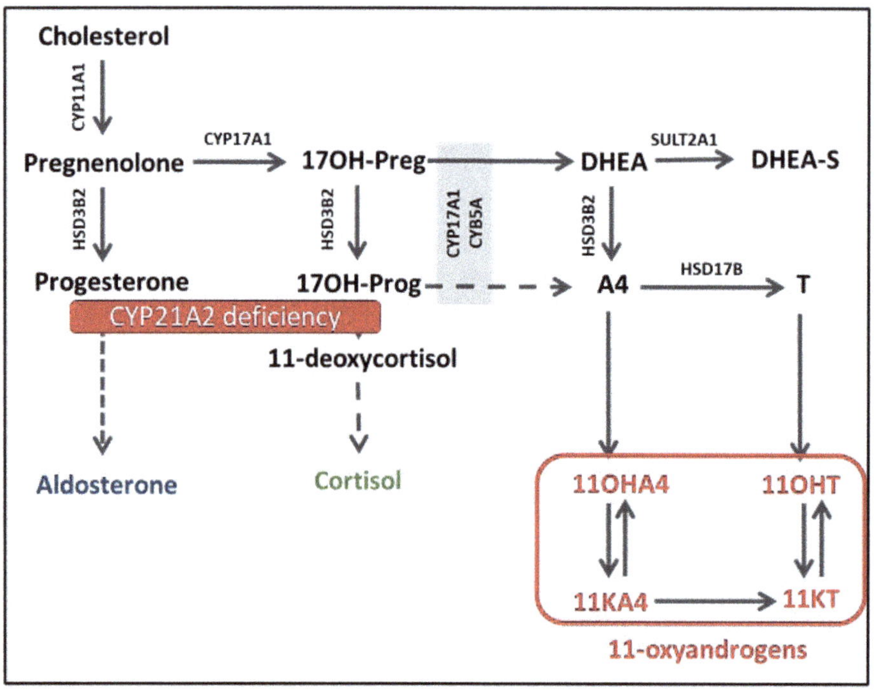

Steroidogenic pathway in 21-hydroxylase deficiency.

CYP11A1, cholesterol side-chain cleavage; HSD3B2, 3β-hydroxysteroid dehydrogenase type 2; CYP17A1, 17α-hydroxylase/17,20-lyase; CYB5A, cytochrome b5 type A; type 2; SULT2A1, sulfotransferase 2A1; 17OHPreg, 17α-hydroxypregnenolone; 17OHProg, 17α-hydroxyprogesterone; DHEA, dehydroepinadrosterone; DHEA-S, DHEA sulfate; A4, androstenedione; T, testosterone; 11OHA4, 11β-hydroxyandrostenedione; 11KA4, 11-ketoandrostenedione; 11OHT, 11β-hydroxytestosterone; 11KT, 11-ketotestosterone. Adapted from Figure 1 in Turcu AF, Nanba AT, Chomic R, et al. *Eur J Endocrinol*, 2016; 174(5): 601-609. © European Society of Endocrinology.

Serum 17-hydroxyprogesterone (Answer B) is expected to be elevated in patients with 21-hydroxylase deficiency, and it represents the basis of the 21-hydroxylase deficiency diagnosis. Normalizing 17-hydroxyprogesterone, however, is not recommended in patients with congenital adrenal hyperplasia, as it is typically achieved at the expense of excessive exogenous glucocorticoid exposure.

In patients with classic 21-hydroxylase deficiency who are not treated adequately, the prolonged and severe ACTH elevation promotes the development of large adrenal myelolipomas and testicular adrenal rest tumors. Adrenal myelolipomas would be notable on cross-sectional abdominal imaging (Answer C), but these are benign masses that do not require routine surgical removal, and thus screening with imaging is not recommended.

Testicular adrenal rest tumors are composed of adrenal-like tissue, typically located within the rete testis. These tumors might obstruct the seminiferous tubules and contribute to infertility. Their size can decrease with adequate glucocorticoid therapy, but if left untreated in the long-term, they can become fibrotic and respond poorly to intensification of glucocorticoid therapy. While surgical removal circumvents enlargement and alleviates pain, fertility is rarely restored. Testicular adrenal rest tumors are detected by testicular ultrasonography (Answer D), and this test should be performed routinely in men with classic 21-hydroxylase deficiency, particularly when suboptimally controlled. This patient probably has testicular adrenal rest tumors, but his gonadal function should be assessed first.

Infertility evaluation for his wife (Answer E) is secondary to his evaluation, particularly given her regular menses and relatively recent successful pregnancy.

Educational Objective

Guide the infertility workup in a man with congenital adrenal hyperplasia who has a normal testosterone concentration.

Reference(s)

Turcu AF, Nanba AT, Chomic R, et al. Adrenal-derived 11-oxygenated 19-carbon steroids are the dominant androgens in classic 21-hydroxylase deficiency. *Eur J Endocrinol.* 2016;174(5):601-609. PMID: 26865584

Turcu AF, Mallappa A, Elman MS, et al. 11-Oxygenated androgens are biomarkers of adrenal volume and testicular adrenal rest tumors in 21-hydroxylase deficiency. *J Clin Endocrinol Metab.* 2017;102(8):2701-2710. PMID: 28472487

Speiser PW, Arlt W, Auchus RJ, et al. Congenital adrenal hyperplasia due to steroid 21-hydroxylase deficiency: an Endocrine Society clinical practice guideline. *J Clin Endocrinol Metab.* 2018;103(11):4043-4088. PMID: 30272171

36 ANSWER: A) Genetic predisposition

Although the patient is this vignette does not have retinopathy or neuropathy, there has been a reduction in estimated glomerular filtration rate. Recently, the role of genetics and epigenetics in the development and progression of diabetic kidney disease has been confirmed. Of patients with diabetic kidney disease, 22% have a pathogenic variant associated with kidney disease on next-generation sequencing. Most persons with diabetic kidney disease experience a progressive decline in kidney function. However, in 1 cohort, approximately 15% of patients with diabetic kidney disease experienced a rapid decline over 3 to 6 years. First-degree relatives of patients at an increased risk more often also experienced rapid decline (odds ratio, 1.92; 95% CI, 1.19-3.09). This patient has had a steep decline in kidney function (glomerular filtration rate decreasing from 61 to 34 mL/min per 1.73 m^2) despite improved glycemic control (hemoglobin A_{1c} improving from 10.0% to 7.5% [86 to 58 mmol/mol]). With this patient's strong family history of type 2 diabetes and kidney disease, a genetic predisposition to diabetic kidney disease (Answer A) is the most likely explanation.

The approach to this patient should include a full urinalysis (as was done) and a thorough history to exclude other causes such as nephrotoxic medications (lithium, nonsteroidal anti-inflammatory drugs, herbal supplements), history of cancer, or possible obstruction. After a thorough physical examination to exclude signs of volume overload or depletion, new skin lesions, or abnormal pulses, initial laboratory assessment includes a complete blood cell count, serum calcium measurement, urine culture (if urinalysis is suggestive of infection), urine microscopy, and spot urine protein-to-creatinine ratio or 24-hour urine protein. This patient's urinalysis and all other laboratory data were normal aside from his kidney function and moderately increased albuminuria.

Although heart failure (Answer B) can cause decreased kidney perfusion with resultant abnormal kidney function, this patient does not have any symptoms of heart failure or cardiovascular history to suggest an increased risk.

Metformin toxicity (Answer C) is unlikely because metformin is not nephrotoxic, and his estimated glomerular filtration rate is greater than 30 mL/min per 1.73 m^2.

While his hemoglobin A_{1c} value is higher than goal, it has significantly improved since his diagnosis, so suboptimal glycemic control (Answer D) is an unlikely cause. In persons without a genetic predisposition to rapid renal decline, the median rate of glomerular filtration loss is –0.7 mL/min per 1.73 m^2 per year, whereas in those with a genetic predisposition, the median rate of glomerular filtration loss is –8.0 mL/min per 1.73 m^2 per year.

His blood pressure is slightly higher than goal and he may have stage 1 hypertension (Answer E); however, one is unable to make this diagnosis based on a single blood pressure measurement.

Educational Objective

Describe the genetic susceptibility of diabetic nephropathy.

Reference(s)

Frodsham SG, Yu Z, Lyons AM, et al. The familiality of rapid renal decline in diabetes. *Diabetes.* 2019;68(2):420-429. PMID: 30425064

Lazaro-Guevara J, Fierro-Morales J, Wright AH, et al. Targeted next-generation sequencing identifies pathogenic variants in diabetic kidney disease. *Am J Nephrol.* 2021;52(3):239-249. PMID: 33774617

37 ANSWER: A) Anabolic therapy with a PTH receptor agonist

Osteoporosis is common in transplant candidates preceding transplant because of a variety of disease-related factors and adverse effects of medications such as glucocorticoids. Additionally, bone density declines rapidly in the first year after transplant, especially in heart or lung transplant recipients. Medications used as immunosuppressive agents such as glucocorticoids and tacrolimus may further contribute to bone loss. The glucocorticoid effect on bone is proportional to dosage. Rapid bone mineral density decline after transplant emphasizes the potential benefit of early treatment. The ideal time to address bone health in transplant recipients is before transplant. Data are limited regarding which therapeutic option after transplant is most beneficial.

In this patient with very low bone mineral density, new compression fractures, and a medication regimen that puts her at high risk, potent anabolic therapy such as a PTH receptor agonist (Answer A) would be appropriate, although there are not extensive studies specifically in the transplant population. However, compared with bisphosphonates, PTH receptor agonists such as teriparatide produce greater improvement in bone mineral density and fracture risk reduction in the general osteoporosis population and when treating glucocorticoid-induced osteoporosis. For example, in the VERO trial (Effects of Teriparatide and Risedronate on New Fractures in Postmenopausal Women With Severe Osteoporosis), 1360 postmenopausal women with vertebral fractures were randomly assigned to receive teriparatide or weekly risedronate. Compared with risedronate, teriparatide reduced the risk for both vertebral and clinical fractures in women with multiple moderate or 1 severe vertebral compression fracture. In another trial by Saag et al, 428 adults treated with glucocorticoids were randomly assigned to receive teriparatide or daily alendronate for 18 months. Bone mineral density at the lumbar spine (the primary outcome) increased more after teriparatide than after alendronate treatment (7.2 ± 0.7% vs 3.4 ± 0.7%, $P < 0.001$). The total number of fractures in the study were small, and while the number of new clinical nonvertebral fractures did not differ between groups, fewer patients developed new morphometric vertebral compression fractures after teriparatide (0.6%) than after alendronate (6.1%).

Oral bisphosphonates (Answer C) have demonstrated preservation of or improvement in bone mineral density after transplant (and also in the setting of glucocorticoid-induced osteoporosis), but this patient has both moderate gastroesophageal reflux symptoms and a hiatal hernia, which renders oral bisphosphonates a less than optimal choice. In addition, the presence of severe osteoporosis in a patient on glucocorticoid therapy warrants anabolic therapy based on current guidelines.

The magnitude of calcitonin's (Answer B) effect on bone mineral density is limited and unlikely to prevent fractures in this patient at high risk.

Resistance exercises (Answer E) have been demonstrated to be beneficial for bone mineral density after transplant but when combined with oral bisphosphonates.

The dosage of immunosuppressive agents such as glucocorticoids (Answer D) should be determined based on the dosage necessary to prevent or treat rejection rather than using the bone effect as the primary factor. Other potential treatment options for this patient at high risk of fractures could be denosumab or intravenous bisphosphonates. Although a possible increased risk of infection in this immunosuppressed patient (denosumab) and concern over further decline in kidney function (bisphosphonate) given the presence of chronic kidney disease should also be considered.

Educational Objective

Diagnose and treat osteoporosis in the setting of organ transplant.

Reference(s)

Shoback D, Rosen CJ, Black DM, Cheung AM, Murad MH, Eastell R. Pharmacological management of osteoporosis in postmenopausal women: an Endocrine Society guideline update. *J Clin Endocrinol Metab.* 2020;105(3):dgaa048. PMID: 32068863

Braith RW, Conner JA, Fulton MN, et al. Comparison of alendronate vs alendronate plus mechanical loading as prophylaxis for osteoporosis in lung transplant recipients: a pilot study. *J Heart Lung Transplant.* 2007;26(2):132-137. PMID: 17258146

Ebeling PR. Approach to the patient with transplantation-related bone loss. *J Clin Endocrinol Metab.* 2009;94(5):1483-1490. PMID: 19420272

Geusens P, Marin F, Kendler DL, et al. Effects of teriparatide compared with risedronate on the risk of fractures in subgroups of postmenopausal women with severe osteoporosis: the VERO trial. *J Bone Miner Res.* 2018;33(5):783-794. PMID: 29329484

Saag KG, Shane E, Boonen S, et al. Teriparatide or alendronate in glucocorticoid-induced osteoporosis. *N Engl J Med.* 2007;357(20):2028-2039. PMID: 18003959

38 ANSWER: C) Oral glucose tolerance test with serum GH measurements

Although this patient's pituitary tumor was initially considered an incidental finding during investigation by the neurology service, it is possible her headache is directly linked to the tumor, especially if somatotroph in origin, as headache is a commonly reported symptom in acromegaly. Her headaches are retro-orbital in nature, which is also consistent with a pituitary origin (the most common site [79%] in one large study of pituitary tumors). MRI shows a poorly enhancing sellar-based mass, which is extending inferiorly through the floor of the sella into the sphenoid sinus. Compared with nonfunctioning pituitary adenomas, GH-secreting adenomas demonstrate a greater propensity for infrasellar extension. In one study, infrasellar growth in isolation was observed in 20% of GH-secreting tumors compared with just 3% of nonfunctioning pituitary adenomas. This patient also has high blood pressure, albeit not at values that would necessarily be expected to be associated with headache, but this could be a manifestation of a somatotroph adenoma.

The IGF-1 concentration is not raised and therefore appears to rule out acromegaly. But there is an important potential confounder in the interpretation of this patient's laboratory results: the oral contraceptive pill. Several studies have shown that serum IGF-1 levels may be suppressed by oral estrogen therapy, as well as in women with acromegaly who receive treatment with selective estrogen receptor modulators (SERMs). This has led to the proposal that oral estrogen or SERM therapy may be a useful adjunct in normalizing serum IGF-1 in women with persistent acromegaly following primary/secondary treatment. The effect is considered to be mediated through peripheral antagonism of GH action, rather than central suppression of GH secretion.

It is also important to recognize that in milder cases of acromegaly (as in this patient) normalization or near-normalization of serum IGF-1, as a consequence of concomitant combined oral contraceptive pill use, may mask the underlying diagnosis. In this context, discontinuation of the pill with subsequent measurement of serum IGF-1 and/or performing an oral glucose tolerance test to assess for GH suppression (Answer C) helps confirm or exclude the diagnosis.

Although Cushing syndrome is an important differential diagnosis to consider, most corticotroph tumors are microadenomas. In addition, screening for autonomous cortisol secretion with the 1-mg overnight dexamethasone-suppression test (as occurred here) while continuing to take the combined oral contraceptive preparation significantly increases the risk of a false-positive result. Oral estrogen triggers a rise in cortisol-binding globulin, leading to false-positive dexamethasone-suppressed serum cortisol in immunoassays, which measure total (as opposed to free) serum cortisol. Therefore, performing a 48-hour (0.5 mg every 6 hours) dexamethasone-suppression test (Answer D) is also not advisable until the pill has been discontinued for 6 weeks. Oral contraceptive pill use also accounts for the suppressed gonadotropin levels in this patient rather than this being a manifestation of hypercortisolism.

Late-night salivary cortisol measurement (Answer B) offers an alternative means of screening for Cushing syndrome, but it is likely to return normal results in this patient, who is more likely to have acromegaly than Cushing disease.

Bilateral inferior petrosal sinus sampling (Answer A) is only required in patients with confirmed ACTH-dependent Cushing syndrome in whom a central source has not been conclusively demonstrated through laboratory and radiologic investigation.

Measurement of serum prolactin in dilution to exclude the "hook effect" (Answer E) should be considered in any patient with a large/giant pituitary macroadenoma in whom serum prolactin is normal or only mildly raised. This ensures that an important treatment option (dopamine agonist therapy) is not inappropriately excluded. However, a recent study of 14 different immunoassay platforms revealed only a single modern assay to be sensitive to the hook effect, suggesting that this is less likely to be a problem for most laboratories. Severe hyperprolactinemia due to a prolactin-secreting adenoma is very unlikely here, especially with a macroadenoma that is smaller than 2 cm in maximum diameter.

Educational Objective

Explain how a combined oral contraceptive preparation can markedly confound interpretation of pituitary function tests.

Reference(s)

Shimon I, Barkan A. Estrogen treatment for acromegaly. *Pituitary.* 2012;15(4):601-607. PMID: 22933045

Cozzi R, Barausse M, Lodrini S, Lasio S, Attanasio R. Estroprogestinic pill normalizes IGF-I levels in acromegalic women. *J Endocrinol Invest.* 2003;26(4):347-352. PMID: 12841543

Duarte FH, Jallad RS, Bronstein MD. Estrogens and selective estrogen receptor modulators in acromegaly. *Endocrine.* 2016;54(2):306-314. PMID: 27704479

39 ANSWER: C) Linagliptin

Chronic kidney disease (CKD) is associated with insulin resistance, a condition that can lead to worsening hyperglycemia. However, as CKD progresses, patients with diabetes may experience a decrease in insulin requirements or even a cessation of insulin therapy, as has the patient in this vignette, due to a reduction of insulin clearance. However, monitoring patients with advanced CKD, and especially those with end-stage kidney disease requiring hemodialysis, can be difficult. Relying on hemoglobin A_{1c} to assess glycemic control can be problematic, as these patients sometimes have anemia or altered red cell turnover because they are also receiving treatment with erythropoiesis-stimulating agents that can alter hemoglobin A_{1c} levels. Hemoglobin A_{1c} levels should be correlated with the reported point-of-care glucose values. When there is a discrepancy, further investigation using other glycemic markers may be needed. In this patient, however, there is a good correlation between hemoglobin A_{1c} and point-of-care glucose values.

Treating patients with advanced CKD/end-stage kidney disease can also be challenging. Although reducing hyperglycemia represents an important management goal, diabetes agents should be carefully used to avoid the risk of hypoglycemia. The patient in this scenario has a mildly elevated hemoglobin A_{1c} value, and a basal-bolus insulin regimen (Answer A) to address this mild hyperglycemia may significantly increase the risk for hypoglycemia. Hypoglycemia is associated with increased morbidity and mortality, especially in this population with frequently coexisting and sometimes undiagnosed cardiovascular disease.

Noninsulin medications could be reasonable alternatives; however, some of these medications cannot be used in patients with diabetes and end-stage kidney disease. Empagliflozin (Answer B) and other SGLT-2 inhibitors are not approved to be used in the setting of end-stage kidney disease and have less glucose-lowering efficacy in patients with a very low estimated glomerular filtration rate.

There are limited data to support the use of semaglutide (Answer D) or other GLP-1 receptor agonists in this population with end-stage kidney disease. GLP-1 receptor agonists could be potentially used among patients with end-stage kidney disease and obesity when weight loss is one of the treatment goals. These medications can induce significant unintentional weight loss, which would be undesirable in this patient with end-stage kidney disease and low BMI. As unintentional weight loss is a manifestation of uremia, this can further lead clinicians to consider that the patient may be having ineffective dialysis sessions. In addition, weight loss and cachexia are significant concerns in patients with end-stage kidney disease, and most of these patients need nutritional support to maintain or promote weight gain rather than weight loss.

DPP-4 inhibitors such as linagliptin (Answer C) are glucose-lowering medications that can be used in patients with mild hyperglycemia. For patients with CKD, and especially end-stage kidney disease, these medications have 2 important advantages. First, DPP-4 inhibitors do not cause hypoglycemia, which makes them extremely useful in these patients who are particularly vulnerable to low glucose values. Second, these medications are relatively safe in patients with CKD. More significantly, and specifically for linagliptin, this medication is only minimally excreted in the urine. Thus, linagliptin does not require dosage adjustment in patients with worsening kidney function.

There is ongoing discussion about the appropriate glycemic targets in patients with underlying comorbidities. Clinical practice guidelines recommend individualized targets and, in some situations, higher hemoglobin A_{1c} target values in individuals with certain underlying medical conditions, mainly because of concerns about hypoglycemia. Hypoglycemia can have a marked effect in patients with CKD/end-stage kidney disease and possible underlying undiagnosed cardiovascular disease. However, for this patient, a medication with no hypoglycemic properties can be prescribed to achieve better glycemic control with minimal additional risk. Thus, adding no new medications (Answer E) is not an appropriate option.

Educational Objective

Recommend medical treatment options in patients with end-stage kidney disease and type 2 diabetes mellitus.

Reference(s)

McGill JB, Sloan L, Newman J, et al. Long-term efficacy and safety of linagliptin in patients with type 2 diabetes and severe renal impairment: a 1-year, randomized, double-blind, placebo-controlled study. *Diabetes Care.* 2013;36(2):237-244. PMID: 23033241

40

ANSWER: E) Topical testosterone replacement

This man has clear-cut organic primary hypogonadism due to (unexplained) testicular pathology and is symptomatic. He has mild anemia, reduced muscle bulk, and osteopenia, features that are, in the absence of other causes, consistent with longstanding, suboptimally treated hypogonadism even preceding his myocardial infarction. Hypogonadism-associated reduced muscle bulk and osteopenia take months to years to manifest. Indeed, previous treatment (testosterone enanthate, 200 mg intramuscularly monthly) was inadequate; the usual dosage is 150 to 200 mg every 2 weeks. Even then, use of testosterone esters (testosterone enanthate or cypionate) leads to nonphysiologic peaks and valleys in serum testosterone concentrations. While there is no evidence that such peaks and troughs are associated with increased cardiovascular risk compared with transdermal testosterone treatment, there is some evidence that, in older men, testosterone ester treatment is associated with a higher risk of erythrocytosis (a potential but not proven cardiovascular risk factor) compared with transdermal preparations. Moreover, injectable testosterone may be associated with hematoma risk given dual antiplatelet therapy (although this is uncommon in clinical practice). Testosterone is indicated to treat his severe hypogonadism. For the reasons discussed, topical therapy (Answer E) with the appropriate contact precautions (to avoid skin-to-skin transfer to other people) is a good option, as it can be titrated to the desired serum testosterone concentration.

Effects of testosterone treatment on cardiovascular outcomes remain unknown because there are currently no published primary endpoint clinical trials evaluating cardiovascular outcomes (eg, major adverse cardiac events). One such study (TRAVERSE [ClinicalTrials.gov Identifier: NCT03518034]) is currently underway. In some observational studies, increased serum testosterone has been associated with a decreased risk of cardiovascular events, but these studies may be confounded by low testosterone reflecting unmeasured comorbidities that themselves increase cardiovascular risk. Retrospective studies of testosterone treatment have suggested either reduced risks of cardiovascular events, neutral effects, or increased risks; such retrospective studies have significant methodologic shortcomings, including confounding by indication (ie, preferential treatment of healthier men) and time-related biases. Clinical trials of testosterone treatment have likewise been mixed, with one study in older men with mobility limitations reporting an increased risk of cardiovascular events while there was no increased risk in a similar trial in frail older men. Of note, all the evidence discussed stems from men with age-related reductions in serum testosterone, and men with organic hypogonadism have been excluded from randomized controlled trials, including TRAVERSE, given that it is generally considered unethical to subject men with organic hypogonadism (the only currently FDA-supported indication for testosterone treatment) to placebo therapy. While current Endocrine Society guidelines recommend against testosterone therapy in men with uncontrolled heart failure, myocardial infarction, or stroke within the last 6 months, this recommendation refers to men with age-related hypogonadism, in whom the benefit-to-risk ratio of testosterone treatment may be different from that in men with established hypogonadism. Thus, concerns regarding cardiovascular risk may be a reason not to offer testosterone treatment to men with age-related testosterone reductions, in whom low testosterone may be a consequence of comorbidities (especially obesity, the so-called eugonadal sick syndrome) rather than a rectifiable contributor to ill health. However, the situation is different in clear-cut organic hypogonadism such as in this vignette, where withholding testosterone replacement would have adverse effects on sexual function, energy levels, and musculoskeletal health.

After discussion and a shared decision-making process that included his cardiologist (noting that results of a cardiac stress test 1 month after the deployment of his coronary stent were normal), testosterone treatment was started. He had marked symptom improvement, including normalization of libido and erectile function and improved quality of life.

Untreated hypogonadism is associated with reduced response to phosphodiesterase-5 inhibitor treatment (Answer D), and these agents would not be first-line therapy for erectile dysfunction in this man. Moreover, phosphodiesterase-5 inhibitor treatment would not address his other clinical features of hypogonadism. This medication class would be an option should erectile dysfunction persist despite testosterone treatment.

Clomiphene (a selective estrogen-receptor modulator) (Answer C) and aromatase inhibitors (Answer A) are used by some practitioners to increase serum testosterone because both agents inhibit the estradiol-mediated negative feedback on GnRH and gonadotropin secretion. However, these agents are ineffective for organic hypogonadism, especially primary hypogonadism, where gonadotropins are already elevated. While both agents can increase serum testosterone in men with functional suppression of the central hypothalamic-pituitary-gonadal axis, there is no evidence that this leads to clinical benefit, and aromatase inhibitors may further reduce bone mineral density.

Although cholecalciferol (Answer B) may be indicated because of this patient's osteopenia, it would not improve his hypogonadal symptoms.

Educational Objective

Treat established hypogonadism (organic hypogonadism) with testosterone and explain why the benefits outweigh the hypothetical cardiac risks.

Reference(s)

Bhasin S, Brito JP, Cunningham GR, et al. Testosterone therapy in men with hypogonadism: an Endocrine Society clinical practice guideline. *J Clin Endocrinol Metab.* 2018;103(5):1715-1744. PMID: 29562364

Jayasena CN, Lok Tung Ho C, Bhasin S. The effects of testosterone treatment on cardiovascular health. *Endocrinol Metab Clin N Am.* 2022;51(1):109-122. PMID: 35216710

Park K, Ku JH, Kim SW, Paick J-S. Risk factors in predicting a poor response to sildenafil citrate in elderly men with erectile dysfunction. *BJU Int.* 2005;95(3):366-370. PMID: 15679795

41 ANSWER: C) Genetic testing

Primary aldosteronism and Cushing syndrome should be suspected in patients with early-onset hypertension and hypokalemia. In this patient, screening for primary aldosteronism showed undetectable renin on 2 occasions; the plasma aldosterone concentration was considerably higher when tested in the morning vs the afternoon value. A second important element in this patient's history is the development of profound hypokalemia with hydrochlorothiazide use. These 2 features, along with the young age at hypertension onset, are suggestive of familial hyperaldosteronism type 1, also known as glucocorticoid remediable aldosteronism (GRA).

GRA is an autosomal dominant disorder caused by a chimeric gene composed of the promoter region of the *CYP11B1* gene and the coding sequences of *CYP11B2* gene. Steroid 11β-hydroxylase (CYP11B1) is expressed in the zona fasciculata of the adrenal cortex, where it catalyzes the conversion of 11-deoxycortisol to cortisol. Aldosterone synthase (CYP11B2) is expressed in the zona glomerulosa, and it executes the last steps in aldosterone synthesis. CYP11B1 is regulated by ACTH, while CYP11B2 function is controlled primarily by renin, although it also responds acutely to ACTH. In patients with GRA, aldosterone secretion occurs in the zona fasciculata, under the governance of ACTH, and it follows the ACTH circadian rhythm, with higher concentrations in the early morning than in the evening.

Patients with GRA are prone to marked hypokalemia following thiazide diuretic use because of an increase in sodium delivery to the distal nephron. Hemorrhagic strokes caused by ruptured intracranial aneurysms are common in individuals with GRA. Affected persons produce elevated amounts of 18-hydroxycortisol and 18-oxocortisol, due to the combined action of 17α-hydroxylase (CYP17A1) and CYP11B2 in the zona fasciculata. Elevations of these steroids support the diagnosis.

Reflecting its regulation by ACTH, aldosterone synthesis is suppressed by dexamethasone in patients with GRA. A 1-mg dexamethasone-suppression test (Answer B) can be used for GRA screening, but because this test has a high rate of false-positive results, genetic testing (Answer C) is required to establish the diagnosis. Patient with GRA can be treated with physiologic dosages of glucocorticoids or mineral corticoid receptor antagonists.

A captopril challenge test (Answer A) and oral salt-loading test (Answer E) are used to confirm primary aldosteronism in patients with positive screening. Confirmatory testing is not necessary in patients with hypertension, a plasma aldosterone concentration greater than 20 ng/dL (>554.8 pmol/L), undetectable renin, and hypokalemia.

Measurement of 24-hour urinary cortisol (Answer D) and dexamethasone-suppression testing (Answer B) are valuable for the diagnosis of endogenous Cushing syndrome. Because this patient did not display any clinical signs of hypercortisolism, testing for Cushing syndrome has lower priority than testing for primary aldosteronism.

Educational Objective

Identify the clinical features of glucocorticoid-remediable aldosteronism and select appropriate diagnostic tests.

Reference(s)

Rich GM, Ulick S, Cook S, Wang JZ, Lifton RP, Dluhy RG. Glucocorticoid-remediable aldosteronism in a large kindred: clinical spectrum and diagnosis using a characteristic biochemical phenotype. *Ann Intern Med.* 1992;116(10):813-820. PMID: 1567095

Dluhy RG, Lifton RP. Glucocorticoid-remediable aldosteronism. *Endocrinol Metab Clin North Am.* 1994;23(2):285-297. PMID: 8070423

Litchfield WR, New MI, Coolidge C, Lifton RP, Dluhy RG. Evaluation of the dexamethasone suppression test for the diagnosis of glucocorticoid-remediable aldosteronism. *J Clin Endocrinol Metab.* 1997;82(11):3570-3573. PMID: 9360508

42 ANSWER: A) Functional hypothalamic amenorrhea

Functional hypothalamic amenorrhea (Answer A) is caused by suppression of the hypothalamic-pituitary-ovarian axis, and it most commonly occurs secondary to disordered eating, weight loss, excessive exercise, and psychological stress. In functional hypothalamic amenorrhea, GnRH pulsatile secretion from the hypothalamus is suppressed, which reduces LH and FSH. This hypogonadotropic hypogonadism leads to a hypoestrogenic state. In evaluating such patients, obtaining a detailed history is critical and should include eating and physical activity habits, psychosocial stressors, changes in body weight, and chronic illness. The history should also include questions that can rule out other possible explanations for amenorrhea such as prolactinoma (galactorrhea, headaches, visual field defects), polycystic ovary syndrome (acne, hirsutism), and primary ovarian insufficiency (vasomotor symptoms).

This patient is feeling very stressed within her graduate school environment, has lost substantial weight, limits her nutritional intake, and is engaged in intensive physical exercise. In addition, she did not have a withdrawal bleed with progesterone therapy, and pelvic ultrasonography demonstrates a normal uterine lining, which indicates a low estrogen state. Her biochemical evaluation also demonstrates a hypogonadotropic hypoestrogenic state that is consistent with functional hypothalamic amenorrhea and rules out primary ovarian insufficiency (Answer D). Primary ovarian insufficiency is diagnosed by the presence of elevated FSH and low estradiol.

She has no signs or symptoms of pituitary excess or a pituitary adenoma, and laboratory values for the remaining anterior pituitary hormones are within normal limits. Taken together, these findings make the likelihood of a pituitary adenoma (Answer B) much less likely.

Given that findings on pelvic ultrasonography are normal other than mild polycystic ovarian morphology, uterine outflow tract obstruction (Answer E) can be excluded as the cause of secondary amenorrhea.

In some cases, there can be overlap in functional hypothalamic amenorrhea and polycystic ovary syndrome (Answer C), and both are considered diagnoses of exclusion. Given that this woman has no signs of androgen excess, has only mild polycystic ovarian morphology on pelvic ultrasonography, and has a normal antimullerian hormone concentration, polycystic ovary syndrome is less likely than functional hypothalamic amenorrhea. Importantly, the finding of polycystic ovarian morphology on ultrasonography does not diagnose polycystic ovary syndrome. Antimullerian hormone is produced by small antral and preantral ovarian follicles, and there is a strong association between elevated antimullerian hormone and increased antral follicle reserve in the body, as well as with hyperandrogenism. Therefore, antimullerian hormone is thought to be a strong tool to aid in the diagnosis of polycystic ovary syndrome. In this patient, the antimullerian hormone level is normal, further supporting the diagnosis of functional hypothalamic amenorrhea.

In fact, after this woman sought mental health counseling, received counseling from a nutritionist, decreased her intensive physical activity, and gained 11 lb (5 kg), her menses resumed.

Educational Objective

Diagnose and treat functional hypothalamic amenorrhea.

Reference(s)

Gibson MES, Fleming N, Zuijdwijk C, Dumont T. Where have the periods gone? The evaluation and management of functional hypothalamic amenorrhea. *J Clin Res Pediatr Endocrinol.* 2020;12(Suppl 1):18-27. PMID: 32041389

Gordon CM, Ackerman KE, Berga SL, et al. Functional hypothalamic amenorrhea: an Endocrine Society clinical practice guideline. *J Clin Endocrinol Metab.* 2017;102(5):1413-1439. PMID: 28368518

Klein DA, Paradise SL, Reeder RM. Amenorrhea: a systematic approach to diagnosis and management. *Am Fam Physician.* 2019;100(1):39-48. PMID: 31259490

Wang JG, Lobo RA. The complex relationship between hypothalamic amenorrhea and polycystic ovary syndrome. *J Clin Endocrinol Metab.* 2008;93(4):1394-1397. PMID: 18230664

43

ANSWER: B) Administer a dose of NPH insulin at bedtime and continue insulin glargine

Use of atypical antipsychotic agents may unmask or precipitate hyperglycemia. Antipsychotic medications have been reported to increase the risk of diabetes through weight gain and directly by adversely affecting insulin sensitivity and secretion. This patient is taking quetiapine, a dopamine antagonist. His worsening glycemic control occurred shortly after initiating this therapy, and his glycemic profile shows that his blood glucose seems to deteriorate most significantly shortly after administration and lasts through the night. He has been taking a large dose of short-acting insulin at 9 AM to manage the hyperglycemia. To address this acute rise in nocturnal blood glucose, initiating a dose of NPH at bedtime and continuing insulin glargine (Answer B) would be most appropriate.

Increasing the dosage of insulin glargine (Answer D) could help to improve nocturnal control/fasting blood glucose. However, it would also have an effect during the rest of the day, when his blood glucose control is usually much better, thereby increasing his risk of hypoglycemia.

Prescribing a sulfonylurea (Answer E) for this patient with latent autoimmune diabetes in adults would not be expected to improve glycemic control because of a reduction or lack of β-cell function.

Administering a dose of short-acting insulin at bedtime (Answer A) would help to address nocturnal hyperglycemia, but its duration of action is shorter than that of NPH, so it would not be effective in improving and maintaining glycemic control through most of the night.

Administering a dose of NPH insulin at bedtime and stopping insulin glargine (Answer C) would be incorrect in this patient with latent autoimmune diabetes in adults and a lack of β-cell function, as evidenced by the undetectable C-peptide in the setting of hyperglycemia. He requires basal insulin throughout the entire 24-hour period, and once-daily NPH insulin at bedtime would not provide this coverage. Another option would be to stop insulin glargine and add a dose of NPH insulin at bedtime and a second dose of NPH insulin in the morning.

Educational Objective

Explain how dopamine antagonist therapy can increase blood glucose concentrations and adjust insulin regimens to address the effect these agents have on glycemic control.

Reference(s)

Holt RIG. Association between antipsychotic medication use and diabetes. *Curr Diab Rep.* 2019;19(10):96. PMID: 31478094

Koller EA, Weber J, Doraiswamy PM, Schneider BS. A survey of reports of quetiapine-associated hyperglycemia and diabetes mellitus. *J Clin Psychiatry.* 2004;65(6):857-863. PMID: 15291665

Liao TV, Phan SV. Acute hyperglycemia associated with short-term use of atypical antipsychotic medications. *Drugs.* 2014;74(2):183-194. PMID: 24399515

Wu CY, Mitchell SR, Seyfried LS, Quetiapine-induced hyperglycemic crisis and severe hyperlipidemia: a case report and review of the literature. *Psychosomatics.* 2014;55(6):686-691. PMID: 25497507

44

ANSWER: B) Perform thyroid laboratory tests in 3 months

Assessment of thyroid function tests in hospitalized ill patients can be challenging, especially in the intensive care unit. Many of these patients have low serum T_4, T_3, and TSH levels. For many years, this condition was called euthyroid sick syndrome, but it is now referred to as nonthyroidal illness syndrome. Although the current name suggests lack of thyroid dysfunction, there is some evidence that affected patients may have acquired transient central hypothyroidism, which may have a protective effect in severe illness in preventing excess tissue catabolism. Several medications used in the intensive care setting, including dopamine, high-dosage steroids, and dobutamine, can also decrease serum TSH levels. Additionally, cytokines and inflammation can lower serum TSH, possibly by reducing production of hypothalamic thyrotropin-releasing hormone. Whether the thyroid hormone abnormalities are due to physiologic adaptation or pathologic changes remains controversial. Most such patients recover appropriate hypothalamic-pituitary-thyroid axis function after recovering from their illness. Therefore, it is crucial to use clinical judgment and reasoning to diagnose the patient correctly, recommend appropriate treatment, and avoid overtreatment with thyroid hormone supplementation. T_4 and T_3 replacement has been used in patients with nonthyroidal illness, but this practice is controversial.

This patient's thyroid function values are probably related to his current illness rather than an underlying thyroid disorder. Therefore, the best action is to repeat thyroid function tests in 3 months (Answer B) when his condition has improved and he has most likely been discharged from the hospital. If the values are abnormal 3 to 6 months after he has recovered from his illness, additional evaluation should be pursued.

His clinical findings are not consistent with hypothyroidism and his laboratory results are unlikely to be due to central hypothyroidism requiring treatment. Therefore, there is no need to perform pituitary MRI (Answer A).

Thyroid ultrasonography (Answer C) is not indicated, especially given that his thyroid gland is not palpable.

Initiation of levothyroxine (Answer D) or liothyronine (Answer E) in a patient with nonthyroidal illness syndrome is not recommended. Thyroid hormone replacement has not been shown to be beneficial in critically ill patients with low serum T_3 and/or low T_4 concentrations. Furthermore, intravenous triiodothyronine administration in patients undergoing coronary artery bypass graft surgery who have low serum T_3 does not demonstrate any clinical benefit.

Educational Objective

Diagnose and manage nonthyroidal illness syndrome.

Reference(s)

Fliers E, Boelen A. An update on non-thyroidal illness syndrome. *J Endocrinol Invest.* 2021;44(8):1597-1607. PMID: 33320308

Brent GA, Hershman JM. Thyroxine therapy in patients with severe nonthyroidal illnesses and low serum thyroxine concentration. *J Clin Endocrinol Metab.* 1986;63(1):1-8. PMID: 3011834

Chopra IJ. Clinical review 86: euthyroid sick syndrome: is it a misnomer? *J Clin Endocrinol Metab.* 1997;82(2):329-334. PMID: 9024211

Becker RA, Vaughan GM, Ziegler MG, et al. Hypermetabolic low triiodothyronine syndrome of burn injury. *Crit Care Med.* 1982;10(12):870-875. PMID: 7140337

Klemperer JD, Klein I, Gomez M, et al. Thyroid hormone treatment after coronary-artery bypass surgery. *N Engl J Med.* 1995;333(23):1522-1527. PMID: 7477166

Bennett-Guerrero E, Jimenez JL, White WD, D'Amico EB, Baldwin BI, Schwinn DA. Cardiovascular effects of intravenous triiodothyronine in patients undergoing coronary artery bypass graft surgery. A randomized, double-blind, placebo-controlled trial. Duke T3 study group. *JAMA.* 1996;275(9):687-692. PMID: 8594265

45 **ANSWER: C) 24-Hour urinary calcium and creatinine excretion**

The Roux-en-Y gastric bypass is a metabolic surgery that leads to significant weight loss and can improve weight-related comorbidities such as type 2 diabetes, fatty liver disease, hypertension, and sleep apnea. The resultant anatomy bypasses the duodenum and proximal jejunum, which are the predominant sites of active transcellular 1,25-dihydroxyvitamin D–mediated calcium uptake. Although calcium can be absorbed passively throughout the rest of the intestine, fractional calcium absorption decreases from 33% preoperatively to 7% postoperatively when assessed using the dual stable isotope method in patients who have undergone Roux-en-Y gastric bypass and are on adequate supplementation of vitamin D (goal concentration >30 ng/mL [74.9 nmol/L]) and calcium (1200 mg daily). Patients who have undergone Roux-en-Y gastric bypass often require higher amounts of calcium supplementation in divided doses throughout the day to enhance calcium absorption. Additionally, these patients are at risk for enteric hyperoxaluria. Calcium-containing supplements bind dietary oxalate and reduce oxalate absorption and enteric hyperoxaluria. Citrated calcium salts are preferred following Roux-en-Y gastric bypass because of hypochlorhydria resulting from a low-acid environment secondary to creation of a gastric pouch.

Calcium and vitamin D malabsorption after Roux-en-Y gastric bypass can contribute to the development of secondary hyperparathyroidism. In addition to calcium and vitamin D malabsorption and rapid weight loss, secondary hyperparathyroidism increases fracture risk in this patient population.

In a patient who has undergone Roux-en-Y gastric bypass surgery, measuring 24-hour urinary calcium and creatinine excretion (Answer C) is the best test to guide adequate calcium and vitamin D intake. This patient had low 24-hour urinary calcium excretion, and increasing her calcium and vitamin D supplementation improved her PTH concentration.

Bone alkaline phosphatase (Answer A) is a marker of bone formation, and its elevation may be seen in the setting of suspected primary or secondary hyperparathyroidism or osteomalacia. However, the alkaline phosphatase value would not provide further information on the etiology of secondary hyperparathyroidism in this case.

Similarly, a parathyroid sestamibi scan (Answer D) is not necessary because this patient has secondary hyperparathyroidism and not primary or tertiary hyperparathyroidism, which are indications for parathyroidectomy.

Low serum magnesium (Answer E) is associated with hypocalcemia and can impair both the secretion and action of PTH. Thus, the typical clinical scenario associated with hypomagnesemia is hypocalcemia and hypoparathyroidism, not hyperparathyroidism.

Measuring 1,25-dihydroxyvitamin D (Answer B) would not provide additional information, as the conversion of 25-hydroxyvitamin D to its active form is not affected by Roux-en-Y gastric bypass and would not explain the elevated PTH concentration.

Educational Objective

Identify secondary hyperparathyroidism as a complication of Roux-en-Y gastric bypass.

Reference(s)

Schafer AL, Weaver CM, Black DM, et al. Intestinal calcium absorption decreases dramatically after gastric bypass surgery despite optimization of vitamin D status. *J Bone Miner Res.* 2015;30(8):1377-1385. PMID: 25640580

Hewitt S, Sovik TT, Aasheim ET, et al. Secondary hyperparathyroidism, vitamin D sufficiency, and serum calcium 5 years after gastric bypass and duodenal switch. *Obes Surg.* 2013;23(3):384-390. PMID: 23015268

46 ANSWER: E) Recommend discontinuation of cannabis

The absence of abdominal symptoms between the reported episodes of diabetic ketoacidosis makes evaluation for diabetic gastroparesis (Answer B) unlikely to explain this patient's presentation (hyperglycemia and ketosis but not clearly acidotic).

Similarly, cross-sectional imaging of the abdomen and pelvis (Answer C) would not be expected to yield a finding that would explain his recurrent hospitalizations.

A proton-pump inhibitor (Answer D), although likely to be prescribed, would not be expected to reduce recurrent hospitalizations.

While the recurrent admissions for diabetic ketoacidosis raise the possibility of medication nonadherence, his overall glycemic control according to hemoglobin A_{1c} values does not suggest he is having issues with medication access. Assessing his pharmacy dispensation history (Answer A) is not likely to help address the current clinical issue.

In contrast, cannabis use has been associated with acute presentations suggestive of diabetic ketoacidosis, but with laboratory evaluation showing ketosis without acidosis. This phenomenon begins with nausea in the mornings that progresses to vomiting later in the day, followed by the development of ketosis. One retrospective study reviewed patients with type 1 diabetes seen in an emergency department with a diagnosis code of diabetic ketoacidosis. The authors documented that while β-hydroxybutyrate levels were similarly elevated in patients who used cannabis and in patients who did not, pH and bicarbonate levels were significantly lower in those who did not use cannabis. In this setting, cannabis users had pH and bicarbonate values that were not characteristic of diabetic ketoacidosis. This may be related to known respiratory changes that occur with cannabis use or metabolic alkalosis associated with vomiting. This issue is clinically important, as treatment decisions are often made based on these parameters. In a sense, the cannabis use "masks" diabetic ketoacidosis. Therefore, practitioners should be vigilant for excessive cannabis use in persons presenting with diabetic ketoacidosis but whose pH and bicarbonate levels are not low. Cannabis use, particularly long-term use of higher-potency formulations, is associated with a cyclical vomiting syndrome that may cause metabolic alkalosis. Cessation of cannabis use (Answer E) is the best recommendation for this patient with type 1 diabetes.

Educational Objective

Diagnose hyperglycemic ketosis and cannabinoid hyperemesis syndrome and explain how this condition can mask diabetic ketoacidosis.

Reference(s)

Hennessy A. Cannabis masks diabetic ketoacidosis. *BMJ Case Rep.* 2011;2011:bcr0220102716. PMID: 22679145

Kinney GL, Akturk HK, Taylor DD, Foster NC, Shah VN. Cannabis use is associated with increased risk for diabetic ketoacidosis in adults with type 1 diabetes: findings from the T1D Exchange Clinic Registry. *Diabetes Care.* 2020;43(1):247-249. PMID: 31628116

Akturk HA, Snell-Bergeon J, Kinney GL, Champakanath A, Monte A, Shah VN. Differentiating diabetic ketoacidosis and hyperglycemic ketosis due to cannabis hyperemesis syndrome in adults with type 1 diabetes. *Diabetes Care.* 2022;45(2):481-483. PMID: 34880067

47 **ANSWER: C) Increased bone mineral density**

The expected physical changes with estrogen therapy in transgender women include breast growth and tenderness, changes in body fat distribution, and cessation of erections. However, such therapy can pose some risks, so it is imperative that the clinician counsel patients regarding these risks.

There is a significantly increased risk of thromboembolism with estrogen therapy. In a report by van Kesteren et al of 816 female transgender patients, the risk for thromboembolism was nearly 20-fold higher (not lower [Answer A]) compared with risk in cis-men.

Estradiol therapy changes the lipid profile and increases (not decreases [Answer B]) triglycerides. In persons with preexisting hypertriglyceridemia, oral estrogen therapy can precipitate pancreatitis.

In one of the largest cross-sectional studies of transgender women receiving estrogen therapy, Gooren et al reported no apparent increased risk of breast cancer (Answer D) compared with risk in cis-men and cis-women.

The risk of prostate cancer appears to be decreased, not increased (Answer E), in transgender women treated with estrogen.

Several studies have reported that transgender women have lower bone mineral density than age-matched cis-gender male patients. The reason for this is unclear, but some experts speculate that lower vitamin D levels and/or less physical activity could contribute. In a meta-analysis by Singh-Ospina et al, estrogen therapy in transgender female patients led to an increase in lumbar spine bone mineral density (Answer C) 12 months and 24 months after initiation of therapy. Although testosterone is important for skeletal maturation and bone mineral density maintenance, estrogen has been confirmed to play a more dominant role in the skeleton than testosterone in both males and females. Despite an increase in bone mineral density, fracture risk remains higher in older transgender women compared with risk in cis-men, as reported in a cross-sectional study by Wiepjes et al.

Educational Objective

Determine the physiologic changes that occur with gender-affirming estrogen therapy.

Reference(s)

Hembree WC, Cohen-Kettenis P, Delemarre-van de Waal HA, et al; Endocrine Society. Endocrine treatment of transsexual persons: an Endocrine Society clinical practice guideline. *J Clin Endocrinol Metab.* 2009;94(9):3132-3154. PMID: 19509099

van Kesteren PJ, Asscheman H, Megens JA, Gooren LJ. Mortality and morbidity in transsexual subjects treated with cross-sex hormones. *Clin Endocrinol (Oxf).* 1997;47(3):337-342. PMID: 9373456

Goldenberg NM, Wang P, Glueck CJ. An observational study of severe hypertriglyceridemia, hypertriglyceridemic acute pancreatitis, and failure of triglyceride-lowering therapy when estrogens are given to women with and without familial hypertriglyceridemia. *Clin Chim Acta.* 2003;332(1-2):11-19. PMID: 12763274

Gooren LJ, van Trotsenburg MA, Giltay EJ, van Diest PJ. Breast cancer development in transsexual subjects receiving cross-sex hormone treatment. *J Sex Med.* 2013;10(12):3129-3134. PMID: 24010586

Van Caenegem E, Taes Y, Wierckx K, et al. Low bone mass is prevalent in male-to-female transsexual persons before the start of cross-sex hormonal therapy and gonadectomy. *Bone.* 2013;54(1):92-97. PMID: 23369987

Stevenson MO, Tangpricha V. Osteoporosis and bone health in transgender persons. *Endocrinol Metab Clin North Am.* 2019;48(2):421-427. PMID: 31027549

Singh-Ospina N, Maraka S, Rodriguez-Gutierrez R, et al. Effect of sex steroids on the bone health of transgender individuals: a systematic review and meta-analysis. *J Clin Endocrinol Metab.* 2017;102(11):3904-3913. PMID: 28945851

Wiepjes CM, de Blok CJ, Staphorsius AS, et al. Fracture risk in trans women and trans men using long-term gender-affirming hormonal treatment: a nationwide cohort study. *J Bone Miner Res.* 2020;35(1):64-70. PMID: 31487065

48 ANSWER: A) Calculate his Fibrosis-4 (FIB-4) score

This patient has type 2 diabetes mellitus, obesity, hyperlipidemia, and elevated liver enzymes. In patients with type 2 diabetes and elevated liver enzymes, the best next step is evaluation for metabolic dysfunction-associated steatotic liver disease (formerly termed nonalcoholic fatty liver disease). The easiest method in the clinical setting is to calculate the Fibrosis-4 (FIB-4) score (Answer A), which uses age, AST, ALT, and platelets to assign a risk score for possible fibrosis (*see equation*).

$$\text{FIB-4} = \text{age (years)} \times [\text{AST (U/L)}/\sqrt{(\text{PLT } [10^9/\text{L}])} \times \text{ALT (U/L)}]$$

A FIB-4 score less than 1.3 is deemed low risk for fibrosis, 1.3 to 2.67 is intermediate risk, and greater than 2.67 is high risk for hepatic fibrosis.

The FIB-4 is not valid for persons 35 years and younger. If the FIB-4 score is high, referral to gastroenterology is warranted for further evaluation of possible high-grade hepatic fibrosis and cirrhosis. Low FIB-4 scores require optimization of metabolic risk factors and periodic reassessment of risk. Intermediate FIB-4 scores should be evaluated with imaging (liver stiffness measurement by elastography) or the enhanced liver fibrosis blood test to further characterize overall hepatic fibrosis/cirrhosis risk. In one study, the prevalence of hepatic steatosis and fibrosis in persons with type 2 diabetes was 70% and 21%, respectively, as determined by liver elastography.

While MRI-based screening (Answer C) is more accurate than the FIB-4 score in assessing liver fibrosis, it is not the first recommended screening method because of cost and limited availability.

Although lifestyle intervention (Answers D and E) is recommended as prevention and treatment of metabolic dysfunction-associated steatotic liver disease, it is not the best next step in evaluating this patient's elevated liver enzymes and overall risk for hepatic fibrosis and cirrhosis.

Stopping statin therapy or decreasing the dosage (Answer B) is not recommended in the setting of mildly elevated liver enzymes. In fact, persons with diabetes mellitus and metabolic dysfunction-associated steatotic liver disease are at high risk for cardiovascular disease and their risk factors should be optimized.

Educational Objective

Evaluate for metabolic dysfunction-associated steatotic liver disease.

Reference(s)

Lomonaco R, Godinez Leiva E, et al. Advanced liver fibrosis is common in patients with type 2 diabetes followed in the outpatient setting: the need for systematic screening. *Diabetes Care.* 2021;44(2):399-406. PMID: 33355256

Kanwal F, Shubrook JH, Younossi Z, et al. Preparing for the NASH epidemic: a call to action. *Diabetes Care.* 2021;44(9):2162-2172. PMID: 34312182

Cusi K, Isaacs S, Barb D, et al. American Association of Clinical Endocrinology clinical practice guideline for the diagnosis and management of nonalcoholic fatty liver disease in primary care and endocrinology clinical settings: co-sponsored by the American Association for the Study of Liver Diseases (AASLD). *Endocr Pract.* 2022;28(5):528-562. PMID: 35569886

49 ANSWER: C) Setmelanotide

Although obesity is generally considered a polygenic disease, certain monogenic forms of obesity are important to recognize. Monogenic obesity typically presents earlier in life and is often characterized by hyperphagia and abnormalities of other organ systems. However, some patients with syndromic forms of obesity are only identified in adulthood, often when they are seen for comorbidities associated with their particular genetic condition.

The patient in this vignette has Bardet-Biedl syndrome, a rare autosomal recessive ciliopathy characterized by obesity, polydactyly, kidney dysfunction, and retinal dystrophy. There are currently 26 recognized biallelic loss-of-function pathogenic variants associated with this condition. Bardet-Biedl syndrome might first be suspected in a fetus with structural kidney disease and polydactyly. Central obesity, which is present in approximately 90% of patients with this condition, usually develops in the first year of life even though birth weight is typically normal. Eye-related symptoms such as decreased visual acuity, photophobia, and loss of color discrimination may not be present until children are school-aged.

Patients with Bardet-Biedl syndrome develop hyperphagia in large part due to impairments in the melanocortin-4 receptor (MC4R) pathway. Setmelanotide (Answer C) is an MC4R agonist. In a phase 3 randomized, double-blind, placebo-controlled trial, participants with Bardet-Biedl syndrome receiving setmelanotide lost approximately 8% body weight in 1 year without the need to change diet or exercise routines. The most commonly reported adverse events were hyperpigmentation of the skin and hair, injection site reactions, nausea, and spontaneous penile erections. In 2022, the US FDA approved setmelanotide for weight management in patients with Bardet-Biedl syndrome who are older than 6 years. Setmelanotide is therefore the best option in this case. Setmelanotide is also approved for weight management in patients older than 6 years who have proopiomelanocortin (POMC) deficiency, PCSK1 deficiency, or leptin receptor deficiency.

Hypogonadism is associated with Bardet-Biedl syndrome, and testosterone (Answer E) could be considered in addition to, but not instead of, setmelanotide therapy.

Recombinant leptin therapy (Answer A) is only effective in the treatment of patients with congenital or acquired generalized lipodystrophy and congenital leptin deficiency, which this patient does not have.

Neither GH (Answer D) nor a GLP-1 receptor agonist (Answer B) would address the underlying disorder, which is hyperphagia secondary to Bardet-Biedl syndrome. GH therapy is used in the management of children with Prader-Willi syndrome.

Educational Objective

Diagnose monogenic forms of obesity that present in adulthood.

Reference(s)

Haws RM, Gordon G, Han JC, Yanovski JA, Yuan G, Stewart MW. The efficacy and safety of setmelanotide in individuals with Bardet-Biedl syndrome or Alström syndrome: phase 3 trial design. *Contemp Clin Trials Commun.* 2021;22:100780. PMID: 34013094

50 ANSWER: B) Prescribe propranolol

Immune checkpoints have a critical role in regulating immune function by inhibiting the proliferation, function, and survival of T cells. Immune checkpoint inhibitors, including those that antagonize the cytotoxic T-lymphocyte antigen-4 (CTLA-4) and programmed cell death protein-1 (PD-1) pathways, are approved for the treatment of patients with advanced malignancies and yield immune-mediated anticancer effects.

Endocrine immune-related adverse events are common in the context of immune checkpoint inhibitor therapy. Thyroid dysfunction is the most common endocrine immune-related adverse event, and it occurs most often with combination therapy (anti-CTLA-4 and anti-PD-1/PD-L1 therapy) followed by anti-PD-1 monotherapy. Thyrotoxicosis is seen in 3% of patients treated with a single immune checkpoint inhibitor and in up to 8% of patients treated with combination therapy. The presence of TPO or thyroglobulin antibodies is associated with the development of thyroid immune-related adverse events, including thyrotoxicosis.

The patient described in this vignette presents with thyrotoxicosis after receiving 2 cycles of nivolumab (PD-1 inhibitor) followed by 1 cycle with nivolumab/ipilimumab (CTLA-4 inhibitor). This is consistent with the observation that most patients who experience this immune-related adverse event develop thyrotoxicosis within 3 months of initiating an immune checkpoint inhibitor. Symptoms of thyroid dysfunction are often relatively mild, with fatigue and weight changes predominating, and appear out of proportion to the extreme laboratory perturbations that may be observed. The frankly elevated free T_4 level in combination with the normal T_3 value reported in this vignette is more consistent with thyroiditis than with Graves disease. Conversely, in Graves disease, the measured T_3 to T_4 ratio often exceeds 20. The etiology of immune checkpoint inhibitor–related thyrotoxicosis in most patients is a destructive thyroiditis, which is thought to be mediated by the actions of cytotoxic T cells. A self-limited thyrotoxic phase lasting 3 to 6 weeks is followed by hypothyroidism in approximately three-quarters of cases. Immune checkpoint inhibitor–related Graves disease is rare.

Although more research is needed, several studies have associated endocrine immune-related adverse events with improved cancer responses to immunotherapy. Interruption of immunotherapy generally does not affect the course of endocrine immune-related adverse events and is usually not necessary. Therefore, discontinuing nivolumab/ipilimumab (Answer A) is incorrect.

As destructive thyroiditis is a much more common etiology of thyrotoxicosis than Graves disease in the setting of immunotherapy, initial treatment with a β-adrenergic blocker alone such as propranolol (Answer B) is recommended to manage tachycardia and adrenergic symptoms. Prescribing propranolol and prednisone (Answer D) is incorrect. This would be appropriate medical management for subacute thyroiditis unresponsive to nonsteroidal anti-inflammatory drugs. Subacute thyroiditis generally presents with fever, thyroid pain and tenderness, and thyrotoxicosis after a viral infection, which is inconsistent with the clinical presentation described in this vignette.

Prescribing methimazole in addition to propranolol (Answer C) or referring for radioactive iodine therapy (Answer E) would be appropriate management options for Graves disease but would be ineffective for thyrotoxicosis related to thyroiditis. As such, neither choice is the appropriate initial management option for immune checkpoint inhibitor–related thyrotoxicosis unless the patient has clinical, laboratory, or imaging findings suggestive of Graves disease.

Educational Objective

Recommend the most appropriate initial management of immunotherapy-related thyrotoxicosis.

Reference(s)

Al Ashi SI, Thapa B, Flores M, et al. Endocrine toxicity and outcomes in patients with metastatic malignancies treated with immune checkpoint inhibitors. *J Endocr Soc.* 2021;5(8):bvab100. PMID: 34195529

Barroso-Sousa R, Barry WT, Garrido-Castro AC, et al. Incidence of endocrine dysfunction following the use of different immune checkpoint inhibitor regimens: a systematic review and meta-analysis. *JAMA Oncol.* 2018;4(2):173-182. PMID: 28973656

Brancatella A, Lupi I, Montanelli L, et al. Management of thyrotoxicosis induced by PD1 or PD-L1 blockade. *J Endocr Soc.* 2021;5(9):bvab093. PMID: 34337277

Hattersley R, Nana M, Lansdown AJ. Endocrine complications of immunotherapies: a review. *Clin Med (Lond).* 2021;21(2):e212-e222. PMID: 33762389

Muir CA, Clifton-Bligh RJ, Long GV, et al. Thyroid immune-related adverse events following immune checkpoint inhibitor treatment. *J Clin Endocrinol Metab.* 2021;106(9):e3704-e3713. PMID: 33878162

51 **ANSWER: E) Romosozumab > zoledronate > drug holiday**

Osteoporosis cannot be cured by current medications, and patients at very high fracture risk, such as the one in this vignette, will likely need long-term therapy. The treatment sequence must consider both the patient's current fracture risk and each drug's mechanism of action. The prescriber should consider not only what happens when the drug is being used, but also what happens metabolically when the drug is stopped and any modulating effects of subsequent therapy. Some clinical trials have assessed bone mineral density response in patients previously treated with another class of agents (usually historical bisphosphonate treatment followed by a new agent), and some have evaluated a specific sequence of 2 or more agents (eg, teriparatide followed by a bisphosphonate). However, few studies have prospectively evaluated different treatment sequences for osteoporosis drugs. The DATA-Switch trial is a notable example of the latter (using teriparatide or denosumab in either order sequentially or in combination).

The optimal duration of bisphosphonate therapy remains uncertain. However, because of the long skeletal half-life of bisphosphonates and prolonged effect on bone turnover and fracture risk reduction as demonstrated in clinical trials, drug holidays are considered after 3 to 5 years of bisphosphonate treatment, depending on the posttreatment assessment of the patient's fracture risk. Drug holidays involve cessation of all osteoporosis medications for a period (to be distinguished from switching to a different therapy), and the optimal duration of a drug holiday also remains uncertain. Importantly, compared with bisphosphates, all other osteoporosis medications (both anabolic and antiresorptive) have a more rapid cessation of effect, so they are not considered for drug holidays. Any therapy sequence that includes a drug holiday should have a bisphosphonate as the last medication before the drug holiday.

Given this patient's fracture risk, treatment with the most potent available anabolic medication (romosozumab, a monoclonal antibody to the endogenous bone formation inhibitor sclerostin) followed by an antiresorptive medication before considering a drug holiday would optimize bone mineral density improvement (Answer E). For patients at high risk of fracture, evidence supports initial therapy with an anabolic agent followed by an antiresorptive agent, for both bone mineral density improvements and fracture risk reduction. In Answer A, an anabolic agent is used first followed by the antiresorptive denosumab, which is an appropriate sequence. There is evidence from the DATA-Switch trial that treating with teriparatide followed by denosumab leads to better bone density gains than treating with denosumab followed by teriparatide. In fact, when switching from denosumab to teriparatide (Answer C), bone density at the hip declines significantly rather than increasing. However, in Answer A, denosumab is stopped without a subsequent antiresorptive agent. This would result in a rapid rebound increase in bone resorption, which is associated with decreases in bone mineral density and, in some studies, with vertebral fractures. Therefore, denosumab should not just be stopped for a drug holiday. Unfortunately, switching to a bisphosphonate after denosumab may not always protect against the rebound increase in bone resorption and loss of bone mineral density.

Answer B is suboptimal because prior treatment with a bisphosphonate may blunt the magnitude of bone mineral density response to subsequent anabolic agents such as PTH receptor agonists. However, many payors will not cover anabolic agents without a patient first experiencing treatment failure with an antiresorptive agent. The more important limitation of Answers B and D is that the anabolic agent is followed immediately by a drug holiday, during which time bone density is expected to decrease because of lack of subsequent antiresorptive therapy.

Educational Objective

Describe the expected effects of sequential treatment with osteoporosis medications.

Reference(s)

Leder BZ, Tsai JN, Uihlein AV, et al. Denosumab and teriparatide transitions in postmenopausal osteoporosis (the DATA-Switch study): extension of a randomised controlled trial. *Lancet.* 2015;386(9999):1147-1155. PMID: 26144908

Curtis EM, Reginster J-Y, Al-Daghri N, et al. Management of patients at very high risk of osteoporotic fractures through sequential treatments. *Aging Clin Exp Res.* 2022;34(4):695-714. PMID: 35332506

Makras P, Appelman-Dijkstra NM, Papapoulos SE, et al. The duration of denosumab treatment and the efficacy of zoledronate to preserve bone mineral density after its discontinuation. *J Clin Endocrinol Metab.* 2021;106(10):e4155-e4162. PMID: 33978745

McClung MR, Bolognese MA, Brown JP, et al. A single dose of zoledronate preserves bone mineral density for up to 2 years after a second course of romosozumab. *Osteoporos Int.* 2020;31(11):2231-2241. PMID: 32623487

52 ANSWER: B) Engage in resistance exercise before starting aerobic exercise

This patient has hypoglycemia during aerobic exercise. In persons with insulin-requiring diabetes, this is due to (1) an inability of current regimens to match the normal physiologic decrease in insulin, (2) increased insulin absorption due to increased subcutaneous blood flow, (3) increased muscle uptake of glucose due to insulin-independent GLUT4 trafficking to the cell membranes during muscle contraction, and (4) impaired counterregulatory hormone responses that may depend on the duration of exercise.

The approach to adjusting insulin administration and carbohydrate consumption is based on whether exercise will be conducted in within 90 to 120 minutes of consuming a meal (so-called high insulin state) or several hours after a meal (so-called low insulin state). In general, exercise is recommended to be done in a low insulin state. However, if exercise is to be conducted soon after eating, reducing the preexercise meal bolus by 30% to 50% (Answer E) would be reasonable. However, because this patient does not exercise during a "high insulin state," such a recommendation would be incorrect as it would needlessly expose the patient to postprandial hyperglycemia.

Similarly, consumption of 45 to 60 g of carbohydrates before exercise (Answer A) is an excessive quantity. Of note, consumption of 15 to 30 g of carbohydrates per hour during exercise is suggested to prevent hypoglycemia that occurs during exercise of this duration. For longer-duration exercise, higher amounts of carbohydrates are needed.

Consumption of fat and protein (Answer C) can lead to postprandial hyperglycemia, which may adversely affect exercise performance.

Interestingly, resistance exercise (Answer B) is associated with a slight increase in blood glucose. Although the mechanism is not fully elucidated, this phenomenon is believed to be due to increased circulating levels of counterregulatory hormones and metabolites that reduce glucose uptake into muscle. Studies suggest that resistance training done before aerobic exercise is associated with improved glucose stability through the exercise period and less hypoglycemia during subsequent aerobic exercise. Therefore, among the choices, engaging in resistance training before aerobic exercise would be the most reasonable step to alleviate this patient's hypoglycemia.

Educational Objective

Advise appropriate measures to mitigate hypoglycemia that occurs soon after commencing aerobic exercise in persons with type 1 diabetes mellitus.

Reference(s)

Riddell MC, Gallen IW, Smart CE, et al. Exercise management in type 1 diabetes: a consensus statement. *Lancet Diabetes Endocrinol.* 2017;5(5):377-390. PMID: 28126459

53 ANSWER: D) Referral to psychology for counseling on alcohol overuse

This patient has alcohol-induced hypercortisolism. Nontumoral hypercortisolism, previously called pseudo-Cushing syndrome, can be challenging to diagnose and treat. Nontumoral hypercortisolism can present with or without suggestive clinical manifestations. Conditions in the first category include alcohol abuse and withdrawal, depression and other neuropsychiatric disorders, uncontrolled type 2 diabetes, polycystic ovary syndrome, chronic kidney disease, and glucocorticoid resistance. Conditions without the classic manifestations of hypercortisolism include chronic intense exercise, starvation, or anorexia nervosa. Mechanistically, paraventricular nuclei activation and decreased sensitivity to glucocorticoid feedback have been involved. Unlike tumoral Cushing syndrome, patients with nontumoral hypercortisolism rarely experience progression of manifestations or involvement of multiple organs and systems.

Nontumoral hypercortisolism due to alcohol use is characterized by facial rounding, muscle weakness and wasting, centripetal fat distribution (even in absence of weight gain), striae, and hypertension.

All screening tests can be abnormal in nontumoral hypercortisolism (low-dose dexamethasone suppression, late-night salivary cortisol, and urinary free cortisol). Mechanisms of hypercortisolism include hypothalamic-pituitary-adrenal axis activation, induction of the 11β-hydroxysteroid dehydrogenase type 1 enzyme, and impaired cortisol clearance (the latter from hepatic dysfunction). In this patient, urinary free cortisol was probably spuriously elevated in the context of polyuria. ACTH concentrations can be high-normal or elevated.

Management of nontumoral hypercortisolism is cumbersome and entails close clinical surveillance, repeated screening tests for hypercortisolism, and treatment of the primary condition when possible. In this case, the patient's clinical and biochemical findings normalized after he engaged in counseling and was able to achieve long-term alcohol abstinence (Answer D). Of note, recent alcohol withdrawal may still be associated with abnormal cortisol values.

This patient has hypogonadism due to alcoholism and is at risk for osteoporosis. However, testosterone initiation (Answer E) is not the next step. Instead, this patient should receive counseling and appropriate support to achieve alcohol abstinence with reassessment of his testosterone concentration.

Referral to neurosurgery for transsphenoidal removal of the pituitary adenoma (Answer C) is incorrect because the patient has a small pituitary incidentaloma, which occurs in up to 38% of the general population who undergo brain MRI. Most pituitary microincidentalomas do not enlarge or require any treatment. Although most cases of Cushing disease are caused by microadenomas, biochemical testing has not been completed.

Similarly, inferior petrosal sinus sampling (Answer B) is not indicated in the absence of biochemical confirmation of ACTH-dependent Cushing syndrome.

High-dose dexamethasone-suppression testing (Answer A) has a low accuracy to distinguish pituitary from ectopic ACTH-dependent Cushing syndrome. Also, this patient does not yet have biochemical confirmation of this diagnosis. Dynamic tests with corticotropin-releasing hormone or desmopressin stimulation may be helpful because many patients with nontumoral hypercortisolism have a flat cortisol and ACTH response.

Educational Objective

Diagnose and manage alcohol-induced hypercortisolism.

Reference(s)

Fleseriu M, Auchus R, Bancos I, et al. Consensus on diagnosis and management of Cushing's disease: a guideline update. *Lancet Diabetes Endocrinol.* 2021;9(12):847-875. PMID: 34687601

Nieman LK. Diagnosis of Cushing's syndrome in the modern era. *Endocrinol Metab Clin North Am.* 2018;47(2):259-273. PMID: 29754631

Findling JW, Raff H. Diagnosis of endocrine disease: differentiation of pathologic/neoplastic hypercortisolism (Cushing's syndrome) from physiologic/non-neoplastic hypercortisolism (formerly known as pseudo-Cushing's syndrome). *Eur J Endocrinol.* 2018;178(3):L1-L2. PMID: 28179447

Scaroni C, Albiger NM, Palmieri S, et al; Altogether to Beat Cushing's Syndrome (ABC) Study Group. Approach to patients with pseudo-Cushing's states. *Endocr Connect.* 2020;9(1):R1-R13. PMID: 31846432

54 ANSWER: C) Hypoadrenalism

Tiredness, lethargy, and weight loss may be attributable to active tuberculosis, and this patient has palpable cervical lymphadenopathy which could point to this. However, she has now received 6 weeks of quadruple therapy with evidence of clinical improvement (diminished night sweats), and it is important to consider other possible causes, including: (1) development of a second endocrinopathy or other condition associated with polyglandular autoimmune syndrome type 2 and (2) the impact of tuberculosis therapy, including its effects on the patient's longstanding hypoadrenalism.

Polyglandular autoimmune syndrome type 1 is also referred to as autoimmune polyendocrinopathy-candidiasis-ectodermal dystrophy (APECED) and is caused by pathogenic variants in the autoimmune regulatory gene (*AIRE*), which is located on chromosome 21q22. APECED is inherited in an autosomal recessive manner. The prevalence of various manifestations is shown in *box 1.*

Box 1. Manifestations of Polyglandular Autoimmune Syndrome Type 1

Endocrine manifestations	
Hypoparathyroidism	80%-90%
Adrenal insufficiency	60%-80%
Primary hypogonadism	10%-50%
Hypothyroidism	10%-20%
Type 1 diabetes mellitus	1%-10%
Hypopituitarism	≤2%
Nonendocrine manifestations	
Chronic mucocutaneous candidiasis	70%-100%
Malabsorption syndromes	~20%
Alopecia totalis or areata	~20%
Pernicious anemia	~15%
Chronic active hepatitis	~10%
Vitiligo	<5%

Polyglandular autoimmune syndrome type 2 is much more prevalent than type 1, and primary adrenal insufficiency is its principal manifestation (see *box 2*).

Box 2. Manifestations of Polyglandular Autoimmune Syndrome Type 2.

Endocrine manifestations	
Adrenal insufficiency	up to 100%
Autoimmune thyroid disease	70%-75%
Type 1 diabetes mellitus	40%-60%
Primary hypogonadism	5%-50%
Nonendocrine manifestations	
Vitiligo	<5%
Other*	<1%

*Alopecia, pernicious anemia, myasthenia gravis, immune thrombocytopenia purpura, Sjögren syndrome, rheumatoid arthritis, celiac disease.

This patient's hemoglobin A_{1c} value is in the prediabetes range, which makes it unlikely that hyperglycemia (Answer B) is the cause of her tiredness, lethargy, and weight loss. Additionally, there is no mention of other clinical features such as increased thirst or frequent urination. However, her hemoglobin A_{1c} will require careful monitoring, and she should be counseled on instituting appropriate lifestyle interventions, as her BMI is 29.8 kg/m^2.

Although the TPO-antibody titer is raised and she has a small symmetric goiter, the pattern of thyroid function test results (mildly subnormal TSH with low-normal free T_4) is not suggestive of primary autoimmune thyroid dysfunction and is more likely to reflect the changes seen in nonthyroidal illness. Serum free T_4 may be normal or low in T_3 thyrotoxicosis (Answer D), but in this case the TSH is not fully suppressed. In addition, T_3 thyrotoxicosis is most commonly seen in the context of nonautoimmune nodular thyroid disease.

Vitamin B_{12} insufficiency (Answer E) may coexist with primary hypoadrenalism in autoimmune polyendocrine syndrome type 2, but this patient's mean corpuscular volume is not raised, her anemia is mild, and she has no features of neurological dysfunction.

Both rifampicin and isoniazid are recognized causes of drug-induced hemolytic anemia (Answer A), but this is unlikely to fully explain the clinical features, especially considering the relatively mild anemia. However, it would be prudent to consider screening for other indicators of hemolysis (eg, serum bilirubin, lactate dehydrogenase, haptoglobins, reticulocyte count, blood smear, direct antiglobulin test) if no other cause is identified or if the anemia becomes more marked.

Rifampicin is a potent inducer of cytochrome P450 3A4 (CYP3A4), a key enzyme regulating hydrocortisone metabolism. As a result, patients who are receiving a fixed-dosage glucocorticoid regimen for adrenal replacement are at significant risk of developing hypoadrenalism (Answer C) when commencing treatment with rifampicin. Here, the patient's clinical symptoms and mild hyponatremia rapidly resolved when her hydrocortisone replacement was doubled. Although fludrocortisone shows close structural similarity to cortisol, there remains a paucity of data on the pathways governing its metabolism. However, it is sensible to also monitor for underreplacement when commencing treatment with agents that induce the CYP3A family of enzymes. In this patient, no adjustment to the fludrocortisone dosage was necessary.

Educational Objective

Explain how rifampicin and other potent CYP3A4 enzyme-inducing agents can trigger hypoadrenalism in patients receiving fixed dosages of glucocorticoid replacement.

Reference(s)

Thijs E, Wierckx K, Vandecasteele S, Van den Bruel A. Adrenal insufficiency, be aware of drug interactions! *Endocrinol Diabetes Metab Case Rep.* 2019;2019:19-0062. PMID: 31581123

Bornstein SR, Allolio B, Arlt W, et al. Diagnosis and treatment of primary adrenal insufficiency: an Endocrine Society clinical practice guideline. *J Clin Endocrinol Metab.* 2016;101(2):364-389. PMID: 26760044

55

ANSWER: C) Oocyte donation and in vitro fertilization

This woman presents with signs and symptoms of spontaneous primary ovarian insufficiency. In the evaluation of primary ovarian insufficiency, it is recommended to order karyotype analysis. In this patient's case, her primary ovarian insufficiency is due to Turner syndrome. Fragile X premutation and autoimmune oophoritis have been ruled out, as has hyperprolactinemia and thyroid dysfunction. Turner syndrome is a disorder in females characterized by absence of all or part of a normal second sex chromosome that leads to primary or hypergonadotropic hypogonadism and infertility. Turner syndrome is associated with short stature; endocrine and metabolic disorders such as autoimmune thyroid disease, type 1 diabetes mellitus, and inflammatory bowel disease; and congenital heart disease, including coarctation of the aorta and bicuspid aortic valve.

Given that spontaneous fertility is rare among individuals with Turner syndrome, physicians should discuss reproductive options with their patients. Gamete transfer with donor oocytes (Answer C) has been attempted in women with Turner syndrome with a success rate equal to that of other infertile women receiving such treatments. Other options include adoption or using a gestational carrier. Prior to considering in vitro fertilization, a careful cardiac evaluation with transthoracic echocardiography and cardiac CT/MRI is required given that cases of aortic dissection and subsequent death have been reported during pregnancy in women with Turner syndrome. Clomiphene citrate (Answer A), letrozole (Answer B), and pulsatile GnRH therapy (Answer E) are ovulation induction agents and are effective for women with ovulatory infertility. However, they are not helpful in women with ovarian insufficiency.

While persistent ovarian function may be present in young women with Turner syndrome, as they age there is rapidly decreasing ovarian reserve. Therefore, egg retrieval is not likely to help this patient conceive. Neither is ovarian drilling (Answer D), which is a potential surgical treatment for anovulatory, infertile women with polycystic ovary syndrome that is unresponsive to clomiphene citrate.

Women with Turner syndrome require screening throughout life. Such screening includes 25-hydroxyvitamin D measurement every 3 to 5 years and annual thyroid function tests, lipid panel, liver function tests, and hemoglobin A_{1c} measurement.

Educational Objective

Explain fertility management in patients with primary ovarian insufficiency, specifically for women with Turner syndrome.

Reference(s)

Gravholt CH, Viuff MH, Brun S, Stochholm K, Andersen NH. Turner syndrome: mechanisms and management. *Nat Rev Endocrinol.* 2019;15(10):601-614. PMID: 31213699

Gravholt CH, Anderson NH, Conway GS, et al; International Turner Syndrome Consensus Group. Clinical practice guidelines for the care of girls and women with Turner syndrome: proceedings from the 2016 Cincinnati International Turner Syndrome Meeting. *Eur J Endocrinol.* 2017;177(3):G1-G70. PMID: 28705803

Sybert VP, McCauley E. Turner's syndrome. *N Engl J Med.* 2004;351(12):1227-1238. PMID: 15371580

56 ANSWER: B) Glimepiride

Sulfonylureas are known to be associated with increasing cardiovascular risk, as initially shown in the University Group Diabetes Program, which reported an increase in cardiovascular mortality with tolbutamide therapy. Accordingly, with the advent of new antidiabetes agents, particularly SGLT-2 inhibitors and GLP-1 receptor agonists, which have demonstrated cardiovascular risk reduction, sulfonylureas are less commonly used in this population, particularly given the risk of hypoglycemia with these agents. However, because of cost, intolerability, or contraindications to other therapies, initiation of sulfonylurea therapy may be sometimes necessary.

First-generation sulfonylureas (eg, chlorpropamide, tolbutamide) are not commonly available or used. Compared with second-generation sulfonylureas, they have a longer duration of action. First-generation sulfonylureas also have an increased risk for hypoglycemia (chlorpropamide) and other adverse effects such as hyponatremia, disulfiram-like effects (chlorpropamide), and increased cardiovascular risk (tolbutamide, in findings from the University Group Diabetes Program).

Sulfonylurea metabolites are renally excreted. Some of these metabolites, such as those of glyburide, are active or have weak hypoglycemic activity. Accordingly, in patients with chronic kidney disease, glipizide and glimepiride are preferred formulations because glipizide is shorter-acting than glyburide and both are metabolized by the liver and primarily excreted in the urine as inactive metabolites. When a decision has been made to treat with a sulfonylurea, a shorter-duration sulfonylurea (eg, glipizide, gliclazide [not available in the United States]) or one with relatively lower risk for hypoglycemia (eg, glimepiride) is preferred.

In patients with established cardiovascular disease, glimepiride (Answer B) is the best sulfonylurea. Glimepiride, compared with linagliptin in the CAROLINA CVOT, did not increase cardiovascular risk despite the higher frequency of hypoglycemia observed with glimepiride. Given that linagliptin was demonstrated to be safe in patients with cardiovascular disease in the CARMELINA trial, one can infer that glimepiride, based on the CAROLINA findings, is also safe from a cardiovascular standpoint. Accordingly, when a sulfonylurea must be used in patients with cardiovascular disease, the best option is glimepiride.

Given the cardiovascular safety data available with glimepiride, use of an alternative sulfonylurea, such as glipizide (Answer C) or chlorpropamide (Answer A), which lack cardiovascular safety data, would not be the best choice. Likewise, using tolbutamide (Answer E) or glyburide (Answer D), which have been reported to increase the risk of adverse cardiovascular outcomes, would not be advised in patients with established cardiovascular disease.

Educational Objective

Identify which sulfonylurea is safe and preferred for patients with cardiovascular disease.

Reference(s)

Meinert CL, Knatterfud GL, Prout TE, Klimt CR. A study of the effects of hypoglycemic agents on vascular complications in patients with adult-onset diabetes. II. Mortality results. *Diabetes.* 1970;19(Suppl):789-830. PMID: 4926376

Rosenstock J, Perkovic V, Johansen OE, et al; CARMELINA Investigators. Effect of linagliptin vs placebo on major cardiovascular events in adults with type 2 diabetes and high cardiovascular and renal risk: the CARMELINA Randomized Clinical Trial. *JAMA.* 2019;321(1):69-79. PMID: 30418475

Rosenstock J, Kahn SE, Johansen OE, et al; CAROLINA Investigators. Effect of linagliptin vs glimepiride on major adverse cardiovascular outcomes in patients with type 2 diabetes: the CAROLINA Randomized Clinical Trial. *JAMA.* 2019;322(12):1155-1166. PMID: 31536101

Ghosh S, Mukhopadhyay P, Pandey P, Chatterjee P. Cardiovascular safety of glimepiride: an indirect comparison from CAROLINA and CARMELINA. *Diab Vasc Dis Res.* 2020;17(6):1479164120973653. PMID: 33213193

57 **ANSWER: D) Starting a moderate-intensity exercise program, aiming for 200 minutes weekly**
Maintaining long-term weight loss is a challenge for many people. Physiologic adaptations that are designed to restore body weight, such as a reduction in energy expenditure and changes in appetite-regulating peripheral hormonal signals, occur in response to weight loss. These hormonal adaptations can persist for long periods and can be difficult to overcome. Over time, such biological settings promote weight regain.

Exercise is a mainstay of successful long-term weight maintenance, no matter how the initial weight loss occurred. Data from the National Weight Control registry, which is the largest prospective investigation of long-term successful weight-loss maintenance, show that almost all successful weight maintainers increase their physical activity, with 90% exercising on average for about an hour per day. In a systematic review of several weight-control registries, an increase in physical activity was the most consistent positive correlate of weight-loss maintenance. When patients who have lost weight cannot maintain a physical activity routine, such as the patient in this vignette, weight regain is common. For this patient to continue losing weight, starting a moderate-intensity exercise program (Answer D) would be most effective. No one type of physical activity has been shown to be superior to another; however, physical activity of at least moderate intensity is typically necessary to maintain weight loss. The patient in this vignette has difficulty walking and may benefit from non–weight-bearing aerobic or resistance exercises.

The ideal macronutrient composition of a long-term weight maintenance diet is unknown. Consuming adequate protein is important to ensure optimal satiety signaling, but increasing high-quality protein consumption alone (Answer A) is not expected to promote additional weight loss. Current evidence supports a dietary plan during the weight-maintenance phase that is consistent with personal preferences.

Additional caloric restriction is the intended effect of both an appetite suppressant (Answer E) or bariatric surgery (Answer B). This patient reports consuming an average of 1800 calories per day and is not losing weight despite this caloric count being lower than predicted basal energy needs. This scenario can arise when the basal energy expenditure by predictive equation overestimates true basal energy expenditure (as can be seen in weight-reduced individuals) or if the patient's self-report of energy intake is inaccurate. In either case, additional caloric restriction can lead to short-term weight loss, but this is unlikely to ensure long-term weight maintenance in the absence of a physical activity program.

Behavioral modification (Answer C) is a useful adjunct to any weight-management program, but in this patient's scenario it is less likely to be as beneficial as starting a moderate-intensity exercise program.

Educational Objective

Describe the limitations of caloric restriction alone for the purpose of weight maintenance and the importance of physical exercise after large body-weight fluctuations.

Reference(s)

Catenacci VA, Grunwald GK, Ingebrigtsen JP, et al. Physical activity patterns using accelerometry in the National Weight Control Registry. *Obesity (Silver Spring).* 2011;19(6):1163-1170. PMID: 21030947

Paixão C, Dias CM, Jorge R, et al. Successful weight loss maintenance: a systematic review of weight control registries. *Obes Rev.* 2020;21(5):e13003. PMID: 32048787

58 ANSWER: D) Start a β-adrenergic blocker

COVID-19 vaccines and boosters have been recommended since their development after the start of the pandemic. Rare cases of subacute thyroiditis have been reported following COVID-19 vaccination (attenuated and inactive vaccines). Vaccines may exert protective effects by increasing immune tolerance but may also facilitate a pathologic immune response. Several hypotheses have been described to explain the development of subacute thyroiditis after COVID vaccination: (1) the adjuvant in the vaccine may cause autoimmune/inflammatory syndrome; (2) antibodies against SARS-CoV-2 proteins could cross-react with several tissue antigens, including thyroid antigens such as TPO (this could represent a mechanism for immune-mediated complications both after SARS-CoV-2 infections and SARS-CoV-2 vaccination); and (3) the vaccine may cause direct injury to the thyroid gland. Genetic susceptibility seems to have a role in the pathogenesis, as subacute thyroiditis is often associated with certain HLA haplotypes, in particular HLA-B*35.

While vaccination remains the best available tool in combatting the COVID-19 pandemic, clinicians should be aware of potential effects of the COVID-19 vaccine on the thyroid gland. In most cases, symptoms of thyroiditis appear in the first few days after vaccination. In addition to subacute thyroiditis, cases of Graves disease have been reported after individuals have received COVID vaccines or contracted COVID-19 infection.

This patient's symptoms of overt hyperthyroidism and neck tenderness started after COVID vaccination. She had biochemical findings of hyperthyroidism and her thyroid scan confirmed thyroiditis (absence of active thyroid tissue). Subacute thyroiditis is managed with use of nonsteroidal anti-inflammatory drugs (NSAIDs) and β-adrenergic blockers (Answer D) during the inflammatory thyrotoxic phase and subsequently with levothyroxine if the patient develops symptomatic hypothyroidism, as with any form of subacute thyroiditis. Corticosteroids may be considered in patients with moderate-to-severe pain who do not respond to NSAID treatment. Given that this patient has palpitations, she requires a β-adrenergic blocker to decrease sympathetic override, including palpitations, anxiety, and tremor. For her neck tenderness, NSAID treatment should be offered and if this does not alleviate the pain, short-term steroid therapy may be required. Thyroiditis is a self-limiting illness. Therefore, it improves over time and follow-up laboratory tests are helpful in detecting illness resolution. However, laboratory tests should be ordered 4 to 6 weeks after the initial diagnosis (not 1 week after [Answer C]).

Radioiodine treatment (Answer A) or antithyroid drugs (Answer E) would be inappropriate in patients with thyroiditis.

Thyroid-stimulating immunoglobulin (Answer B) is not necessary, as she has had a thyroid scan that demonstrates no active thyroid tissue.

Educational Objective

Identify COVID-19 vaccination as a risk factor for subacute thyroiditis.

Reference(s)

Franquemont S, Galvez J. Subacute thyroiditis after mRNA vaccine for Covid-19. *J Endocr Soc.* 2021;5:A956-A957.

Ippolito S, Gallo D, Rossini A, et al. SARS-CoV-2 vaccine-associated subacute thyroiditis: insights from a systematic review. *J Endocrinol Invest.* 2022;45(6):1189-1200. PMID: 35094372

Nyulassy S, Hnilica P, Buc M, Guman M, Hirschova V, Stefanovic J. Subacute (de Quervain's) thyroiditis: association with HLA-Bw35 antigen and abnormalities of the complement system, immunoglobulins and other serum proteins. *J Clin Endocrinol Metab.* 1977;45(2):270-274. PMID: 885992

59 ANSWER: B) Reduced risk of breast cancer recurrence

Bisphosphonates are often used in women with breast cancer to block bone mineral density loss caused by aromatase inhibitors and to reduce skeletal-related events (pathologic fractures, surgical fixation, and need for pain medications) from bone metastases. Another unexpected benefit of bisphosphonates in this population of patients is a reduced risk of breast cancer recurrence (Answer B) and mortality. This benefit appears to apply only to postmenopausal women with early-stage breast cancer. This was demonstrated in the 2015 Early Breast Cancer Trialists Collaborative Group Trial that reported bisphosphonates reduced the relative risk of breast cancer recurrence by 18%.

There is no evidence that bisphosphonate treatment increases muscle mass (Answer A) or reduces risk of falls (Answer D). Radiation therapy increases the risk of osteosarcoma, but no evidence exists that bisphosphonates mitigate this risk (Answer C). Although bisphosphonates may reduce the bone turnover caused by osteoarthritis, no evidence exists that these medications reduce the symptoms of osteoarthritis (Answer E).

Educational Objective

Recognize that antiresorptive medications reduce the risk of breast cancer recurrence.

Reference(s)

Early Breast Cancer Trialists' Collaborative Group (EBCTCG). Adjuvant bisphosphonate treatment in early breast cancer: meta-analyses of individual patient data from randomised trials. *Lancet.* 2015;386(10001):1353-1361. PMID: 26211824

O'Carrigan B, Wong MH, Willson ML, Stockler MR, Pavlakis N, Goodwin A. Bisphosphonates and other bone agents for breast cancer. *Cochrane Database Syst Rev.* 2017;10(10):CD003474. PMID: 29082518

60 **ANSWER: A) Add ezetimibe, 10 mg daily**

In patients who have had a transient ischemic attack or stroke, the risk of recurrent stroke is quite high, and it is important to institute aggressive secondary prevention strategies. The Stroke Prevention by Aggressive Reduction of Cholesterol Level (SPARCL) trial has shown the benefit of high-intensity statin therapy (atorvastatin, 80 mg daily) to reduce the risk of recurrent stroke. It has therefore been a common practice to prescribe high-intensity statin therapy for patients who have had a transient ischemic attack or atherogenic stroke regardless of achieved LDL-cholesterol concentration. A more recent study examined the strategy of treating to a target LDL-cholesterol concentration less than 70 mg/dL (<1.81 mmol/L) or 90 to 110 mg/dL (2.33-2.85 mmol/L) using a statin, ezetimibe, or both (Treat Stroke to Target study). There was 22% relative risk reduction of atherosclerotic cardiovascular disease (ASCVD) events, including stroke, in the group treated to achieve an LDL-cholesterol concentration below 70 mg/dL (<1.81 mmol/L) (achieved LDL-cholesterol value was 65 mg/dL [1.68 mmol/L]). This patient has had a recent transient ischemic attack and was unable to tolerate atorvastatin, 80 mg daily, in the past. Adding ezetimibe (Answer A) would be reasonable to achieve an LDL-cholesterol concentration less than 70 mg/dL (<1.81 mmol/L) rather than trying to increase the atorvastatin dosage (Answer C) or recommending no medication changes (Answer D).

Adding icosapent ethyl (Answer B) to statin therapy in individuals at high risk who have elevated triglyceride levels has also been shown to reduce ASCVD risk in the REDUCE-IT trial. However, patients enrolled in that trial had either established ASCVD or diabetes and other risk factors. The median baseline LDL-cholesterol concentration in the trial was 75 mg/dL. Data supporting a primary LDL-cholesterol reduction strategy are stronger for the type of patient presented in this vignette, and this is preferred over adding icosapent ethyl. For prevention of stroke, intensive LDL-cholesterol lowering should be the primary target.

This patient has prediabetes, and there is little evidence that metformin therapy (Answer E) reduces the risk of long-term complications, including stroke and other ASCVD events.

Educational Objective

Identify the appropriate LDL-cholesterol target concentration for stroke prevention.

Reference(s)

Amarenco P, Bogousslavsky J, Callahan A 3rd, et al; Stroke Prevention by Aggressive Reduction in Cholesterol Levels (SPARCL) Investigators. High-dose atorvastatin after stroke or transient ischemic attack. *N Engl J Med.* 2006;355(6):549-559. PMID: 16899775

Amarenco P, Kim JS, Labreuche J, et al; Treat Stroke to Target Investigators. A comparison of two LDL cholesterol targets after ischemic stroke. *N Engl J Med.* 2020;382(1):9. PMID: 31738483

61 **ANSWER: C) Measure the urine albumin-to-creatinine ratio**

The first report of a patient developing neuropathy characterized by burning pain after initiating insulin therapy was published in 1933. The pain resolved after insulin was discontinued and it recurred after insulin was re-started. Assuming this phenomenon was an allergy to insulin, it was labeled "insulin neuritis." Subsequently, over many decades, there have been numerous case reports of painful neuropathy developing after rapid glycemic control in the setting of insulin treatment. Within the last 20 years, it has been recognized that painful neuropathy may develop after rapid glucose control, even in persons with type 2 diabetes and those treated with oral hypoglycemic agents and severe dietary restriction. Therefore, *treatment-induced neuropathy of diabetes* (TIND) is the term that has been suggested to refer to this clinical syndrome. Studies suggest that development of TIND is related to the rate at which hemoglobin A_{1c} decreases. For example, if hemoglobin A_{1c} decreases by 2% over 3 months, risk of TIND is 10%. If hemoglobin A_{1c} decreases by 5% over 3 months, risk of TIND is 90%. TIND is characterized by pain, allodynia, and hyperalgesia. Autonomic symptoms are also common, although they are often unrecognized because of the degree of pain.

Microvascular complications can progress rapidly in the setting of TIND. In one cohort, Gibbons et al described that only 17% of patients had microalbuminuria and all had normal kidney function, but within 1 year after the onset of TIND, 83% had microalbuminuria and 8% had developed end-stage kidney disease requiring hemodialysis. Generally, gradual improvement in neuropathic pain severity and distribution occurs over 1.5 to 3 years. This is accompanied by improvement in intraepidermal nerve fiber density over 8 years. Recurrence of TIND has been reported in those who have additional trends of hyperglycemia with subsequent rapid improvement in glycemic control.

While guidelines suggest that screening for microalbuminuria (Answer C) be done 5 years after diagnosis, given that microalbuminuria is recognized with increased frequency after the onset of TIND, it would be very reasonable to assess for microalbuminuria now.

TIND is not an allergy to a particular insulin formulation and therefore changing this patient's regimen to insulin detemir and insulin aspart (Answer A) is not appropriate.

Similarly, TIND can occur even in patients taking sulfonylureas, so changing his regimen to oral hypoglycemic agents (Answer B) is not expected to be helpful. Beyond this, the patient has type 1 diabetes, so oral hypoglycemic agents are not appropriate.

Anecdotes suggest that permissive hyperglycemia may lead to recovery from neuropathic symptoms. In patients with type 1 diabetes, long-term stable and good glycemic control is associated with better recovery. Therefore, relaxation of hemoglobin A_{1c} targets to 8.0% to 8.5% (Answer E) should not be pursued.

Performing no additional diagnostic testing or treatment changes (Answer D) would not be appropriate given his increased risk of other microvascular complications.

Educational Objective

Diagnose treatment-induced neuropathy in patients with diabetes mellitus and explain what is known about its epidemiology.

Reference(s)

Gibbons CH. Treatment induced neuropathy of diabetes. *Curr Diab Rep.* 2017;17(12):127. PMID: 29064042

Gibbons CH, Freeman R. Treatment-induced neuropathy of diabetes: an acute, iatrogenic complication of diabetes. *Brain.* 2015;138(Pt 1):43-52. PMID: 25392197

62 ANSWER: D) Primary adrenal insufficiency

Nonspecific gastrointestinal symptoms, including nausea, vomiting, abdominal pain, and anorexia, are typical of adrenal insufficiency. Additional symptoms of adrenal insufficiency include fatigue, weight loss, and generalized weakness. Because these symptoms are shared by a variety of other pathologies, the diagnosis of adrenal insufficiency is frequently delayed.

Several clinical features distinguish primary from secondary adrenal insufficiency:

1. **Elevated ACTH** ACTH is cleaved from the prohormone pro-opiomelanocortin along with other peptides such as melanocyte-stimulating hormone. Excess melanocyte-stimulating hormone causes hyperpigmentation, which is often generalized, but it can also be more prominent in areas of friction (elbows, knees, etc), mucosae, and scars. Examining these areas is particularly important in patients with darker skin complexion.
2. **Electrolyte abnormalities** Primary adrenal insufficiency is characterized by both cortisol and aldosterone deficiency. Aldosterone synthesis is physiologically regulated via renin, which is preserved in secondary adrenal insufficiency. Hyponatremia, hyperkalemia, and mild hyperchloremic acidosis are due to mineralocorticoid deficiency.

Hypercalcemia occurs only rarely in patients with adrenal crisis. Factors contributing to hypercalcemia include bone resorption, increased reabsorption of calcium in the proximal tubule, and volume contraction. Persons with secondary adrenal insufficiency can have hypercalcemia. Eosinophilia can also be observed in individuals with cortisol deficiency. Hypoglycemia is rare in affected adults, but it can be seen in infants with adrenal insufficiency.

This patient has oral hyperpigmentation, electrolyte abnormalities suggestive of mineralocorticoid deficiency, and hypothyroidism (presumably autoimmune), all suggestive of primary adrenal insufficiency (Answer D). Patients with secondary adrenal insufficiency (Answer E) have inappropriately normal or low ACTH and hence no hyperpigmentation. Because their aldosterone production is preserved, patients with secondary adrenal insufficiency do not develop hyperkalemia and hyponatremia unless they have other concomitant pathologies.

Type 1 diabetes and diabetic ketoacidosis (Answer A) can also develop in patients with an autoimmune predisposition, but this patient has a normal glucose concentration and normal anion gap metabolic acidosis.

Hyperthyroidism (Answer B) can lead to decreased appetite and weight loss but would not explain the remaining signs and symptoms present in this patient. The mildly suppressed TSH could be due to his recent weight loss, requiring a reduction in levothyroxine dosage.

Recreational marijuana use is increasingly common. Chronic marijuana users (Answer C) might experience symptoms such as cyclic abdominal pain, vomiting, and/or nausea, which are often relieved by hot showers.

Educational Objective

Diagnose primary adrenal insufficiency and distinguish it from secondary adrenal insufficiency based on clinical presentation.

Reference(s)

Hahner S, Ross RJ, Arlt W, et al. Adrenal insufficiency. *Nat Rev Dis Primers.* 2021;7(1):19. PMID: 33707469

63 ANSWER: B) Right lobectomy

The 2015 American Thyroid Association management guidelines for adult patients with thyroid nodules and differentiated thyroid cancer changed the surgical management for patients with the diagnosis of differentiated thyroid cancer. Prior to these published guidelines, most patients with differentiated thyroid cancer would have undergone total thyroidectomy with central neck dissection followed by radioiodine treatment. Based on the 2015 American Thyroid Association management guidelines, patients with an FNA-proven diagnosis of differentiated thyroid cancer with a nodule up to 4 cm may undergo lobectomy if there is no extrathyroidal extension and no clinical evidence of lymph node metastases. In addition, there has been a shift away from widespread use of radioiodine therapy. Recent guidelines recommend radioiodine treatment for patients deemed to be at high risk according to the American Thyroid Association guidelines and for some patients at intermediate risk. Radioiodine treatment is not recommended for patients at low risk.

This patient probably has low-risk thyroid cancer because her tumor is smaller than 4 cm without extrathyroidal extension identified on ultrasonography and she has no clinical evidence of lymph node metastases. Right lobectomy (Answer B) can be recommended as initial therapy. Therefore, total thyroidectomy (Answer C), total thyroidectomy followed by radioiodine treatment (Answer D), and total thyroidectomy with central neck dissection (Answer E) would be inappropriate.

Radiofrequency ablation (Answer A) is incorrect because this nodule is large and has been proven to be thyroid cancer. Radiofrequency ablation can be performed in benign thyroid nodules (after 2 negative FNA biopsies) to reduce the size of the nodule and for curative or palliative purposes in the setting of recurrent thyroid cancer in the thyroidectomy bed and cervical node metastases.

Educational Objective

Recommend appropriate thyroid surgery based on thyroid nodule size and FNA biopsy result.

Reference(s)

Haugen BR, Alexander EK, Bible KC, et al. 2015 American Thyroid Association management guidelines for adult patients with thyroid nodules and differentiated thyroid cancer: the American Thyroid Association Guidelines Task Force on Thyroid Nodules and Differentiated Thyroid Cancer. *Thyroid.* 2016;26(1):1-133. PMID: 26462967

Kim J-H, Baek JH, Lim HK, et al. 2017 Thyroid radiofrequency ablation guideline: Korean Society of Thyroid Radiology. *Korean J Radiol.* 2018;19(4):632-655. PMID: 29962870

64 ANSWER: C) Continue metformin, stop empagliflozin, stop NPH insulin, start rapid-acting insulin with evening and morning meals

Fasting during the month of Ramadan is one of the pillars of Islam, the religion practiced by approximately one-quarter of the world's population. During Ramadan, no food or drink consumption is allowed between sunrise and sunset and physical activity is typically reduced overall.

A religious fast is one form of time-restricted eating (TRE). A TRE pattern of 16:8, for example, is one where calories are consumed during an 8-hour time window, while fasting is observed for the remaining 16 hours of the day. TRE as an eating pattern is gaining popularity because of its proven benefits for weight loss and glycemic control. Any alteration in eating habits affects blood glucose values, and diabetes pharmacotherapy should be modified accordingly.

The patient in this vignette is on metformin, an SGLT-2 inhibitor (empagliflozin), and NPH insulin twice daily. Several studies have demonstrated the safety of SGLT-2 inhibitors during Ramadan, but careful patient education is needed regarding hydration during permissible hours, the potential risk for volume contraction (particularly in warmer climates), and the potential for diabetic ketoacidosis. Elderly patients in particular should be cautious with continued use of SGLT-2 inhibitors during fasting, and therefore stopping this class of medications in this patient is appropriate. Metformin dosing does not need to be adjusted during fasting. She could benefit from rapid-acting insulin in the evening and in the morning (ie, when she eats [Answer C]).

Stopping basal insulin and relying on metformin and empagliflozin alone (Answer D) may be enough for patients at low risk for hyperglycemia or those who are willing to check blood glucose values more frequently. However, in this patient with a hemoglobin A_{1c} value of 8.1% (65 mmol/mol), there is a risk of unrecognized hyperglycemia if the frequency of blood glucose self-monitoring is not increased.

Although a reduction in the NPH insulin dosage would be reasonable, discontinuing metformin in this situation is not necessary and continuing empagliflozin is not recommended (Answer B). Likewise, continuing with the prefasting doses of NPH insulin (Answer A) is likely to precipitate hypoglycemia.

Stopping NPH insulin, empagliflozin, and metformin and using rapid-acting insulin as needed for hyperglycemia 3 times daily (Answer E) is not the best answer because the patient does not need to discontinue metformin during fasting, and correcting hyperglycemia alone is not optimal for glycemic control.

Educational Objective

Manage diabetes medications when a patient is following a time-restricted eating pattern.

Reference(s)

Ibrahim M, Davies MJ, Ahmad E, et al. Recommendations for management of diabetes during Ramadan: update 2020, applying the principles of the ADA/EASD consensus. *BMJ Open Diabetes Res Care.* 2020;8(1):e001248. PMID: 32366501

Shao Y, Lim GJ, Chua CL, et al. The effect of Ramadan fasting and continuing sodium-glucose co-transporter-2 (SGLT2) inhibitor use on ketonemia, blood pressure and renal function in Muslim patients with type 2 diabetes. *Diabetes Res Clin Pract.* 2018;142:85-91. PMID: 29802956

65 ANSWER: D) Recommend insulin pump initiation

Achieving a hemoglobin A_{1c} value less than 7.0% (<53 mmol/mol) should be the goal for adults with diabetes who have no significant underlying comorbidities. Therefore, recommending no regimen changes (Answer E) is inappropriate for this patient with a hemoglobin A_{1c} value of 7.6% (60 mmol/mol). Achieving this goal can be difficult, even for motivated patients. Patients with type 1 diabetes have a significant degree of insulin deficiency and, as a result, they depend on exogenous insulin.

Developing hyperglycemia in the mornings (fasting hyperglycemia) is a well-described phenomenon. It usually occurs between 2 AM and 8 AM and is believed to be caused by the diurnal secretion of different hormones, mainly GH. Fasting hyperglycemia cannot be corrected because of underlying insulin deficiency.

Reviewing glycemic patterns is considerably easier with continuous glucose monitoring (CGM) devices. These systems measure glucose values every 5 minutes and provide comprehensive information about glycemic control, revealing glycemic trends in different periods. This is especially true at night, as identifying nocturnal hypoglycemia and hyperglycemia without CGM can be problematic. Without CGM devices, patients must wake during the night and perform point-of-care glucose measurements. The dawn phenomenon can be easily identified with CGM. As seen in the graph, this patient starts to experience rising hyperglycemia after 3 AM, and it progressively worsens.

Notably, she reports that she eats her first meal between 11:30 AM and 1:00 PM. As a result, her hyperglycemia is not postprandial. However, clinicians should be careful when evaluating fasting hyperglycemia, as they must ensure that the patient does not have a late meal or bedtime snack. To consider the dawn phenomenon, the hyperglycemia needs to (1) occur at least 4 hours after the previous meal or snack and (2) occur overnight (usually after 3 AM).

The dawn phenomenon can be better managed by initiating continuous subcutaneous insulin infusion (insulin pump therapy) (Answer D). One of the major limitations of multiple daily insulin injections is that the patient is receiving a "fixed" amount of basal insulin over a 24-hour period. As a result, if basal insulin needs to be increased or decreased during different periods, this cannot be achieved. In contrast, insulin pumps can modify the basal rate during different periods. This patient needs to receive a lower dose of basal insulin between 12 AM and 4 AM and then higher doses after 4 AM. Currently, new hybrid closed-loop systems are available that can self-adjust basal rates accordingly. Although an insulin pump can be a great solution for many patients with diabetes, some requirements must be met. One of the most important is that the patient should have the mental capacity and the willingness to manage their insulin pump independently. Patients should also be comfortable with carbohydrate counting, as they will still need to manage bolus insulin with meals.

As the dawn phenomenon is an example of fasting hyperglycemia, increasing the prandial insulin doses with meals (Answer C) will not help. This case of hyperglycemia is unrelated to meals and the focus should be to prevent the hyperglycemia that occurs overnight.

Increasing the basal insulin glargine dosage (Answer B) is the usual initial approach to address fasting hyperglycemia in patients with diabetes who receive multiple daily insulin injections. However, this patient's CGM report shows that she has overnight (12 AM to 4 AM) glucose values close to or even in the hypoglycemia range. Therefore, increasing basal insulin is not the best management because it may increase nocturnal hypoglycemia. Decreasing the basal insulin dosage (Answer A) may reduce the risk of hypoglycemia; however, it would also cause more hyperglycemia.

Educational Objective

Describe the role of and indication for continuous subcutaneous insulin infusion in patients with type 1 diabetes mellitus with severe dawn phenomenon.

Reference(s)

Deckert T, Lorup B. Regulation of brittle diabetics by a pre-planned insulin infusion programme. *Diabetologia.* 1976;12(6):573-579. PMID: 1001846

Carroll MF, Schade DS. The dawn phenomenon revisited: implications for diabetes therapy. *Endocr Pract.* 2005;11(1):55-64. PMID: 16033737

66 **ANSWER: D) Medical therapy with the steroidogenesis inhibitor osilodrostat**

When transsphenoidal resection of ACTH-secreting microadenomas is performed by expert neurosurgeons, biochemical remission is expected in 80% to 91% of patients. Therapeutic choices for patients with persistent hypercortisolism include reoperation, radiation, and medical treatment. Treatment should be individualized based on clinical, histologic, biochemical, and radiologic factors. Remission rates for reoperation are lower (59%) compared with remission rates after initial surgery according to a recent meta-analysis, and risk of hypopituitarism is higher with reoperation. Stereotactic radiation achieves biochemical remission in approximately 74% of patients in the first 8 years of follow-up (according to a recent meta-analysis) and is associated with hypopituitarism in 25% to 50% (higher in patients with longer follow-up). Medical treatment has achieved significant progress in recent years with several classes of medications approved by the US FDA for Cushing disease: steroidogenesis inhibitors (osilodrostat and levoketoconazole), somatostatin receptor ligands (pasireotide), and cortisol receptor blockers (mifepristone). Additional medications also used in treatment of Cushing syndrome are ketoconazole and metyrapone, which are non–FDA-approved for this indication. All patients taking medications for hypercortisolism must be educated about manifestations of corticoadrenal insufficiency and should carry rescue glucocorticoids. Tumor growth can occur, especially in patients taking medications that do not target the tumor, and imaging surveillance is necessary in all patients. Monitoring the QT interval on electrocardiography is necessary in patients taking pasireotide and levoketoconazole. Frequent drug-drug interactions can occur with levoketoconazole and mifepristone (eg, substrates, inhibitors or inducers of CYP3A4 isoenzymes).

Osilodrostat (Answer D) is a potent 11β-hydroxylase inhibitor that was shown to normalize urinary free cortisol in 77% to 86% of patients with Cushing disease in 2 phase 3 randomized trials. Due to the site of steroidogenesis inhibition, testosterone levels usually increase in both sexes during therapy. This makes osilodrostat a good option in this patient who also has hypogonadism. Some women receiving osilodrostat experience worsening of hirsutism. Hypokalemia and hypertension can occur due to increased mineralocorticoid precursors. Levoketoconazole was evaluated in a phase 3 open-label, nonrandomized, single-arm trial in adult patients with Cushing syndrome. After dosage titration, 31% of patients achieved normal urinary free cortisol levels. The most common adverse effects were nausea (32%) and headache (28%). ALT concentrations more than 3 times above the upper normal limit reversibly increased in 11% patients. Because of levoketoconazole's ability to block multiple adrenal enzymes, treated women usually experience improved hirsutism and acne, and men experience a decrease in testosterone levels with resulting hypogonadism and gynecomastia.

Pasireotide (not an option here) binds with higher affinity to the somatostatin receptor type 5, which is usually abundantly expressed in ACTH-secreting tumors. Phase 3 trials have documented biochemical efficacy (ie, normalized urinary free cortisol) in 15% to 26% of patients treated with subcutaneous pasireotide and in 40% of those treated with long-acting release pasireotide. In a recent meta-analysis, tumor shrinkage was demonstrated in approximately 30% of patients with functioning ACTH-secreting pituitary adenomas. Pasireotide is associated with risk of new or worsening hyperglycemia in two-thirds of patients with Cushing disease. Mechanisms entail decreased incretin and insulin secretion. Treatment with metformin or incretin-based therapies is usually successful, but some patients require insulin. In this case, the patient does not have a visible residual tumor and reports diabetes in 2 first-degree family members, which makes pasireotide a less attractive option than steroidogenesis inhibitors.

Inferior petrosal sinus sampling (Answer B) is recommended for patients with biochemical confirmation of ACTH-dependent hypercortisolism if imaging shows either a small adenoma or no adenoma. In this case, this test was completed preoperatively. However, this procedure would not be recommended at this time because the patient has histologic confirmation of an ACTH-secreting adenoma.

While radiotherapy (Answer E) can be used as adjuvant therapy for persistent or recurrent postoperative hypercortisolism or for residual tumor growth, this patient had a small tumor at presentation, which was not visualized postoperatively. Imaging surveillance 6 to 12 months after initiation of steroidogenesis inhibitors is recommended.

The cortisol receptor blocker mifepristone (Answer C) was approved for patients with hyperglycemia and Cushing syndrome. A phase 3 open-label study indicated that 60% of patients had a reduction of 25% or more from baseline in area under the curve for glucose during oral glucose tolerance testing, along with improved insulin resistance, weight, and waist circumference. Diastolic blood pressure improved in 38% of patients. During treatment, cortisol levels cannot be used as a marker of drug efficacy and are expected to increase. This patient has a normal glucose concentration, which means mifepristone should not be used.

If testosterone concentrations remain low despite normalization of cortisol, screening for osteoporosis and initiating testosterone replacement (Answer A) would be appropriate.

Educational Objective

Treat persistent hypercortisolism after transsphenoidal surgery for Cushing disease.

Reference(s)

Gadelha M, Bex M, Feelders RA, et al. Randomized trial of osilodrostat for the treatment of Cushing disease. *J Clin Endocrinol Metab.* 2022;107(7):e2882-e2895. PMID: 35325149

Fleseriu M, Pivonello R, Elenkova A, et al. Efficacy and safety of levoketoconazole in the treatment of endogenous Cushing's syndrome (SONICS): a phase 3, multicentre, open-label, single-arm study. *Lancet Diabetes Endocrinol.* 2018;7(11):855-865. PMID: 31542384

Fleseriu M, Auchus R, Bancos I, et al. Consensus on diagnosis and management of Cushing's disease: a guideline update. *Lancet Diabetes Endocrinol.* 2021;9(12):847-875. PMID: 34687601

Perez-Vega C, Ramos-Fresnedo A, Tripathi S, et al. Treatment of recurrent and persistent Cushing's disease after first transsphenoidal surgery: lessons learned from an international meta-analysis. *Pituitary.* 2022;25(3):540-549. PMID: 35508745

Tritos NA, Biller BMK. Advances in the medical treatment of Cushing's disease. *Endocrinol Metab Clin North Am.* 2020;49(3):401-412. PMID: 32741479

67 **ANSWER: B) Fluoride**

Skeletal fluorosis is a rare disorder associated with toxic exposure to fluoride-containing agents (Answer B). In many parts of the world, elevated fluoride concentrations in groundwater used as a drinking source lead to high prevalence of this condition. Other sources include accidental exposures from inhalation or skin absorption of industrial cleaning agents and refrigerants, drinking fluoride-containing mouthwashes, and a newer disturbing pattern of "huffing" computer keyboard aerosolized cleaners containing difluoroethane. Voriconazole, an antifungal medication, contains 3 fluoride atoms comprising 16% of the medication's mass. In reported cases of voriconazole-induced skeletal fluorosis, most patients were taking the medication for at least 6 months.

With toxic exposure, fluoride substitutes for hydroxide groups of hydroxyapatite in bone to form fluorapatite. Given the relatively long half-life of the mineral component of bone, the skeletal half-life of fluoride is also long, in the range of many years. For reasons not understood, fluoride is a strong stimulus for bone formation leading to a pattern of osteosclerosis. Despite a higher bone mass, evidence suggests that patients with skeletal fluorosis have a higher fracture rate.

Symptoms of skeletal fluorosis include bone pain and the formation of exostoses, defined areas of new bone formation on existing bone, as well as calcified ligamentous attachments. Signs include elevated alkaline phosphatase, indicating new bone formation, and secondary hyperparathyroidism from a negative calcium balance of the marked increase in new bone formation and calcium mobilization into the skeleton. Radiologic findings include evidence of periostitis and long-bone exostoses. Nuclear medicine bone scans often find a global increase in scintigraphic uptake, and DXA bone density scans often identify very high bone density. Skeletal fluorosis is diagnosed by detecting a high serum fluoride level.

Cadmium toxicity (Answer A) is a relatively rare disorder with reported cases due to accidental occupational exposure, food sources in areas with high soil concentrations, and cigarette smoke. Bone disease can occur with cadmium toxicity and is linked to increased fracture risk and lower bone mineral density. Hyperparathyroidism, marked increases in alkaline phosphatase, periostitis, and thickened bone cortices are not associated with cadmium toxicity.

Elevated vitamin B_{12} (Answer E) is not associated with periostitis.

Elevated serum tryptase (Answer C) often occurs in systemic mastocytosis, a neoplastic accumulation of bone marrow mast cells. Low bone mineral density and mixed lytic/sclerotic bone lesions are often detected, features that the described patient does not have.

Vitamin A toxicity (Answer D) can have marked effects on osteoclast activation, leading to lower bone mineral density, increased fracture risk, and non–PTH-mediated hypercalcemia due to rapid calcium mobilization from the skeleton. Although periostitis has been reported with vitamin A toxicity, this patient does not have other features of this condition.

Educational Objective

Identify voriconazole as a cause of skeletal fluorosis.

Reference(s)

Cook FJ, Seagrove-Guffey M, Mumm S, et al. Non-endemic skeletal fluorosis: causes and associated secondary hyperparathyroidism (case report and literature review). *Bone.* 2021;145:115839. PMID: 33418099

Tucci JR, Whitford GM, McAlister WH, et al. Skeletal fluorosis due to inhalation abuse of a difluoroethane-containing computer cleaner. *J Bone Miner Res.* 2017;32(1):188-195. PMID: 27449958

Moon WJ, Scheller EL, Suneja A, et al. Plasma fluoride level as a predictor of voriconazole-induced periostitis in patients with skeletal pain. *Clin Infect Dis.* 2014;59(9):1237-1245. PMID: 24992954

68 **ANSWER: D) Recommend no change to current therapy**

Total thyroidectomy with neck dissection should be performed by experienced surgeons to prevent complications, including postoperative hypoparathyroidism, hoarseness due to recurrent laryngeal nerve damage, and, less frequently, Horner syndrome. Horner syndrome is caused by interruption of the sympathetic pathway that supplies the neck, eyes, and head. This complication is very rare (0.2% after thyroidectomy).

Horner syndrome is characterized by ptosis, myosis, and anhidrosis on one side of the face due to damage of the ipsilateral cervical sympathetic chain. Some patients may have a vascular dilation on the other side of the face characterized by red skin. Operations that can cause Horner syndrome include thyroid and parathyroid surgery, drainage of a retropharyngeal or parapharyngeal abscess, excision of a cervical schwannoma, sympathectomy, removal of paragangliomas, removal of cervical ganglioneuromas, and cervical lymph node dissection. This syndrome can develop within the first week after surgery. The close anatomical relationship between the thyroid and the sympathetic trunk and the middle cervical ganglion makes these structures susceptible to damage during thyroidectomy, especially with neck dissection. This complication can happen after postoperative hemorrhage compressing the cervical sympathetic chain, ischemia-induced neural damage, stretching of the cervical sympathetic chain by lateral retractor, and damage to the communication between the cervical sympathetic chain and the recurrent laryngeal nerve during its localization. Once Horner syndrome occurs after thyroid surgery, it can be permanent in 70% of cases. Recovery occurs in 30% of patients within 5 to 15 months after surgery. There is no specific treatment for Horner syndrome occurring after thyroidectomy with neck dissection. Furthermore, pancoast tumor (apical lung tumor) can cause ipsilateral Horner syndrome via pressure on the brachial plexus.

This patient has developed Horner syndrome following lateral neck dissection for thyroid cancer recurrence. Given that there is no specific treatment, recommending no changes to her current therapy (Answer D) is appropriate. Performing additional diagnostic testing, including neck CT (Answer B) or orbit CT (Answer C), is unnecessary.

In addition, there is no reason to refer this patient to ophthalmology (Answer E) because the etiology of Horner syndrome is related to her lateral neck dissection.

She does not have Graves eye disease, and there is no role for steroid administration (Answer A).

Educational Objective

Diagnose Horner syndrome as a complication of lateral modified neck dissection in patients with thyroid cancer.

Reference(s)

Seneviratne SA, Kumara DS, Drahaman AMP. Horner's syndrome: an unusual complication of thyroidectomy: a case report. *J Med Case Reports.* 2016;10(1):300. PMID: 27784321

Gonzalez-Aguado R, Morales-Angulo C, Obeso-Aguera S, Longarela-Herrero Y, García-Zornoza R, Acle Cervera L. Horner's syndrome after neck surgery. *Acta Otorrinolaryngol Esp.* 2012;63(4):299-302. PMID: 22502736

Sapalidis K, Florou M, Tsopouridou K, et al. Horner's syndrome: an uncommon complication of thyroidectomy and selective lateral neck dissection. *Curr Health Sci J.* 2019;45(1):111-115. PMID: 31297271

69 ANSWER: A) Asfotase alfa

This patient has hypophosphatasia as evidenced by very low total alkaline phosphatase in the absence of other causes such as antiresorptive therapy or glucocorticoid treatment. Hypophosphatasia is due to pathogenic variants in the gene encoding tissue nonspecific alkaline phosphatase (*ALPL*), an enzyme that cleaves pyrophosphate, the accumulation of which impairs bone mineralization. This patient also has an elevated vitamin B_6 level (while not on B_6 vitamin supplementation), which is a marker of alkaline phosphatase enzyme impairment. B_6 is also a substrate for tissue nonspecific alkaline phosphatase. Although most of her symptoms have occurred in adulthood, her medical history supports the suspicion that disease manifestations began in childhood in the form of fractures. The clinical picture of hypophosphatasia can vary, including a severe and life-threatening perinatal form, childhood appearance of rickets (with low alkaline phosphatase), adult fractures, joint and other musculoskeletal symptoms, and odontohypophosphatasia (which may occur in combination with other features or as a phenotype limited only to apparent dentition abnormalities). With odontohypophosphatasia, there is early deciduous tooth loss by the entire root, although some affected patients go on to develop other musculoskeletal symptoms as adults. Adults with hypophosphatasia may be asymptomatic with low alkaline phosphatase or have recurrent stress fractures (which may include the proximal femur), calcium pyrophosphate joint disease, and mobility limitations. Adults with hypophosphatasia often have normal bone mineral density.

Asfotase alfa (Answer A) is an enzyme replacement therapy for alkaline phosphatase that improves bone mineralization. In children with the severe form of hypophosphatasia, this therapy improves skeletal mineralization, pulmonary function due to restoration of costal bone mineralization, and survival. Although there is not a trial in adults sufficiently powered to demonstrate reduced fracture risk, asfotase alfa does increase lumbar spine bone mineral density and improve mobility, and it may provide some improvement in fracture healing. Whether enzyme replacement therapy alters the joint symptoms or dental phenotype in adults is unknown.

Treatment of hypophosphatasia has been challenging in adults because of limited responsiveness to standard medications for osteoporosis, such as bisphosphonates (Answer D) or teriparatide (Answer E) regarding improvement in bone mineral density or fracture response. In addition, patients with hypophosphatasia are at risk for atypical femur fractures, even without antiresorptive therapy, and case reports suggest that antiresorptive agents may increase this risk further.

Treatment with calcium and vitamin D (Answer C) is also not likely to alter fracture risk in this patient population. Patients with hypophosphatasia often have mild elevations in serum calcium and phosphate attributed to the impaired mineralization of bone, and treatment with calcium and vitamin D may increase the risk for hypercalciuria and nephrocalcinosis.

Burosumab (Answer B) is an FGF-23 antibody used to treat X-linked hypophosphatemia and will not address the mineralization defect in hypophosphatasia. Furthermore, this patient's phosphate value is high-normal with low alkaline phosphatase, while in persons with X-linked hypophosphatemia, phosphate is low and alkaline phosphatase is typically normal or high.

Asfotase alfa circulates after injection, and it will be detected by the alkaline phosphatase activity assay on routine laboratory testing, giving the appearance of extreme elevations. Informing patients and their providers of this phenomenon can help avoid unnecessary evaluation in the event of an abnormal value. Alkaline phosphatase concentrations should not be used for monitoring or dosage adjustment.

Educational Objective

Diagnose and treat hypophosphatasia.

Reference(s)

Seefried L, Dahir K, Petryk A, et al. Burden of illness in adults with hypophosphatasia: data from the global hypophosphatasia patient registry. *J Bone Miner Res.* 2020;35(11):2171-2178. PMID: 32654183

Lefever E, Witters P, Gielen E, et al. Hypophosphatasia in adults: clinical spectrum and its association with genetics and metabolic substrates. *J Clin Densitom.* 2020;23(3):340-348. PMID: 30655187

Genest F, Rak D, Petryk A, Seefried L. Physical function and health-related quality of life in adults treated with asfotase alfa for pediatric-onset hypophosphatasia. *JBMR Plus.* 2020;4(9):e10395. PMID: 32995696

Kishnani PS, Rockman-Greenberg C, Rauch F, et al. Five-year efficacy and safety of asfotase alfa therapy for adults and adolescents with hypophosphatasia. *Bone.* 2019;121:149-162. PMID: 30576866

Kishnani PS, Rush ET, Arundel P, et al. Monitoring guidance for patients with hypophosphatasia treated with asfotase alfa. *Mol Genet Metab.* 2017;122(1-2):4-17. PMID: 28888853

70 ANSWER: E) Weight loss and spironolactone

This patient meets all 3 diagnostic criteria for polycystic ovary syndrome based on the 2003 Rotterdam criteria. Two of the 3 following findings must be present to diagnose polycystic ovary syndrome: (1) oligoovulation and/or anovulation, (2) clinical and/or biochemical signs of hyperandrogenism, (3) polycystic ovaries (≥12 follicles measuring 2 to 9 mm in diameter and/or an ovarian volume >10 mL in at least 1 ovary on ultrasonography). In addition to menstrual irregularities, hyperandrogenism, and polycystic ovaries, metabolic issues are very common in women with polycystic ovary syndrome. Affected women have a higher risk of insulin resistance, glucose intolerance, type 2 diabetes, dyslipidemia, sleep apnea, and cardiovascular disease.

To address this patient's concerns of androgen excess symptoms and irregular menstrual cycles, first-line therapy would be a combined oral contraceptive pill (Answer A). This treatment would suppress LH secretion and thereby suppress ovarian androgen production by theca cells, while also increasing levels of hepatic SHBG, which would then lower free androgen serum levels. However, the patient has tried combined oral contraceptive pills in the past and was unable to tolerate this treatment. In addition, according to the US Medical Eligibility Criteria for Contraceptive Use (2016), combined oral contraceptive users who smoke cigarettes are at increased risk for cardiovascular disease compared with risk of nonsmokers, although it is thought that the advantages outweigh the theoretical or proven risks. Moreover, this patient has obesity (BMI = 35.1 kg/m^2), and research has demonstrated that women with obesity who use combined oral contraceptives are at higher risk for venous thromboembolism. Therefore, while not an absolute contraindication, caution should be exercised.

Spironolactone would also help her hirsutism and acne and is considered second-line treatment for symptoms of androgen excess. Spironolactone is an aldosterone receptor antagonist that also acts as an antagonist to the androgen receptor, thereby blocking the effect of androgens. Used in combination with weight loss (Answer E), she could benefit her overall metabolic profile, and this is the best recommendation for her. She has obesity (BMI = 35.1 kg/m^2), hyperlipidemia, and prediabetes. This patient would greatly benefit from lifestyle modifications to decrease her overall lifetime risk of cardiometabolic disease. While weight loss alone would improve her risk of cardiometabolic disease, it would not adequately treat her hirsutism and symptoms of androgen excess. Importantly, patients who are engaging in sexual behavior that places them at risk for pregnancy must be counseled that while on an antiandrogen (spironolactone), contraception must be used. If this would have applied to this patient, an intrauterine device may have been considered both as a contraceptive and as protection for the uterus from unopposed estrogen exposure seen in women with polycystic ovary syndrome.

Laser hair removal (Answer C) involves a photothermal reaction that causes damage to the hair follicle. Without managing this patient's androgen excess, the result of laser hair removal could be poor and she would likely require more sessions to achieve the desired effect. Therefore, most clinicians experienced in managing polycystic ovary syndrome would recommend to first decrease and/or block androgen excess prior to laser hair removal.

Dexamethasone (Answer B) is not recommended for treatment of polycystic ovary syndrome, even if a patient has clinical signs of androgen excess. It is recommended in the treatment of classic congenital adrenal hyperplasia with 21-hydroxylase deficiency, which she does not have.

Metformin (Answer D) can increase the number of ovulatory menstrual cycles in women with polycystic ovary syndrome. However, it does not effectively treat androgen excess (acne, hirsutism, hair loss), which is one of this patient's main concerns.

Educational Objective

Recommend treatment for irregular menses and hyperandrogenism in a woman with polycystic ovary syndrome.

Reference(s)

Bhat YJ, Bashir S, Nabi N, Hassan I. Laser hair treatment in hirsutism: an update. *Dermatol Pract Concept*. 2020;20;10(2):e2020048. PMID: 32363110

Curtis KM, Tepper NK, Jatlaoui TC, et al. U.S. Medical Eligibility Criteria for Contraceptive Use, 2016. *MMWR Recomm Rep*. 2016;65(3):1-103. PMID: 27467196

Legro RS, Arslanian SA, Ehrmann DA, et al; Endocrine Society. Diagnosis and treatment of polycystic ovary syndrome: an Endocrine Society clinical practice guideline. *J Clin Endocrinol Metab*. 2013;98(12):4565-4592. PMID: 24151290

Martin KA, Chang RJ, Ehrmann DA, et al. Endocrine Society. Evaluation and treatment of hirsutism in premenopausal women: an Endocrine Society clinical practice guideline. *J Clin Endocrinol Metab*. 2008;93(4):1105-1120. PMID: 18252793

Randeva HS, Tan BK, Weickert MO, et al. Cardiometabolic aspects of the polycystic ovary syndrome. *Endocr Rev*. 2012;33(5):812-841. PMID: 22829562

71 ANSWER: C) Start pioglitazone

Persons with type 2 diabetes are at increased risk of metabolic dysfunction-associated steatotic liver disease (formerly termed nonalcoholic fatty liver disease), which can progress to cirrhosis. Aggressive management of metabolic risk factors and reversal of steatotic disease are required to reduce overall cardiovascular morbidity and mortality. This patient has already implemented aggressive lifestyle intervention, successfully losing 6% of her body weight. Additional medical therapy can be added to reduce her overall risk of cirrhosis. GLP-1 receptor agonists and pioglitazone (Answer C) are the only diabetes medications that have been effective in the treatment of metabolic dysfunction-associated steatotic liver disease or nonalcoholic steatohepatitis. Pioglitazone is effective in treating nonalcoholic steatohepatitis (odds ratio, 3.22; 95% CI, 2.17-4.79, for resolution) and reversal of fibrosis at any stage (odds ratio, 1.66; 95% CI, 1.12-2.47). Adverse effects of pioglitazone include weight gain, heart failure in those with cardiac disease, increased risk of fracture, and bladder cancer. GLP-1 receptor agonists (liraglutide and semaglutide) delay progression of metabolic dysfunction-associated steatotic liver disease and have the added benefit of weight loss. A GLP-1 receptor agonist would be a reasonable alternative for this patient, but it was not offered as a choice.

Given that her weight loss has plateaued, continuing with lifestyle changes (Answer A) would not further reduce her risk for cirrhosis.

Insulin (Answer B) and DPP-4 inhibitors (Answer D) would improve glycemic control but have no additional benefit in treating nonalcoholic steatohepatitis.

Vitamin E (Answer E) has not been effective in treating nonalcoholic steatohepatitis in patients with type 2 diabetes. Overall, the data are mixed, and no study has shown improvement in fibrosis. However, vitamin E has been effective in treating steatohepatitis in patients without type 2 diabetes.

Educational Objective

Recommend medications with proven efficacy to treat metabolic dysfunction-associated steatotic liver disease in patients with type 2 diabetes mellitus.

Reference(s)

Cusi K, Orsak B, Bril F, et al. Long-term pioglitazone treatment for patients with nonalcoholic steatohepatitis and prediabetes or type 2 diabetes mellitus: a randomized trial. *Ann Intern Med.* 2016;165(5):305-315. PMID: 27322798

Musso G, Cassader M, Paschetta E, Gambino R. Thiazolidinediones and advanced liver fibrosis in nonalcoholic steatohepatitis: a meta-analysis. *JAMA Intern Med.* 2017;177(5):633-640. PMID: 28241279

Cusi K, Isaacs S, Barb D, et al. American Association of Clinical Endocrinology clinical practice guideline for the diagnosis and management of nonalcoholic fatty liver disease in primary care and endocrinology clinical settings: co-sponsored by the American Association for the Study of Liver Diseases (AASLD). *Endocr Pract.* 2022;28(5):528-562. PMID: 35569886

72 ANSWER: A) Add evinacumab (monoclonal antibody to ANGPTL3)

This patient has features suggestive of homozygous familial hypercholesterolemia. Both parents have hypercholesterolemia, and his maximum untreated LDL-cholesterol concentration is greater than 400 mg/dL (>10.36 mmol/L). While heterozygous familial hypercholesterolemia is not an uncommon disorder (incidence of 1 in 250), the homozygous form is much rarer. Previously, it was estimated to occur in 1 in 1 million persons, but it is now recognized to be more prevalent, with an approximate incidence of 1 in 250,000. Homozygous familial hypercholesterolemia is associated with very early aggressive atherosclerotic cardiovascular disease (ASCVD), and it should be managed with effective lipid-lowering therapy from a young age. The condition can be caused by biallelic pathogenic variants in the gene encoding the LDL receptor, defective apolipoprotein B, or activating pathogenic variants in the *PCSK9* gene. There are a few rare autosomal recessive variants. Patients with complete loss of LDL-receptor function are particularly difficult to treat with poor response to pharmacotherapy. Early initiation of statin therapy with the addition of ezetimibe and PCSK9 inhibitors is the initial approach. However, this strategy is rarely successful in achieving the desired LDL-cholesterol concentration less than 100 mg/dL (<2.59 mmol/L) for primary prevention or less than 70 mg/dL (<1.81 mmol/L) for secondary prevention. In the past, a 50% reduction in LDL cholesterol from baseline was considered a reasonable goal, but with the advent of novel therapies, aiming for lower LDL-cholesterol values is desirable.

One such recently developed therapeutic option is evinacumab (Answer A), a monoclonal antibody to ANGPTL3 that is an inhibitor of plasma lipases. The exact mechanism by which it lowers LDL cholesterol, especially in patients without functional LDL receptors, is not clear but may involve decreased synthesis of LDL particles through its action on endothelial lipase. A nearly 50% reduction in LDL cholesterol has been observed in patients with both severe refractory hypercholesterolemia and homozygous familial hypercholesterolemia who were on maximally tolerated statin therapy and PCSK9 inhibitors. Based on these studies, the US FDA approved evinacumab for the treatment of homozygous familial hypercholesterolemia as an adjunct to other lipid-lowering therapies in individuals older than 12 years. It is administered either intravenously (15 mg/kg every 4 weeks) or subcutaneously (300-450 mg every 1 to 2 weeks) and would likely be the most effective and convenient next step in this patient's management.

Another relatively new option for LDL-cholesterol lowering is small interfering RNA therapy, inclisiran (Answer B), which decreases PCSK9 production and therefore increases LDL-receptor activity. However, there is no evidence to suggest that it has greater efficacy than monoclonal antibodies targeting PCSK9, which this patient is currently taking (evolocumab). Its main advantage over the PCSK9 monoclonal antibodies is the decreased frequency of administration (every 3 to 6 months). There is no benefit to combining inclisiran with PCSK9 monoclonal antibodies. The mechanism of action of different LDL cholesterol–lowering drugs is summarized in the *table*.

Table. Mechanism of Action of Different Cholesterol-Lowering Drugs

Medication	Mechanism of action
Statin	Inhibition of HMG CoA reductase, leading to decreased endogenous cholesterol biosynthesis and subsequent increase in hepatic LDL receptor expression
Ezetimibe	Decreased cholesterol absorption by inhibiting NPC1L1 receptors on the intestinal cells ultimately leading to decreased intrahepatic cholesterol concentration and up-regulation of hepatic LDL receptor expression
Bile acid binding resin	Decreased bile acid pool leading to decreased intrahepatic cholesterol concentration and up-regulation of hepatic LDL receptor expression
Bempedoic acid	Inhibition of ATP citrate lyase, leading to decreased endogenous cholesterol biosynthesis and subsequent increase in hepatic LDL receptor expression
PCSK9 monoclonal antibody	Inhibition of PCSK9 activity leading to increased recycling of LDL receptors and more efficient clearing of circulating LDL particles
PCSK9 siRNA (Inclisiran)	Inhibition of PCSK9 synthesis and activity leading to increased recycling of LDL receptors and more efficient clearing of circulating LDL particles
ANGPTL3 monoclonal antibody (evinacumab)*	Decreased synthesis of VLDL and LDL particles through unclear mechanisms
Apo B ASO (mipomersen)*	Antisense oligonucleotide to apolipoprotein B leading to decreased synthesis of VLDL and subsequently LDL particles
Lomitapide*	Inhibitor of microsomal triglyceride transfer protein leading to decreased synthesis of VLDL and subsequently LDL particles

* Approved for use in patients with homozygous familial hypercholesterolemia only.

Biweekly LDL apheresis (Answer E) would certainly effectively lower LDL cholesterol, and it has been shown to reduce ASCVD events in patients with familial hypercholesterolemia, although not in a controlled trial. However, LDL apheresis is considerably more labor intensive and demanding on patients and should be considered after all pharmacological options have been tried.

Changing atorvastatin to a potentially more effective statin, rosuvastatin (Answer C), is unlikely to cause a significant change, especially in patients on PCSK9 inhibitor therapy.

Not making any changes to current therapy in a patient with an LDL-cholesterol concentration of 146 mg/dL (3.78 mmol/L) (Answer D) would not be appropriate in this young patient.

Educational Objective

Prescribe evinacumab as a novel treatment option for patients with homozygous familial hypercholesterolemia.

Reference(s)

Raal FJ, Rosenson RS, Reeskamp LF, et al; ELIPSE HoFH Investigators. Evinacumab for homozygous familial hypercholesterolemia. *N Engl J Med.* 2020;383(8):711-720. PMID: 32813947

Rosenson RS, Burgess LJ, Ebenbichler CF, et al. Evinacumab in patients with refractory hypercholesterolemia. *N Engl J Med.* 2020;383(24):2307-2319. PMID: 33196153

Aguilar-Salinas CA, Gómez-Díaz RA, Corral P. New therapies for primary hyperlipidemia. *J Clin Endocrinol Metab.* 2022;107(5):1216-1224. PMID: 34888679

73 ANSWER: C) Serum estradiol measurement

This patient's clinical presentation, laboratory values, and history of maternal virilization during pregnancy are typical of congenital estradiol deficiency due to aromatase deficiency. Thus, measuring estradiol (Answer C) is the best next step. Male aromatase deficiency is a rare autosomal recessive disorder due to pathogenic variants in the aromatase gene and is instructive, as it illuminates the physiological role of estrogens in men. Of note, a similar phenotype has been reported in men with inactivating pathogenic variants in the gene encoding the estrogen receptor α; however, maternal virilization during pregnancy does not occur when male fetuses have estrogen receptor α variants. Moreover, in contrast to men with aromatase gene variants, men with estrogen receptor α pathogenic variants do not respond to estradiol treatment. The clinical phenotype in aromatase-deficient men demonstrates that estrogens are pivotal for epiphyseal closure (note tall stature, delayed bone age), acquisition of peak bone mass (note low bone mineral density for age), and regulation of fat mass and glucose-lipid metabolism (note evidence of central adiposity, dyslipidemia, and insulin resistance—ie, features of metabolic syndrome). This phenotype is replicated in mice with targeted deletion in the aromatase gene. Notably, elegant experimental studies in healthy young men receiving GnRH analogue therapy (to reduce gonadal steroids) with testosterone add-back and aromatase inhibitor treatment (to reduce estradiol production) have likewise concluded that some aspects of male hypogonadism (reduced bone mass, central adiposity and metabolic syndrome) are mediated by estradiol deficiency rather than by testosterone deficiency. Therefore, in men with hypogonadism, testosterone replacement (which provides the substrate for aromatization to estradiol and for 5α-reduction to dihydrotestosterone) has also been referred to as providing "3 hormones in 1." Men with estradiol deficiency lack negative central feedback of estradiol on the male gonadal axis, hence explaining the elevated gonadotropin and testosterone concentrations.

Observations of men with aromatase deficiency have also illustrated the importance of placental aromatase to protect the mother (and the female fetus) from excess androgen exposure, by catalyzing the conversion of fetal adrenal androgens to estrogens. Placental aromatase deficiency explains the transient virilization of the mother during pregnancy and also explains why female babies with pathogenic variants in the aromatase gene present with ambiguous genitalia due to masculinization of the urogenital sinus and external genitalia. Because of absence of ovarian aromatase, affected females present with progressive virilization during puberty and polycystic ovaries but have no signs of estrogen action. In men with aromatase deficiency, estradiol treatment leads to rapid skeletal maturation with epiphyseal fusion, marked increase in bone density, and amelioration of metabolic syndrome.

This patient has no stigmata of Cushing syndrome, so ACTH and cortisol measurement (Answer A) is not the best next step.

Likewise, given the absence of clinical androgen excess, there is no indication to measure DHEA-S (Answer B), an adrenal testosterone precursor. DHEA-S measurement is rarely helpful unless a virilizing adrenal tumor or a cortisol-producing adrenal adenoma is suspected (in which case, DHEA-S will be high or low, respectively).

Serum 17-hydroxyprogesterone measurement (Answer D) is a screening test for congenital adrenal hyperplasia, and there is no reason to suspect this condition.

While tall stature and insulin resistance can be associated with acromegaly, there are no other clinical features of GH excess in this vignette. Therefore, serum IGF-1 and GH measurement (Answer E) is not the best investigation.

Educational Objective

Diagnose male estradiol deficiency due to rare aromatase deficiency and explain the importance of estrogens in male health.

Reference(s)

Morishima A, Grumbach MM, Simpson ER, Fisher C, Qin K. Aromatase deficiency in male and female siblings caused by a novel mutation and the physiological role of estrogens. *J Clin Endocrinol Metab.* 1995;80(12):3689-3698. PMID: 8530621

Finkelstein JS, Lee H, Leder BZ, et al. Gonadal steroid-dependent effects on bone turnover and bone mineral density in men. *J Clin Invest.* 2016;126(3):1114-1125. PMID: 26901812

Russell N, Grossmann M. Mechanisms in endocrinology: estradiol as a male hormone. *Eur J Endocrinol.* 2019;181(1):R23-R43. PMID: 31096185

74 **ANSWER: E) Refer for right thyroid lobectomy**

This 33-year-old woman has primary hyperparathyroidism. Serum calcium is elevated in the context of high serum PTH, low-normal serum phosphate, urinary calcium excretion greater than 200 mg/24 h, and a urine calcium-to-creatinine clearance ratio of 0.02 [urine calcium × serum creatinine] / [serum calcium × urine creatinine]. There is no evidence of secondary hyperparathyroidism (normal kidney function, vitamin D status). Parathyroidectomy is indicated given the patient's young age.

According to the Fifth International Workshop for the Management of Primary Hyperparathyroidism, parathyroidectomy is currently indicated for asymptomatic patients who have 1 or more the following:

1. Serum calcium >1 mg/dL (>0.3 mmol/L) above the upper normal limit
2. Bone mineral density by DXA <2.5 at any site or imaging evidence of vertebral fracture
3. Creatinine clearance <60 mL/min per 1.73 m^2
4. 24-hour urinary calcium >250 mg/24 h (>6.3 mmol/d) in women or >300 mg/24 h (>7.5 mmol/d) in men
5. Imaging evidence of nephrolithiasis or nephrocalcinosis
6. Age <50 years

The only revision in these criteria since those issued from the Fourth International Workshop is a lower urinary calcium threshold for surgery.

The typical location of the superior and inferior parathyroid glands is along the posterior surface of the thyroid gland, while ectopic locations include intrathymic, mediastinal, paraesophageal, intrathyroidal, submandibular, and within the carotid sheath. Although uncommon, occurring at an incidence of 1% to 6%, intrathyroidal parathyroid adenoma should be considered in the differential diagnosis of a thyroid nodule, especially in the context of hyperparathyroidism. This patient has concordant ultrasonographic and nuclear medicine parathyroid localization studies demonstrating a parathyroid adenoma within the right thyroid lobe. In this case, the use of dual isotope imaging with both ^{123}I and ^{99m}Tc sestamibi allowed for the intrathyroidal parathyroid adenoma to be more easily recognized on parathyroid scintigraphy. On ultrasonography, intrathyroidal parathyroid adenomas are characteristically hypoechoic solid nodules with clearly defined borders, increased vascularity, and polar feeding vessels originating from the superior or inferior thyroid artery, as demonstrated in this case (*see image, yellow arrow*). Other imaging modalities that can be used for preoperative localization include triple-phase CT with contrast, also referred to as "4D" CT, and fluorocholine PET/CT.

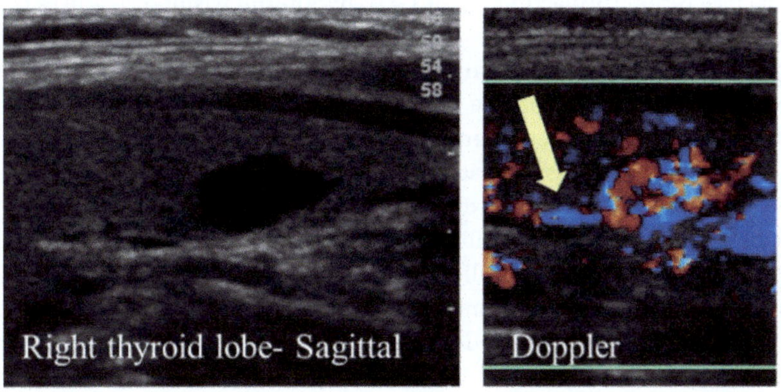

Ultrasound-guided FNA of the right thyroid nodule (Answer D) is not needed given the imaging findings characteristic of parathyroid adenoma. FNA may be considered in cases when the diagnosis is unclear based on imaging. However, cytologic distinction between thyroid and parathyroid lesions can be challenging. Parathyroid aspirates may demonstrate "naked" nuclei, papillary fragments with fibrovascular cores, and microfollicular architecture. A PTH washout of the FNA aspirate can confirm the diagnosis of parathyroid adenoma, as can thyroid molecular diagnostic testing. In clinical scenarios when parathyroid carcinoma is suspected (eg, presentation with parathyroid crisis, palpable neck mass), FNA is contraindicated.

Parathyroidectomy is indicated for this young patient. Preoperative imaging studies have identified a single parathyroid adenoma within the right thyroid lobe. As such, referral for right thyroid lobectomy is recommended (Answer E). However, it is also important to note that testing for a genetic cause of primary hyperparathyroidism should be considered in younger patients such as this one. Recent data suggest that as many as 10% of patients younger than 45 years with apparent sporadic primary hyperparathyroidism harbor a germline pathogenic variant in a gene associated with a familial form of this disorder, including multiple endocrine neoplasia type 1, multiple endocrine neoplasia type 2, and familial hyperparathyroidism.

Performing DXA (Answer B) and kidney ultrasonography (Answer C) should be considered in the initial workup of asymptomatic hyperparathyroidism. However, for this young patient in whom surgery is already indicated, neither DXA nor kidney imaging is likely to affect her immediate management.

Remeasuring calcium, albumin, and creatinine in 6 months (Answer A) is not appropriate given the unequivocal indication for parathyroidectomy.

Educational Objective

Consider intrathyroidal parathyroid adenoma in the differential diagnosis of a thyroid nodule.

Reference(s)

Bilezikian JP, Khan AA, Silverberg SJ, et al; International Workshop on Primary Hyperparathyroidism. Evaluation and management of primary hyperparathyroidism: summary statement and guidelines from the Fifth International Workshop. *J Bone Miner Res.* 2022;37(11):2293-2314. PMID: 36245251

Shi C, Guan H, Qi W, et al. Intrathyroidal parathyroid adenoma: diagnostic pitfalls on fine-needle aspiration: two case reports and literature review. *Diagn Cytopathol.* 2016;44(11):921-925. PMID: 27392021

Wei Zhao, Ruigang Lu, Li Yin, et al. The value of preoperative and intraoperative ultrasound in the localization of intrathyroidal parathyroid adenomas. *J Invest Surg.* 2022;35(4):752-757. PMID: 34167410

75 ANSWER: D) Pituitary adenoma

TSH-secreting pituitary adenomas (thyrotropinoma, TSHoma) (Answer D) are among the rarest of the anterior pituitary tumors (1%-2% of all pituitary adenomas), with an estimated prevalence of 2 to 3 per million population. Although historical reports have suggested a predominance of macroadenomas (often with parasellar invasion), microadenomas are increasingly described, and occult tumors, analogous to those found in Cushing disease, are now recognized. TSH-secreting pituitary adenomas present with symptoms and signs of thyrotoxicosis (as in this case), hormonal cosecretion (prolactin and/or GH), hypopituitarism, or features of local mass effect (eg, optic chiasm compression).

In a patient with apparent hyperthyroxinemia and nonsuppressed TSH, it is important to review the clinical context for (1) possible confounding medication use (including amiodarone [with impaired T_4 to T_3 conversion], heparin [causing thyroid hormone displacement from binding proteins], or levothyroxine therapy [including nonconcordance]), and (2) intercurrent illness (eg, acute psychiatric disorders).

Next, laboratory assay interference should be excluded. Positive interference in commonly used TSH assays can be caused by heterophilic or antianimal immunoglobulins or macro-TSH. Free thyroid hormone measurements may be falsely elevated in the presence of heterophilic or antiiodothyronine antibodies and with altered binding proteins (eg, familial dysalbuminemic hyperthyroxinemia or dystransthyretenimic hyperthyroxinemia). The use of biotin may also result in apparent raised free thyroid hormone levels when measured using a susceptible platform (eg, those that depend on formation of a streptavidin-biotin complex) and, if combined with a susceptible TSH assay (where TSH is artifactually low), may falsely suggest primary hyperthyroidism.

Once true hyperthyroxinemia with nonsuppressed TSH has been confirmed, the challenge is to distinguish a TSH-secreting pituitary adenoma from resistance to thyroid hormone (RTHβ; due to a loss-of-function pathogenic variant in the gene encoding the β isoform of the thyroid hormone receptor). Making this distinction on clinical grounds alone can be challenging, as patients with thyrotropinomas in whom free thyroid hormone levels are only mildly raised may appear relatively asymptomatic, while patients with RTHβ may manifest thyrotoxic features (eg, tachycardia) due to preserved normal TR alpha (TRα) function. It therefore typically depends on:

- Review of historical thyroid function test results and family history if available; documentation of normal thyroid function at an earlier timepoint makes a thyrotropinoma more likely, whereas identification of similar thyroid function abnormalities in other family members favors RTHβ.
- Measurement of SHBG and α subunit; elevated values may be seen in patients with TSH-secreting tumors.
- Genetic screening; 85% to 90% of patients with RTHβ harbor a loss-of-function pathogenic variant in the *THRB* gene.
- Pituitary imaging (MRI, ^{11}C-methionine PET); although demonstration of a pituitary abnormality is strongly suggestive of a thyrotropinoma, pituitary incidentalomas have been reported in RTHβ.
- Depot somatostatin analogue trial (2 to 3 injections); rapid and sustained normalization of thyroid function supports a diagnosis of thyrotropinoma.
- Dynamic tests (thyrotropin-releasing hormone test; liothyronine-suppression test) where available; thyrotropinomas exhibit autonomy with attenuated responses to thyrotropin-releasing hormone stimulation and liothyronine suppression.

In this patient, several features of thyrotoxicosis are evident (menstrual disturbance, heat intolerance, weight loss, resting tachycardia), and the finding of an elevated free T_4 concentration with nonsuppressed TSH and raised SHBG is suggestive of a TSH-secreting pituitary adenoma (Answer D).

Although primary hyperthyroidism (eg, due to Graves disease) (Answer B) is much more common than secondary hyperthyroidism, full suppression of serum TSH (ie, <0.1 mIU/L, and typically <0.03 mIU/L in most modern assays) is expected.

Occasionally, primary adrenal insufficiency (Answer A) presents with menstrual disturbance either as a direct manifestation of hypoadrenalism or as part of a broader polyendocrine syndrome (eg, autoimmune polyglandular syndrome type 2). This patient has several clinical features that could be consistent with Addison disease (weight loss, menstrual disturbance), but there is no significant postural fall in blood pressure, and she has normal secondary sexual characteristics. Thus, further assessment (eg, repeated measurement of 8-AM cortisol or dynamic testing [insulin stress test or cosyntropin stimulation]) would be primarily aimed at excluding or confirming secondary, rather than primary, hypocortisolism.

Significant weight loss and low body weight (Answer C) may cause menstrual dysfunction, but in this patient, weight loss is more likely to be a consequence of a specific underlying endocrine disorder rather than the primary cause.

Premature ovarian insufficiency (Answer E) is expected to be associated with raised gonadotropin concentrations, which is not the case here.

Educational Objective

Differentiate among causes of secondary hypogonadism in a premenopausal woman and explain the steps required to establish a diagnosis of central hyperthyroidism.

Reference(s)

Koulouri O, Gurnell M. TSH-secreting pituitary adenomas. In: Huhtaniemi I, ed. *Encyclopedia of Endocrine Diseases.* 2nd ed. Academic Press; 2018: 261-268.

Bashari W, Senanayake RM, MacFarlane JR, Koulouri O, Gurnell M. Thyroid-stimulating hormone-producing pituitary tumors. In: *DeGroot's Endocrinology.* 8th ed. Robertson RP, ed. Elsevier; 2022.

76 **ANSWER: B) Gastric bypass surgery**

Approximately 42% of adults in the United States have obesity (BMI ≥30 kg/m^2). Comorbidities such as type 2 diabetes, hypertension, hyperlipidemia, and obstructive sleep apnea are recognized to be associated with obesity. Obesity-associated cancers include postmenopausal breast, endometrial or uterine, ovarian, esophageal adenocarcinoma, gallbladder, gastric cardia, colorectal, renal cell, liver, pancreas, thyroid, meningioma, and multiple myeloma.

What remains unclear is whether weight loss, particularly through bariatric surgery, reduces the risk of developing cancer and/or affects cancer-associated mortality. Aminian et al recently reported that among adults with obesity, bariatric surgery compared with no surgery was associated with a significantly lower incidence of obesity-associated cancer and cancer-related mortality. The cumulative incidence of the primary end point (time to incident obesity-associated cancer, a composite of 13 cancer types as the primary end point at 10 years) was 2.9% (95% CI, 2.2%-3.6%) in the bariatric surgery group and 4.9% (95% CI, 4.5%-5.3%) in the nonsurgical control group (absolute risk difference, 2.0% (95% CI, 1.2%-2.7%); adjusted hazard ratio, 0.68 (95% CI, 0.53-0.87; $P = .002$). Cancer-related mortality occurred in 21 patients in the bariatric surgery group and in 205 patients in the nonsurgical control group (incidence rate of 0.6 events vs 1.2 events, respectively, per 1000 person-years). The cumulative incidence of cancer-related mortality at 10 years was 0.8% (95% CI, 0.4%-1.2%) in the bariatric surgery group and 1.4% (95% CI, 1.1%-1.6%) in the nonsurgical control group (absolute risk difference, 0.6% [95% CI, 0.1%-1.0%]; adjusted hazard ratio, 0.52 [95% CI, 0.31-0.88]; $P = .01$).

The risk for the primary end point was assessed separately after Roux-en-Y gastric bypass and sleeve gastrectomy. The median observation time was 6.8 years (interquartile range, 3.4-10.0 years) for Roux-en-Y and 4.6 years (interquartile range, 3.0-6.8 years) for sleeve gastrectomy. Obesity-associated cancer cases by surgery type (Roux-en-Y vs sleeve gastrectomy) were similar during the course of follow-up (hazard ratio, 1.05; 95% CI, 0.66-1.67; $P = .82$). Thus, both Roux-en-Y and sleeve gastrectomy are associated with decreased risk of obesity-related cancer. Of the listed choices, Roux-en-Y gastric bypass (Answer B) is the best recommendation for this patient.

While the incidence of acute pancreatitis in patients undergoing bariatric surgery has been reported to be slightly higher than in the general population (1.04% vs 0.017%), most cases have been clinically mild and managed conservatively with good outcomes.

The dual gastric inhibitory polypeptide/GLP-1 receptor agonist tirzepatide (Answer E) or GLP-1 receptor agonist semaglutide (Answer D) would not be the best choices in a patient concerned about cancer risk associated with antiobesity treatment. These medications have been linked to an increased risk of developing medullary thyroid cancer, specifically in rodents. In addition, these therapies are not recommended for patients with a history of acute pancreatitis.

Bupropion/naltrexone (Answer A) is contraindicated in patients with seizure disorders.

Phentermine/topiramate (Answer C) is contraindicated in patients with glaucoma.

Educational Objective

Assess the risk of cancer associated with bariatric surgery.

Reference(s)

Hales CM, Carroll MD, Fryar CD, Ogden CL. Prevalence of obesity and severe obesity among adults: United states, 2017-2018. *NCHS Data Brief.* 2020;(360):1-8. PMID: 324872284

Lauby-Secretan B, Scoccianti C, Loomis D, Grosse Y, Bianchini F, Straif K; International Agency for Research on Cancer Handbook Working Group. Body fatness and cancer–viewpoint of the IARC Working Group. *N Engl J Med.* 2016;375(8):794-798. PMID: 27557308

Aminian A, Wilson R, Al-Kurd A, et al. Association of bariatric surgery with cancer risk and mortality in adults with obesity. *JAMA.* 2022;327(24):2423-2433. PMID: 35657620

Kumaravel A, Zelisko A, Schauer P, Lopez R, Kroh M, Stevens T. Acute pancreatitis in patients after bariatric surgery: incidence, outcomes, and risk factors. *Obes Surg.* 2014;24(12):2025-2030. PMID: 24972683

77 ANSWER: B) Measure bone-specific alkaline phosphatase

Adynamic bone disease is a complication of chronic kidney disease and is part of the chronic kidney disease–mineral and bone disorder (CKD-MBD) spectrum. Bone histomorphometry demonstrates a lack of osteoblast bone formation and osteoclastic bone resorption, and few, if any, osteoblasts or osteoclasts. Adynamic bone disease is associated with high fracture risk. Adynamic bone disease can be difficult to diagnose definitively in patients with CKD because the routine performance of tetracycline-labeled transiliac bone biopsies is becoming less common. Risks for this condition include higher dosages of vitamin D analogues used to treat secondary hyperparathyroidism to lower PTH and aluminum toxicity, now a rare entity because of less reliance on oral aluminum phosphate binders and the routine water filtration in dialysis centers to remove aluminum in municipal water sources. In patients with stage 5 CKD or end-stage kidney disease receiving renal replacement therapy, a PTH concentration up to 5 times the upper normal limit may be associated with normal bone turnover. This is because the current PTH assays not only measure the active 1-84 protein, but also the 7-84 presumably inactive metabolite that has a longer half-life and is cleared by the kidneys. Moreover, such patients develop a type of PTH resistance that is poorly understood.

The described patient has stage 5 CKD and a PTH concentration of 63 pg/mL (63 ng/L). Although this value is in the normal range, it could, in fact, suggest adynamic bone disease. The 2017 KDIGO (Kidney Disease: Improving Global Outcomes) guidelines recommend a PTH concentration of 2- to 9-fold of the upper normal limit (130-600 pg/mL [130-600 ng/L]). The first step is to confirm the diagnosis before changing medication dosages. Bone-specific alkaline phosphatase (Answer B), like PTH, is a useful bone turnover marker in patients with CKD. Ureña et al reported that serum bone-specific alkaline phosphatase directly correlated well with bone biopsy histomorphometric indices of bone turnover in patients receiving hemodialysis.

Serum C-telopeptide (Answer C), while valuable in assessing bone turnover in patients with normal kidney function, has poor performance in patients with CKD due to renal clearance of this marker.

Prescribing cinacalcet (Answer E) would be incorrect because this medication treats secondary hyperparathyroidism in CKD. The patient's PTH value (in the normal range) is not consistent with secondary hyperparathyroidism.

Increasing the calcitriol dosage (Answer A) would also be inappropriate because this could worsen any suspected adynamic bone disease by further lowering PTH.

Finally, measuring serum 1,25-dihydroxyvitamin D (Answer D) would not be helpful at this point since it is expected to be low in stage 5 CKD. More importantly, it does not have any discriminatory value in the diagnosis of adynamic bone disease.

Educational Objective

Assess bone turnover in a patient with chronic kidney disease.

Reference(s)

Ketteler M, Block GA, Evenepoel P, et al. Executive summary of the 2017 KDIGO chronic kidney disease-mineral and bone disorder (CKD-MBD) guideline update: what's changed and why it matters. *Kidney Int.* 2017;92(1):26-36. PMID: 28646995

Ureña P, Hruby M, Ferreira A, Ang KS, de Vernejoul MC. Plasma total versus bone alkaline phosphatase as markers of bone turnover in hemodialysis patients. *J Am Soc Nephrol.* 1996;7(3):506-512. PMID: 8704118

Vervloet MG, Brandenburg VM; CKD-MBD working group of ERA-EDTA. Circulating markers of bone turnover. *J Nephrol.* 2017;30(5):663-670. PMID: 28502032

78 ANSWER: A) Discontinue mirtazapine

Binge-eating disorder (BED) is defined by consuming an amount of food over a discrete period that is larger than what most people would eat in a similar amount of time and under similar circumstances. There are specific diagnostic criteria for BED, and the severity of the condition is determined by the frequency of binge-eating episodes per week. About 50% of patients with BED are overweight or have obesity.

To meet the *Diagnostic and Statistical Manual 5* diagnostic criteria for BED, each of the following should be present:

Criterion 1: Episodes of binge eating, defined as consuming an amount of food in a discrete period (eg, within 2 hours) that is definitely larger than what most people would eat in a similar amount of time under similar circumstances. This is often associated with a sense of loss of control over how much they are eating and the inability to stop eating.

Criterion 2. Binge-eating episodes are marked by at least 3 of the following:

- Eating more rapidly than normal
- Eating until feeling uncomfortably full
- Eating large amounts of food when not feeling physically hungry
- Eating alone because of embarrassment about the amount of food consumed
- Feeling disgusted with oneself, depressed, or guilty after overeating

Criterion 3. Marked distress regarding binge eating is present.

Criterion 4. Episodes occur, on average, at least once a week for 3 months.

Criterion 5. There is no regular use of inappropriate compensatory behaviors to manage weight, such as purging, fasting, or excessive exercise, and episodes do not occur exclusively in the course of anorexia nervosa, bulimia nervosa, or avoidant/restrictive food intake disorder.

An active eating disorder such as BED is a relative contraindication to pursuing bariatric surgery (Answers B and C). Having an eating disorder before bariatric surgery is predictive of having an eating disorder after bariatric surgery. Current data also suggest poorer long-term weight-loss outcomes after bariatric surgery in patients with an eating disorder. Recognizing and managing eating disorders is important for patients who are seeking bariatric surgery.

When assessing a patient with obesity, any weight-promoting medications that the patient may be taking should be identified and discontinued if possible. In this case, mirtazapine could be contributing to this patient's symptoms of excessive appetite. Therefore, the most appropriate next step is to discontinue mirtazapine (Answer A).

Lisdexamfetamine is FDA-approved for the treatment of moderate to severe BED. Although the patient may fulfill criteria for BED, treatment with lisdexamfetamine (Answer E) should not be considered until his eating behaviors are assessed after mirtazapine is discontinued.

Bupropion is a component of an FDA-approved appetite suppressant, an extended-release combination pill of bupropion and naltrexone. Bupropion-containing medications may be an appropriate choice for patients who are seeking weight management and who have concurrent mood disturbance or who are trying to quit cigarette smoking. Among antidepressant agents, selective serotonin reuptake inhibitors have shown efficacy in patients with BED when used alone or when combined with cognitive behavioral therapy. In this case, starting bupropion (Answer D) without addressing underlying eating behaviors is unlikely to benefit the patient.

Educational Objective

Diagnose and treat binge-eating disorder before referral for bariatric surgery.

Reference(s)

Niego SH, Kofman MD, Weiss JJ, Geliebter A. Binge eating in the bariatric surgery population: a review of the literature. *Int J Eat Disord.* 2007;40(4):349-359. PMID: 17304586

Domecq JP, Prutsky G, Leppin A, et al. Clinical review: drugs commonly associated with weight change: a systematic review and meta-analysis. *J Clin Endocrinol Metab.* 2015;100(2):363-370. PMID: 25590213

79 **ANSWER: D) Initiate semaglutide**

Medical providers frequently encounter patients with type 2 diabetes and severe obesity, such as the patient in this vignette. Obesity is associated with increased mortality and morbidity and an increased risk of diabetes mellitus, dyslipidemia, hypertension, heart failure, coronary artery disease, malignancies, or myoskeletal disease such as osteoarthritis.

Reducing weight may, therefore, have significant health benefits for patients with obesity. Clinicians should consider that they need to treat not only diabetes but also obesity. The use of U500 concentrated insulin is reserved for patients who have severe uncontrolled hyperglycemia and in whom no other medication can be used in its management. This patient probably has severe insulin resistance and increased carbohydrate-nutrition intake with meals, which makes his insulin requirements extremely high. In this vignette, even with the U500 insulin regimen, he is still hyperglycemic as evidenced by his high hemoglobin A_{1c} value. However, increasing the U500 insulin dosage (Answer A) is not the best approach. This patient may have a reduction in hemoglobin A_{1c}, but he may also experience more weight gain because insulin is an anabolic hormone. Another concern in this case is the risk for hypoglycemia. Increasing the U500 insulin dosage confers an increased risk of hypoglycemia, which is more concerning with this extremely potent and highly concentrated type of insulin.

Referring the patient for bariatric surgery (Answer E) would lead to significant weight loss as another way of improving diabetes control. However, because of his medical history, he is considered to be a high-risk candidate for any type of surgery. He has diabetes-related complications, chronic obstructive pulmonary disease requiring home oxygen, and coronary artery disease. More importantly, he recently had coronary artery bypass graft surgery.

Medical treatment may be an alternative to bariatric surgery. GLP-1 receptor agonists can improve glycemic control and induce significant weight loss. Agents from this medication class can slow gastric emptying, inhibit inappropriate postmeal glucagon release, and increase satiety due to their effect on the appetite center in the brain. Semaglutide (Answer D) is one of the most effective GLP-1 receptor agonists. In a meta-analysis that included several trials, semaglutide reduced hemoglobin A_{1c} by up to 1.38% compared with placebo. In addition, semaglutide has increased weight-loss properties at higher dosages. In one of the trials, semaglutide was reported to have induced a 9.6% decrease in weight vs weight loss with placebo. Dosages up to 2.4 mg weekly are recommended in those with severe obesity. Up-titrating semaglutide should be done carefully, as this medication, like others in the same category, can induce nausea and vomiting that may lead to medication discontinuation.

Saxagliptin (Answer C) is a DPP-4 inhibitor. Although these medications have glucose-lowering properties, they are weight-neutral.

Phentermine/topiramate (Answer B) can induce milder weight loss and has no significant glycemic effect. It is also contraindicated in patients with coronary artery disease.

Educational Objective

Determine when to prescribe GLP-1 receptor agonist therapy in patients with obesity and type 2 diabetes mellitus who are on a U500 insulin regimen.

Reference(s)

Davies M, Færch L, Jeppesen OK, et al. Semaglutide 2.4 mg once a week in adults with overweight or obesity, and type 2 diabetes (STEP 2): a randomised, double-blind, double-dummy, placebo-controlled, phase 3 trial. *Lancet.* 2021;397(10278):971-984. PMID: 33667417

Khera R, Murad MH, Chandar AK, et al. Association of pharmacological treatments for obesity With weight loss and adverse events: a systematic review and meta-analysis. *JAMA.* 2016;315(22):2424-2434. PMID: 27299618

Liu X-Y, Zhang N, Chen R, Zhao J-G, Yu P. Efficacy and safety of sodium-glucose cotransporter 2 inhibitors in type 2 diabetes: a meta-analysis of randomized controlled trials for 1 to 2 years. *J Diabetes Complications.* 2015;29(8):1295-1303. PMID: 26365905

Andreadis P, Karagiannis T, Malandris K, et al. Semaglutide for type 2 diabetes mellitus: a systematic review and meta-analysis. *Diabetes Obes Metab.* 2018;20(9):2255-2263. PMID: 29756388

Meyer J, Dresischmeier E, Lehmann M, Phelan J. The effects of adding semaglutide to high daily dose insulin regimens in patients with type 2 diabetes. *Ann Pharmacother.* 2023;57(3):241-250. PMID: 35778801

80

ANSWER: C) Combined oral contraceptive pill (ethinyl estradiol-norelgestromin)

The etiology of hyperprolactinemia is broad and includes physiological factors such as coitus, exercise, lactation, pregnancy, sleep, and stress. Pathologic causes of hyperprolactinemia include pituitary prolactinoma, hypothalamic-pituitary stalk damage, medication-induced hyperprolactinemia, and systemic disorders such as chronic kidney failure and cirrhosis. In this vignette, the elevated prolactin level is likely secondary to a microprolactinoma.

Dopamine agonists (bromocriptine [Answer A] and cabergoline [Answer B]) lower prolactin, decrease tumor size, and restore gonadal function for patients who have symptomatic prolactin-secreting microadenomas or macroadenomas. However, these drugs do not prevent conception. This patient is experiencing oligomenorrhea and headaches, and regular menstrual cycles would be expected to be restored with a dopamine agonist. In contrast, one would not necessarily expect any change in headaches given that they are unlikely to be directly related to her microprolactinoma, but rather to other confounders. Given that this patient has expressly stated that she does not want to get pregnant for at least 4 years, dopamine agonists are not the best choice at this time.

For a woman who does not desire pregnancy and has hyperprolactinemia, the recommendation is to treat with combined oral contraceptives (Answer C) rather than dopamine agonists. A combined oral contraceptive pill would restore estrogen levels that are often low (as in this patient) in the setting of hyperprolactinemia. The elevated prolactin suppresses gonadotropin secretion, thereby leading to a hypoestrogenemic state and either oligomenorrhea or amenorrhea. One must be aware of the stimulatory role of estrogen on prolactin secretion and the potential for estrogen to stimulate prolactinoma growth. However, combined oral contraceptive pills are not contraindicated for a woman with a prolactin-secreting pituitary microadenoma, given that microadenomas rarely grow in the presence of exogenous estrogen therapy.

A progestogen challenge with medroxyprogesterone acetate (Answer E) is not indicated in this vignette given that the etiology of her oligomenorrhea is understood. Vaginal withdrawal bleeding would not be expected because of her low serum estradiol concentration secondary to hyperprolactinemia. In contrast, withdrawal vaginal bleeding would be expected in women with a serum estradiol value greater than 50 pg/mL (>183.6 pmol/L) on average, and this would indicate oligomenorrhea/amenorrhea secondary to chronic estrogenized anovulation. Accordingly, norethindrone (Answer D) would not be the best management approach for this patient because it would not restore estrogen levels (it is a progestin-only pill and does not contain any estrogen). Norethindrone would provide contraception, but it would not address her continued hypoestrogenemic state, which merits treatment.

Educational Objective

Diagnose and manage ovulatory dysfunction due to hyperprolactinemia in a woman who desires contraception.

Reference(s)

Chanson P, Maiter D. The epidemiology, diagnosis and treatment of prolactinomas: the old and the new. *Best Pract Res Clin Endocrinol Metab.* 2019;33(2):101290. PMID: 31326373

Christin-Maitre S, Delemer B, Touraine P, Young J. Prolactinoma and estrogens: pregnancy, contraception and hormonal replacement therapy. *Ann Endocrinol (Paris).* 2007;68(2-3):106-112. PMID: 17540335

Melmed S, Casanueva FF, Hoffman AR, et al; Endocrine Society. Diagnosis and treatment of hyperprolactinemia: an Endocrine Society clinical practice guideline. *J Clin Endocrinol Metab.* 2011;96(2):273-288. PMID: 21296991

81 ANSWER: D) Pulmonary function tests

While the dominant features of osteogenesis imperfecta (OI) are skeletal fragility and resultant skeletal deformities and impairments in range of motion, issues related to other systems contribute to morbidity and mortality. Persons with OI can develop cardiovascular and pulmonary abnormalities, which may present with symptoms of shortness of breath. Pulmonary disease is more common than cardiovascular disease in this patient population. Respiratory failure is a major cause of death in persons with OI, and the hazard ratio for death from pulmonary disease is up to 3 times higher than that of the reference population. Pulmonary function may be affected by restrictive lung disease due to severe kyphoscoliosis and abnormalities of the shape of the rib cage. An altered breathing pattern has been described with rapid and shallow breathing and paradoxical inspiratory movement of the ribs that worsens with age. Additionally, type 1 collagen is a component of the lung parenchyma, and there is evidence that their type 1 collagen abnormality contributes to impaired pulmonary function independently of the thoracic shape in patients with type 3 OI. Patients with OI have decreased vital capacity, as well as restrictive lung disease. In a large study of pulmonary function in patients with OI, forced expiratory volume in one second (FEV_1) and forced vital capacity were lowest in type III and IV OI, and 65% of those with type III OI had impaired FEV_1. The authors also concluded that normalizing for height might underestimate the functional deficit in these patients with varying severity of short stature. In some studies, more than 50% of patients with OI have evidence of restrictive lung disease. Thus, assessing pulmonary function (Answer D) is the most likely way to identify a cause of this patient's symptoms.

Chest radiography (Answer B) can show abnormalities in thoracic shape, pulmonary edema, or infiltrates, as well as cardiomegaly. This patient, however, does not have other associated symptoms.

Echocardiography (Answer C) would detect valve disease, or heart failure, which also occur in persons with OI but at lower rates than pulmonary disease. Procedures such as valve replacements are sometimes indicated. A Canadian study of 109 patients with OI indicated that 3.7% had clinically discernible valve dysfunction. A Danish population study indicated a small but increased risk of mitral valve regurgitation (1.6%) and aortic valve regurgitation (0.9%), atrial fibrillation or flutter (3.4%), and heart failure (4.1%) compared with findings in the general population. A separate study indicated moderate mitral regurgitation in 7.1% of patients with OI. In the Danish study, ischemic cardiovascular disease occurred at a similar rate to that in the reference population. Thus, a stress test (Answer A) is less likely to identify the cause of his symptoms in the absence of other clinical features.

Aortic dilatation is also common in persons with OI, but this would not likely explain his symptoms. Vascular aneurisms or dissections are also possible in persons with OI, but the frequency in studies is too low to estimate risk. Venous Doppler studies (Answer E) may be relevant to detect venous thrombosis and risk for pulmonary embolism. However, patients with OI are noted to have susceptibility to easy bruising and bleeding in general rather than coagulopathy, and this patient has no other signs of venous thrombosis.

Educational objective

Identify pulmonary complications of osteogenesis imperfecta.

Reference(s)

Tam A, Chen S, Schauer E, et al. A multicenter study to evaluate pulmonary function in osteogenesis imperfecta. *Clin Genet.* 2018;94(6):502-511. PMID: 30152014

Storoni S, Treurniet S, Micha D, et al. Pathophysiology of respiratory failure in patients with osteogenesis imperfecta: a systematic review. *Ann Med.* 2021;53(1):1676-1687. PMID: 34569391

Folkestad L, Hald JD, Gram J, et al. Cardiovascular disease in patients with osteogenesis imperfecta - a nationwide, register-based cohort study. *Int J Cardiol.* 2016;225:250-257. PMID: 27741483

LoMauro A, Fraschini P, Pochintesta S, Romei M, D'Angelo MG, Aliverti A. Ribcage deformity and the altered breathing pattern in children with osteogenesis imperfecta. *Pediatr Pulmonol.* 2018;53(7):964-972. PMID: 29766672

Keuning MC, Leeuwerke SJG, van Dijk PR, et al. Prevalence of scoliosis and impaired pulmonary function in patients with type III osteogenesis imperfecta. *Eur Spine J.* 2022;31(9):2295-2300. PMID: 35604455

82 ANSWER: B) Discontinue methimazole

Since the mid-2000s, the number of antithyroid drug prescriptions has increased while the number of radioiodine prescriptions has decreased for the management of Graves disease in the United States. Antithyroid drugs such as methimazole, carbimazole, and propylthiouracil are associated with serious adverse effects, including agranulocytosis and hepatic dysfunction in 0.5% to 1.0% of patients. After 6 case reports of acute pancreatitis associated with methimazole/carbimazole, the European Medicines Agency issued a special warning and an update to the product label in 2019 to include acute pancreatitis as a possible serious adverse effect.

A study from Denmark (1995-2018) assessed acute pancreatitis in patients receiving methimazole/carbimazole (104,873 patients) and propylthiouracil (14,824 patients). Of 39,996 cases of acute pancreatitis, 692 (1.7%) had filled at least 1 prescription of methimazole and 108 (0.3%) had filled at least 1 prescription of propylthiouracil. The analysis yielded an increased risk for acute pancreatitis associated with ongoing methimazole/carbimazole treatment (odds ratio, 1.56; 95% CI, 1.04-2.33) compared with ongoing propylthiouracil treatment (odds ratio, 0.88; 95% CI, 0.26-2.96). Cases of pancreatitis occurred within 3 months of initiating methimazole and recurred sooner with reinitiation of therapy. The risk of developing pancreatitis was not dosage dependent. A retrospective population-based cohort study in Italy showed an increased risk of acute pancreatitis in the first months of methimazole treatment with a probability well below 1%. A case of methimazole-induced pancreatitis 12 days after initiation of methimazole was described in a 72-year-old Japanese woman with Graves disease. Serological HLA typing identified HLA-DRB1*08:03:02, the same HLA haplotype seen in agranulocytosis induced by methimazole and propylthiouracil. Based on the study from Denmark, propylthiouracil can be prescribed for the management of hyperthyroidism in patients with methimazole-associated pancreatitis. However, patients can also be observed if hyperthyroidism is mild, and cholestyramine can be administered to reduce thyroid hormone levels by interfering with enterohepatic circulation and recycling of thyroid hormone. In case of severe hyperthyroidism in patients with methimazole-associated pancreatitis, more definitive treatment such as radioiodine treatment or thyroidectomy can be considered once the pancreatitis improves.

The patient in this vignette is being treated with methimazole. After 8 weeks of methimazole treatment, she has nausea and epigastric pain and generally feels unwell. Her lipase concentration is also elevated. Her clinical and biochemical findings are consistent with pancreatitis. Her triglycerides and liver enzymes are normal, which eliminates other etiologies of acute pancreatitis such as hypertriglyceridemia and gallstones. Because methimazole is known to cause pancreatitis, this medication should be discontinued (Answer B).

Decreasing the methimazole dosage (Answer A) is incorrect, as this medication is the culprit for her pancreatitis and should therefore be discontinued.

Even though performing abdominal CT (Answer D) will be necessary, the best step now is to stop methimazole.

Her symptoms are not consistent with exacerbation of gastroesophageal reflux disease and neither increasing the omeprazole dosage (Answer C) nor ordering an upper endoscopy (Answer E) is necessary.

Educational Objective

Identify pancreatitis as an adverse effect of methimazole.

Reference(s)

Brito JP, Schilz S, Singh Ospina N, et al. Antithyroid drugs-the most common treatment for Graves' disease in the United States: a nationwide population-based study. *Thyroid.* 2016;26(8):1144-1145. PMID: 27267495

Pecere A, Caputo M, Sarro A, et al. Methimazole treatment and risk of acute pancreatitis: a population-based cohort study. *J Clin Endocrinol Metab.* 2020;105(12):dgaa544. PMID: 32813014

Brix TH, Lund LC, Henriksen DP, et al. Methimazole and risk of acute pancreatitis. *Lancet Diabetes Endocrinol.* 2020; 8(3):187-189. PMID: 32035032

Agito K, Manni A. Acute pancreatitis induced by methimazole in a patient with subclinical hyperthyroidism. *J Investig Med High Impact Case Rep.* 2015;3(2):2324709615592229. PMID: 26425645

Yoshimura Y, Tatsushima K, Goshima Y, et al. A case of methimazole-induced acute pancreatitis with an HLA allele causing antithyroid drug-induced agranulocytosis. *J Endocr Soc.* 2022;6(5):bvac038. PMID: 35402762

83 ANSWER: D) Repeat oral glucose tolerance testing, with consumption of 150 g carbohydrate per day for 3 days before testing

This patient had a screening blood test that showed a mildly abnormal fasting glucose level. First, one must consider whether screening for diabetes was reasonable in this young person. Per guidelines from the American Diabetes Association, universal screening for diabetes (ie, regardless of age) should be performed in all asymptomatic persons who are classified as having overweight or obesity (BMI ≥25 kg/m^2 and in those of Asian descent with BMI ≥23 kg/m^2) AND who have 1 or more risk factor for diabetes. Diabetes risk increases at a lower BMI cut-point for Asian Americans, and studies suggest that one-third to one-half of Asian Americans with diabetes are undiagnosed.

Currently, this patient could be categorized as having prediabetes based on the 2-hour plasma glucose value between 140 and 200 mg/dL (7.8 and 11.1 mmol/L) after oral glucose challenge, and this finding has caused anxiety. Of the diagnostic tests for diabetes, the 2-hour plasma glucose measurement after oral glucose challenge is the most sensitive test for identifying persons with diabetes. After performing a screening test, it is recommended that the diagnosis be confirmed by repeating the test on the same sample or on a different date. In recent years, oral glucose tolerance testing has become less frequently used for a variety of reasons, including convenience for patients. However, it is useful to remember that compared with measurement of hemoglobin A_{1c} or fasting plasma glucose, the 2-hour glucose value after a 75-g oral glucose load is likely a more sensitive test for hyperglycemia. Also, hyperglycemia at the 2-hour time point is associated with increased risk for cardiovascular disease, hypertension, dyslipidemia, and microalbuminuria.

Patients should be given important instructions before performing this test. Consumption of a low-carbohydrate diet before oral glucose tolerance testing may result in impaired glucose tolerance in a substantial proportion of individuals, primarily women. The mechanism for this adaptation is not fully understood, but studies suggest reduced first-phase insulin secretion, reduced postload incretin secretion, and decreased insulin sensitivity. The World Health Organization has recommended that 150 g of carbohydrate or more be consumed daily for 3 days before oral glucose tolerance testing. Interestingly, this concept of "hunger diabetes" was recognized in the late 18th century when starving dogs were fed high-carbohydrate diets, which resulted in glycosuria. Even eating a very low-carbohydrate meal for dinner prior to oral glucose tolerance testing has been associated with impaired glucose tolerance. Therefore, this patient should be instructed to consume an adequate amount of carbohydrates before oral glucose tolerance testing (Answer D). In addition, patients should be instructed to eat 3 meals per day, and the last meal of the day should contain 50 g of carbohydrate or more. Indeed, this patient had been consuming less than 50 g of carbohydrate for almost 1 month prior to oral glucose tolerance testing because of the concern generated by her laboratory test results. When oral glucose tolerance testing was repeated after provision of these instructions, results were normal.

Given that the diagnosis of diabetes has not been established, assessing risk for type 1 diabetes with antibodies (Answer E) is not necessary.

Similarly, as the patient's average glycemic control is not in the diabetes range per the test results available, measurement of C-peptide (Answer A) would not be useful.

Fructosamine (Answer B) is used to assess average glycemia over a 2-week period, particularly when hemoglobin A_{1c} testing may be inaccurate. In this patient, there is no reason to suspect that her hemoglobin A_{1c} may be inaccurate, and measurement of fructosamine is not expected to be helpful.

In a patient for whom a diagnosis of diabetes or even impaired glucose tolerance is not established, advising fingerstick glucose measurements at home (Answer C) is a needless burden.

Educational Objective

Determine the risk for developing type 2 diabetes mellitus based on results of typical diagnostic tests.

Reference(s)

ElSayed NA, Aleppo G, Aroda VR, et al. 2. Classification and diagnosis of diabetes: *standards of care in diabetes-2023. Diabetes Care.* 2023;46(Suppl 1):S19-S40. PMID: 36507649

Klein KR, Walker CP, McFerren AL, Huffman H, Frohlich F, Buse JB. Carbohydrate intake prior to oral glucose tolerance testing. J Endocr Soc. 2021;5(5):bvab049. PMID: 33928207

84 ANSWER: A) Abdominal CT with and without contrast

This patient was diagnosed with hypercortisolism during workup for an incidentally detected adrenal nodule during hospital admission for a cardiac ischemic event. Individuals with Cushing syndrome have an increased risk of cardiovascular comorbidities, including coronary artery disease, which represents the first cause of death in this population. While cortisol and ACTH levels can be elevated in acutely ill patients, the outpatient workup confirmed ACTH-dependent Cushing syndrome due to lack of serum cortisol suppression following dexamethasone administration, as well as 2 elevated urinary free cortisol measurements and elevated ACTH.

This patient rapidly developed severe muscle weakness and hypokalemia. Her ACTH was not stimulated after corticotropin-releasing hormone administration, indicating a nonpituitary or ectopic source of ACTH secretion.

CT of the chest and abdomen (Answer A) identified a 6-cm tumor in the pancreatic tail. After tumor resection, the patient's cortisol and ACTH levels decreased below the reference range, confirming ectopic ACTH secretion from a pancreatic neuroendocrine neoplasm. She required hydrocortisone replacement for 18 months.

Laparoscopic removal of the left adrenal gland (Answer D) is incorrect because the adrenal nodule is not responsible for hypercortisolism based on the elevated ACTH concentration. A few cases of ACTH-producing adrenal pheochromocytomas have been reported, but this patient's plasma metanephrine concentration is normal. Her adrenal incidentaloma requires further evaluation with CT without contrast administration (or with washout protocol) to distinguish an adenoma from metastasis.

Transsphenoidal resection of the pituitary adenoma (Answer E) is incorrect because the clinical and biochemical picture, including the flat cortisol and ACTH response to corticotropin-releasing hormone, points toward an ectopic ACTH-producing tumor. In general, a significant increase in ACTH levels is observed in patients with pituitary ACTH-producing adenomas after corticotropin-releasing hormone or desmopressin administration. The mechanism entails expression of corticotropin-releasing hormone and vasopressin receptors on corticotroph pituitary tumor cells. The macroadenoma identified by MRI was a nonfunctioning incidentaloma that did not enlarge during the 3-year interval of follow-up. Imaging surveillance is important is these cases because tumor growth can occur in 24% of pituitary macroincidentalomas.

High-dose dexamethasone-suppression testing (Answer B) does not accurately distinguish between pituitary- and ectopic ACTH-producing tumors, and sufficient clinical and biochemical information in this case points towards a nonpituitary ACTH source.

Inferior petrosal sinus sampling (Answer C) is the gold standard test that correctly distinguishes between pituitary and ectopic ACTH production in most patients with ACTH-dependent hypercortisolism. In this case, the rapidly evolving clinical manifestations of hypercortisolism and the significantly elevated cortisol and ACTH levels strongly suggested ectopic ACTH production. Localization imaging with CT of the chest and abdomen identified a mass that was biopsy-confirmed as neuroendocrine tumor. Inferior petrosal sinus sampling is performed at specialized pituitary centers, while CT is a readily available imaging technique.

Educational Objective

Guide the diagnostic steps in a patient with ACTH-dependent Cushing syndrome and multiple endocrine tumors in the pituitary gland, adrenal glands, and pancreas.

Reference(s)

Hayes AR, Grossman AB. Distinguishing Cushing's disease from the ectopic ACTH syndrome: needles in a haystack or hiding in plain sight? *J Neuroendocrinol.* 2022;34(8):e13127. PMID: 35980277

Fleseriu M, Auchus R, Bancos I, et al. Consensus on diagnosis and management of Cushing's disease: a guideline update. *Lancet Diabetes Endocrinol.* 2021;9(12):847-875. PMID: 34687601

Ferriere A, Tabarin A. Biochemical testing to differentiate Cushing's disease from ectopic ACTH syndrome. *Pituitary.* 2022;25(5):705-708. PMID: 35759056

Govindarajan V, Lu VM, Clarke JE, et al. Positive predictive value and trends of inferior petrosal sinus sampling (IPSS) in diagnosing Cushing disease and ectopic ACTH secretion: a systematic review and meta-analysis. *Clin Neurol Neurosurg.* 2022;220:107350. PMID: 35820339

Yip L, Duh Q-Y, Wachtel H, et al. American Association of Endocrine Surgeons guidelines for adrenalectomy: executive summary. *JAMA Surg.* 2022;e223544. PMID: 35976622

85 ANSWER: E) 24-Hour urinary steroid profile

The patient has numerous clinical features of Cushing syndrome, and results of all 3 screening investigations (dexamethasone-suppressed cortisol, 24-hour urinary free cortisol, and late-night salivary cortisol) are strongly supportive of the diagnosis. In a young woman, the most likely cause is Cushing disease due to an ACTH-secreting pituitary adenoma. In this case, ACTH is completely suppressed, which suggests an adrenal origin. However, unexpectedly, CT shows normal adrenal glands with no evidence of an adrenal adenoma, adrenal carcinoma, adrenal hyperplasia, or nodular adrenal disease.

MRI (Answer B) may permit the identification of adrenal pathology not previously appreciated on CT (eg, in a lean patient in whom the absence of retroperitoneal adipose tissue hinders visualization of the adrenal glands).

However, in this case, the patient has central obesity, and it is unlikely that MRI will reveal a previously unseen adrenal mass.

Adrenal vein sampling (Answer A) is principally used to distinguish unilateral and bilateral causes of primary aldosteronism. Less commonly, it is deployed in ACTH-independent Cushing syndrome in the context of bilateral adrenal lesions to inform surgical decision-making. However, interpretation may be challenging when markers other than serum cortisol (eg, plasma metanephrines) are used to judge the adequacy of adrenal vein cannulation. Adrenal vein sampling is not indicated for this patient given the normal appearance of her adrenal glands on CT.

Another important consideration in this case is the possibility of a misleading plasma ACTH result—meaning the patient actually has ACTH-dependent Cushing syndrome with an artifactually low ACTH value. Preanalytical practices such as inappropriate specimen handling can cause false results when ACTH is measured (eg, maintenance of samples at room temperature, delayed centrifugation/separation of plasma, hemolysis, and excessive use of EDTA can all cause a false decrease in ACTH concentration). Interference in laboratory assay measurement, analogous to that seen with TSH measurement, may also be a cause of false-positive or, less commonly, false-negative ACTH results when using immunoassays. Verification using a second assay with discrete assay architecture or deployment of other methods to exclude interference by heterophilic or antianimal immunoglobulins may be required. In this case, appropriate sample handling and measurement with an alternative assay confirmed undetectable ACTH. However, another important finding in the initial laboratory profile—the very low DHEA-S value—strongly suggests that the suppressed ACTH level would be verified. In ACTH-dependent Cushing syndrome, DHEA-S is typically normal or raised, reflecting the ACTH-dependence of adrenal androgen production.

Other less common causes of ACTH-independent Cushing syndrome include:

- Micronodular adrenal hyperplasia, including Carney complex, a rare disorder characterized by cutaneous and cardiac myxomas, skin pigmentation, primary pigmented nodular adrenocortical disease, acromegaly, large-cell calcifying Sertoli-cell tumors, and thyroid nodules.
- Ectopic receptor expression (eg, gastric inhibitory polypeptide receptor; β-adrenoceptor), which is typically associated with adrenal hyperplasia.

In Carney complex, adrenal irregularity ("string of beads") may be subtle and not appreciated on initial review of anatomical imaging. Further investigation should therefore be considered if there is evidence of other associated clinical features (eg, spotty skin pigmentation and lentigines, cutaneous myxomas, cardiac myxomas, unexplained embolic stroke) or a suggestive family history. In this context, combined low- and high-dose dexamethasone-suppression testing (Liddle test: 0.5 mg dexamethasone every 6 hours for 2 days followed by 2-mg dexamethasone every 6 hours for 2 days) (Answer C) classically shows a paradoxical rise in cortisol in serum or urine. Genetic testing identifies a pathogenic variant in the *PRKAR1A* gene in more than 70% of cases, including 80% of those with primary pigmented nodular adrenocortical disease. The patient in this vignette has no other features to suggest Carney complex.

When faced with a patient with ACTH-independent hypercortisolism in whom adrenal imaging is normal, the possibility of factitious Cushing syndrome due to surreptitious (covert) corticosteroid administration should be considered. Although several synthetic glucocorticoids are not detected in commonly used cortisol immunoassays, others may cross-react to yield abnormal results. For example, prednisolone can lead to spuriously high urinary cortisol levels that may suggest endogenous Cushing syndrome. Similarly, hydrocortisone and cortisone will be detected, but, unlike prednisolone, may yield elevated levels even when using liquid chromatography–tandem mass spectrometry, as they are associated with increased serum cortisol levels after ingestion (as was subsequently confirmed in this case). A careful history should therefore be taken, and a 24-hour urinary steroid profile (Answer E) should be performed. The latter allows documentation of the specific steroid metabolites excreted in the urine, which can help to distinguish between exogenous hydrocortisone usage and endogenous hypercortisolism. In the former, urinary cortisol and its metabolites will be elevated, while other steroid metabolites will be within the normal range or low. In contrast, in endogenous Cushing syndrome, other steroid metabolites will also be elevated due to the overproduction of cortisol precursors. Therefore, a urinary steroid profile that shows elevated levels of only cortisol metabolites, without any abnormalities in other adrenal steroids, would be suggestive of surreptitious hydrocortisone administration as the cause of Cushing syndrome. A 24-hour urinary steroid profile can also help to identify the type of exogenous steroid that is being used if it is not hydrocortisone. Finally, when exogenous glucocorticoid ingestion is sustained over a period, the resulting hypothalamic-pituitary-adrenal–axis suppression can result in adrenal gland atrophy, which is a potentially important clue to the adrenal-independent nature of the hypercortisolism.

A ^{68}Ga-DOTATATE PET/CT scan (Answer D) localizes an ectopic source of ACTH secretion, but it is not indicated in this case because ACTH is undetectable.

Educational Objective

Recognize when factitious Cushing syndrome should be considered during evaluation of a patient with hypercortisolism.

Reference(s)

Pineyro MM, Redes L, De Mattos S, et al. Factitious Cushing's syndrome: a diagnosis to consider when evaluating hypercortisolism. *Front Endocrinol (Lausanne).* 2019;10:129. PMID: 30886602

Donegan DM, Algeciras-Schimnich A, Hamidi O, et al. Corticotropin hormone assay interference: a case series. *Clin Biochem.* 2019;63:143-147. PMID: 30423322

Kamilaris CDC, Faucz FR, Voutetakis A, Stratakis CA. Carney complex. *Exp Clin Endocrinol Diabetes.* 2019;127(2-03):156-164. PMID: 30428497

86 ANSWER: D) Serum SHBG measurement

This young, healthy appearing patient presents with a marked reduction in serum testosterone, without any clinical evidence of androgen deficiency. The initial presentation leading his primary care provider to measure serum testosterone was very nonspecific, and these symptoms have since resolved. While a laboratory error was considered initially, the similar result using liquid chromatography–tandem mass spectrometry makes this extremely unlikely. The clinical picture of eugonadism with very low total testosterone suggests that the non–SHBG-bound testosterone, comprising free testosterone (~2%-4% of total testosterone) and loosely albumin-bound testosterone (considered bioavailable, ~40% of total testosterone) will be normal. Given that direct measurement of free testosterone requires equilibrium dialysis that is not readily available, measuring SHBG (Answer D), which can be used to calculate free testosterone (eg, Vermeulen formula, either provided by the laboratory or using internet calculators) is the best next step. In this patient, serum SHBG was undetectable when measured using 2 different assay platforms. He most likely has inactivating pathogenic variants in the *SHBG* gene. Genetic testing was offered, but the patient declined.

Of note, the patient's parents were from a region in Tasmania that is known for a relatively high degree of consanguinity. In conjunction with other case reports of complete absence of the SHBG protein (usually due to homozygous missense variants in the *SHBG* gene), the clinical phenotype suggests that a lack of serum SHBG does not interfere with male, or female, gonadal function. Instead, gonadal development (and, when tested, spermatogenesis) is normal, and the nonelevated gonadotropins (in the absence of hypothalamic-pituitary pathology) are consistent with pituitary perception of normal sex steroid availability. There is some evidence (mostly from preclinical studies) that SHBG may have biologic actions beyond just being a passive carrier of circulating sex steroids, including actively enhancing cellular sex steroid uptake. This, however, appears to have limited relevance in humans, although it has been speculated that passive diffusion of testosterone alone may be insufficient for target tissues requiring high intracellular concentrations of sex steroids. In a sense, the clinical picture associated with the lack of SHBG is similar to the clinical picture seen in individuals with inactivating variants in the gene encoding cortisol-binding globulin (~80%-90% of cortisol is bound to cortisol-binding globulin), who present with low serum (total) cortisol but lack evidence of glucocorticoid deficiency and have normal ACTH concentrations.

Anabolic steroid use can also be associated with very low—but rarely undetectable—SHBG, especially when nonaromatizable androgens are abused. However, there are no features suggestive of anabolic steroid abuse, such as muscular physique, truncal acne, or small testes. Whether it is ethical to order anabolic steroid testing without informing the patient (Answer E) is highly debatable. Anabolic steroid testing is not standardized across laboratories, and diagnostic precision is uncertain. Patients can easily avoid detection by temporarily pausing anabolic steroid use or by providing someone else's urine sample. In clinical practice, the best "diagnostic test" for anabolic steroid abuse remains to ask the patient directly, and this appears to have reasonably high reliability.

An increase in glucocorticoids or in serum estradiol can cause secondary male hypogonadism due to central (hypothalamic-pituitary) gonadal-axis suppression, but the absence of clinical features of hypogonadism coupled with the absence of clinical features suggesting Cushing syndrome or estrogen excess or make these possibilities unlikely. Thus, measuring serum estradiol (Answer B) or 24-hour urinary cortisol (Answer A) is incorrect.

Serum 17-hydroxyprogesterone measurement (Answer C) is a screening test for congenital adrenal hyperplasia. However, this patient's clinical picture is not consistent with this diagnosis.

Educational Objective

Identify the discrepancy between the clinical picture of eugonadism and a very low total testosterone concentration.

Reference(s)

Vos MJ, Mijnhout GS, Rondeel JMM, Baron W, Groeneveld PHP. Sex hormone binding globulin deficiency due to a homozygous missense mutation. *J Clin Endocrinol Metab.* 2014;99(9):E1798-E1802. PMID: 24937543

Goldman AL, Bhasin S, Wu FCW, Krishna M, Matsumoto AM, Jasuja R. A reappraisal of testosterone's binding in circulation: physiological and clinical implications. *Endocr Rev.* 2017;38(4):302-324. PMID: 28673039

Shankara-Narayana N, Brooker L, Goebel C, Speers N, Handelsman DJ. Reliability of drug history to verify androgen abuse in men. *J Clin Endocrinol Metab.* 2022;107(9):e3790-e3796. PMID: 35661889

87 ANSWER: D) Multiple myeloma

Hypercalcemia of malignancy is an unfortunate complication of common types of cancer, namely breast, lung, lymphoma, and multiple myeloma. Symptoms of moderate to severe hypercalcemia are fatigue, polyuria, and polydipsia. This patient's initial serum calcium concentration is 13.1 mg/dL (3.3 mmol/L) and thus would be classified as moderate hypercalcemia (mild = <12 mg/dL [<3.0 mmol/L], moderate = 12-14 mg/dL [3.0-3.5 mmol/L], severe = >14 mg/dL [>3.5 mmol/L]).

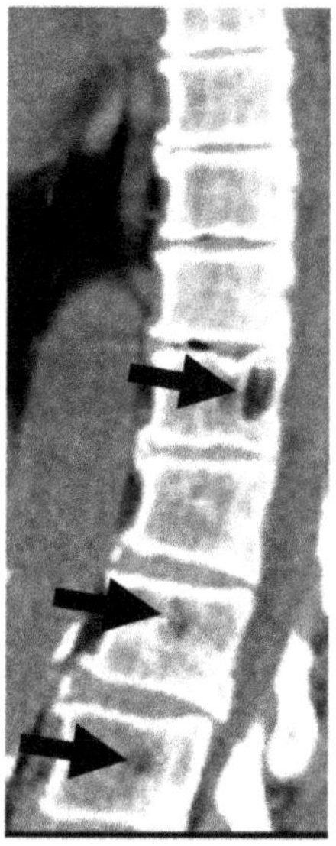

Humoral hypercalcemia of malignancy occurs when cancer cells secrete endocrine factors that cause hypercalcemia. Malignancies such as renal cell and breast cancer can secrete PTHrP, which activates the PTH receptor in a manner similar to primary hyperparathyroidism and leads to hypercalcemia and subsequent hypercalciuria. Other examples of PTH-independent hypercalcemia include the overproduction of 1,25-dihydroxyvitamin D by lymphomas resulting in, in essence, activated vitamin D toxicity. In the described patient, PTH is low, supporting that primary hyperparathyroidism is not the cause of hypercalcemia. Furthermore, serum PTHrP and 1,25-dihydroxyvitamin D are not elevated, so the patient appears not to have humoral hypercalcemia of malignancy.

Cancer cells metastatic to bone often activate osteoblast-dependent bone formation, osteoclast-dependent bone resorption, or a mixture of both. Local osteolysis hypercalcemia is a type of hypercalcemia of malignancy commonly seen with breast, lung, and renal cell cancer metastases. In such cases of rapid bone resorption, the amount of calcium removed from the skeleton can be greater than the capacity of the kidneys to eliminate calcium, which leads to hypercalcemia. The radiographic appearance of lesions is described as osteolytic, with well-defined radiolucent areas on x-ray. This patient's spine CT demonstrates osteolytic lesions (*see image, arrows*).

While osteolytic lesions develop as a consequence of rapid bone osteoclast-dependent bone resorption, osteoblast activity remains high due to the coupling of these 2 bone cells. Nuclear medicine bone scans often detect increased scintigraphic uptake of bone metastasis from breast and lung cancers and renal cell carcinoma. Therefore, metastatic breast cancer (Answer A), metastatic lung cancer (Answer B), and renal cell carcinoma (Answer C) are incorrect because the described patient did not have any focal increases in scintigraphic uptake in the bone scan. NonHodgkin lymphoma can cause humoral hypercalcemia of malignancy by producing 1,25-dihydroxyvitamin D or cause local osteolysis hypercalcemia by producing local osteolytic factors. As with the other cancer types, it would be expected that osteoblast activity would be increased due to expected osteoclast-osteoblast coupling. Therefore, nonHodgkin lymphoma (Answer E) is incorrect.

Hypercalcemia is a common complication of multiple myeloma (Answer D) due to the production of local factors that increase osteoclastic bone resorption. A unique characteristic of multiple myeloma is also the production of factors that suppress osteoblast activity, including the Dickkopf and secreted frizzled-related proteins. Because scintigraphic bone scans detect areas of increased bone formation, scintigraphic scanning is often normal in patients with multiple myeloma. This patient's scintigraphic bone scan does not reveal areas of abnormal uptake. Skeletal x-ray surveys and low-dose whole-body CT therefore have a larger role in identifying osteolytic lesions of multiple myeloma.

The patient described had numerous radiographic osteolytic lesions, especially of the spine and pelvis, but without an increase in scintigraphic uptake. This pattern is most consistent with multiple myeloma.

Educational Objective

Differentiate among the causes of hypercalcemia of malignancy and identify the imaging characteristics of common cancers that cause hypercalcemia of malignancy.

Reference(s)

Clines GA. Mechanisms and treatment of hypercalcemia of malignancy. *Curr Opin Endocrinol Diabetes Obes.* 2011;18(6):339-346. PMID: 21897221

Guise TA, Wysolmerski JJ. Cancer-Associated Hypercalcemia. *N Engl J Med.* 2022;386(15):1443-1451. PMID: 35417639

El-Hajj Fuleihan G, Clines GA, Hu MI, et al. Treatment of hypercalcemia of malignancy in adults: an Endocrine Society clinical practice guideline. *J Clin Endocrinol Metab.* 2023;108(3):507-528. PMID: 36545746

Hillengass J, Moulopoulos LA, Delorme S, et al. Whole-body computed tomography versus conventional skeletal survey in patients with multiple myeloma: a study of the International Myeloma Working Group. *Blood Cancer J.* 2017;7(8):e599. PMID: 28841211

Adamik J, Galson DL, Roodman GD. Osteoblast suppression in multiple myeloma bone disease. *J Bone Oncol.* 2018;13:62-70. PMID: 30591859

88 **ANSWER: E) Recommend psychiatric evaluation for anorexia nervosa**

This patient has severe acquired hypercholesterolemia as evidenced by a previously normal lipid panel. Common causes of acquired hypercholesterolemia are hypothyroidism, Cushing syndrome, nephrotic syndrome, cholestatic liver disease, and certain drugs. While she does have primary hypothyroidism with a TSH value in the upper end of normal, it is very unlikely to be the sole cause of the severe hypercholesterolemia and increasing the levothyroxine dosage (Answer C) is incorrect. She has many classic features of anorexia nervosa, which is well known to cause hypercholesterolemia. She has a low BMI but does not think she is lean or has an eating problem. In addition, she has a low free T_3 value, high cortisol value, and amenorrhea, all of which are commonly seen in anorexia nervosa. In patients with anorexia nervosa, correction of malnutrition usually leads to resolution of hyperlipidemia. It is therefore important to make this diagnosis and start treatment rather than prescribe lipid-lowering therapies (Answers A, B, and D). Thus, recommending psychiatric evaluation (Answer E) is the best next step.

The exact cause of hypercholesterolemia in persons with anorexia is not known, but it may be related to decreased cholesterol and bile acid turnover along with decreased LDL-receptor expression in the liver. Low T_3 could also be contributing to these abnormalities. Increased cholesteryl ester transfer protein activity has also been reported.

While hypercholesterolemia is fairly common in patients with anorexia, it is usually not this severe and the reported total cholesterol concentration is usually in the range of 300 to 400 mg/dL (7.77-10.36 mmol/L), with increases in both LDL and HDL cholesterol. Another contributing factor to hypercholesterolemia in this patient could be her ketogenic diet. Although low-carbohydrate, high-fat diets have been reported to promote weight loss and improve hyperlipidemia, some patients experience marked increases in total cholesterol and triglycerides when they start such diets. The underlying cause for the hyperabsorptive hypercholesterolemia is not clear, but it is important to monitor lipid levels in patients who start ketogenic diets.

The patient was counseled to eat a balanced diet to help with weight gain. Over the next 6 months, she gained 10 lb (4.5 kg), and a repeated lipid panel showed the following values:

Total cholesterol = 202 mg/dL (SI: 5.23 mmol/L)
Triglycerides = 90 mg/dL (SI: 1.02 mmol/L)
HDL cholesterol = 66 mg/dL (SI: 1.71 mmol/L)
LDL cholesterol = 118 mg/dL (SI: 3.06 mmol/L)

Educational Objective

Recognize anorexia nervosa and ketogenic diets as rare causes of severe hypercholesterolemia.

Reference(s)

Ohwada R, Hotta M, Oikawa S, Takano K. Etiology of hypercholesterolemia in patients with anorexia nervosa. *Int J Eat Disord.* 2006;39(7):598-601. PMID: 16791856

Misra M, Klibanski A. Endocrine consequences of anorexia nervosa. *Lancet Diabetes Endocrinol.* 2014;2(7):581-592. PMID: 24731664

Goldberg IJ, Ibrahim N, Bredefeld C, et al. Ketogenic diets, not for everyone. *J Clin Lipidol.* 2021;15(1):61-67. PMID: 33191194

89 **ANSWER: B) Perform ultrasound-guided FNA with rapid on-site evaluation of cytology specimens**
Nondiagnostic thyroid FNA biopsies are those that do not meet established qualitative and quantitative criteria for cytological adequacy (at least 6 groups of 10 or more follicular cells). FNA operator skill, nonuse of ultrasound guidance, poor smear preparation, and certain nodule characteristics (eg, cystic change, fibrosis, increased vascularity, and calcification) can contribute to nondiagnostic results. The risk of malignancy associated with nondiagnostic cytology is estimated to be 5% to 10% according to the revised (2017) Bethesda System for Reporting Thyroid Cytology. Surgical series suggest a much higher rate of malignancy of 17% to 25%; however, these studies overestimate risk due to selection bias (nodules with higher clinical risk tend to be resected). In contrast, a study by Sauter and colleagues that included histology or long-term follow-up as acceptable clinical end points demonstrated a malignancy rate of only 3.5%.

The use of ultrasound guidance is the most important tool to improve diagnostic yield during thyroid FNA. After an initial nondiagnostic FNA, a diagnostic specimen can be obtained in 60% to 80% of cases when repeated biopsy with ultrasound guidance is performed. Therefore, performing neck ultrasonography again in 12 months (Answer A) is not the best next step in the management of this intermediate-risk nodule after 1 nondiagnostic FNA result (2015 American Thyroid Association Risk Stratification System estimated risk 10%-20%). Similarly, referral for right thyroid lobectomy (Answer D) is premature and would not be indicated now for this patient without clinical risk factors for malignancy or compressive symptoms.

When available, rapid on-site evaluation of cytology smears to confirm specimen adequacy (Answer B) during the ultrasound-guided FNA procedure has also been shown to improve diagnostic yield. A 2013 meta-analysis demonstrated a 44% relative risk reduction in the occurrence of nondiagnostic samples with the use of rapid on-site evaluation of cytology smears, as well as a decrease in the number of required needle passes.

Performing repeated FNA with 5 separate needle passes (Answer C) is incorrect. A retrospective study of 121 patients demonstrated that optimal adequacy rates could be achieved with 2 to 3 needle passes and that performing additional passes beyond this point did not significantly improve yield.

Sending the specimen collected during previous FNA for molecular analysis (Answer E) is also incorrect. The performance of molecular diagnostic testing for thyroid nodules with nondiagnostic cytology has not been extensively studied, and testing is not yet approved for this indication. Although mutational testing could have the potential to be informative in samples considered nondiagnostic due to poor preparation or staining, it is much less likely to be useful for specimens with inadequate cellularity. However, some studies have evaluated nondiagnostic cytology specimens for the presence of the *BRAF V600E* pathogenic variant, which could be detected in a subset (10%) of nodules, allowing those to be triaged to surgical management.

Educational Objective

Recommend the next steps in the evaluation of thyroid nodules after initially nondiagnostic ultrasound-guided fine-needle aspiration.

Reference(s)

Cibas ES, Ali SZ. The 2017 Bethesda System for Reporting Thyroid Cytopathology. *Thyroid.* 2017;27(11):1341-1346. PMID: 29091573

Kuzan TY, Canbey Goret C. Comparison of number of passes and cytopathological specimen adequacy for thyroid fine-needle aspiration biopsy in the absence of an on-site pathologist. *Eur Thyroid J.* 2020;9(1):49-54. PMID: 32071902

Sauter JL, Lehrke H, Zhang X, et al. Assessment of The Bethesda System for Reporting Thyroid Cytopathology. *Am J Clin Pathol.* 2019;152(4):502-511. PMID: 31305880

Witt BL, Schmidt RL. Rapid onsite evaluation improves the adequacy of fine-needle aspiration for thyroid lesions: a systematic review and meta-analysis. *Thyroid.* 2013;23(4):428-435. PMID: 23043247

90 **ANSWER: E) MIBG scintigraphy**
Benign adrenal adenomas are commonly homogeneous, well circumscribed, and have attenuation values less than 10 Hounsfield units on unenhanced CT, reflecting their high cholesterol content. For homogeneous tumors with unenhanced attenuation greater than 10 Hounsfield units, delayed contrast washout can be used to differentiate lipid-poor adenomas (contrast medium washout >50% at 10 minutes) from pheochromocytomas or malignant tumors. Hounsfield units and contrast medium washout measurements are not reliable in patients with heterogeneous adrenal masses.

An adrenal mass with high precontrast attenuation and poor contrast washout was noted incidentally in this patient. The differential diagnosis of such a mass includes pheochromocytoma and malignancy (either adrenal cortical carcinoma or metastasis).

This patient has a history of lymphoma, which presented with a set of symptoms that are frequently seen in patients with pheochromocytoma, including headaches, sweating, and weight loss. The first step in distinguishing between a pheochromocytoma and a malignant tumor is measuring metanephrines. This patient had dramatic elevation of plasma normetanephrine, suggestive of a pheochromocytoma. Nevertheless, because recurrent lymphoma was also diagnosed, confirmation of pheochromocytoma was sought to guide therapy for the adrenal mass.

Functional imaging studies that target neuroendocrine tumors are valuable in patients with an uncertain diagnosis, not only to clarify the etiology of indeterminate masses, but also to identify possible extraadrenal metastatic foci. $^{131}I/^{123}I$-MIBG imaging (Answer E) has high specificity for detecting pheochromocytomas and paragangliomas. In 2016, the US FDA approved ^{68}Ga-DOTATATE (Answer A) for imaging well-differentiated neuroendocrine tumors. Gallium 68–labeled high-affinity somatostatin analogues confer excellent spatial resolution in the diagnosis of well-differentiated neuroendocrine tumors, pheochromocytomas, and paragangliomas. The sensitivity of MIBG scintigraphy is lower than that of ^{68}Ga-DOTATATE, particularly in patients with *SDHx* pathogenic variants and in patients with metastatic disease. However, somatostatin receptor expression in lymphomas limits the utility of somatostatin analogue–based imaging in this patient. Focal radiotracer accumulation within the right adrenal mass was observed on ^{123}I MIBG scintigraphy, confirming the diagnosis of pheochromocytoma.

Chromogranin A (Answer B) is a nonspecific biomarker of neuroendocrine tumors, including pheochromocytomas and paragangliomas. Proton-pump inhibitor use leads to chromogranin A elevation, and the effect can be prolonged for months after stopping such antiacids. Thus, chromogranin A measurement would be difficult to interpret in this patient because he takes pantoprazole.

Plasma catecholamines (Answer D) have a high rate of false-positive results, and their measurement is not recommended for pheochromocytoma testing. Twenty-four–hour urinary catecholamines or, when available, plasma methoxytyramine should be measured if a dopamine-secreting pheochromocytoma or paraganglioma is suspected. Urinary metanephrines (Answer C) have a slightly higher specificity than that of plasma metanephrines. Nevertheless, plasma metanephrines are dramatically elevated in this patient, which is in concordance with the dimensions of the mass. False-positive normetanephrine results are suspected in patients taking medications that interfere with their reuptake, such as tricyclic antidepressants or serotonin and norepinephrine reuptake inhibitors. In most such cases, plasma normetanephrine elevation is less than twice the upper normal limit. Hospitalized patients with acute pathology often mount dramatic elevation of both metanephrines and normetanephrine. Isolated elevation of metanephrines is always suggestive of a pheochromocytoma. Phenylethanolamine N-methyltransferase converts norepinephrine to epinephrine, and this enzyme is expressed in the adrenal medulla, but not in paragangliomas.

Educational Objective

Determine when to use functional imaging studies in the differential diagnosis of indeterminate adrenal nodules.

Reference(s)

Sawka AM, Jaeschke R, Singh RJ, Young WF Jr. A comparison of biochemical tests for pheochromocytoma: measurement of fractionated plasma metanephrines compared with the combination of 24-hour urinary metanephrines and catecholamines. *J Clin Endocrinol Metab.* 2003;88(2):553-558. PMID: 12574179

Eisenhofer G, Lenders JWM, Goldstein DS, et al. Pheochromocytoma catecholamine phenotypes and prediction of tumor size and location by use of plasma free metanephrines. *Clin Chem.* 2005;51(4):735-744. PMID: 15718487

Ruuska T, Ramirez Escalante Y, Vaittinen S, et al. Somatostatin receptor expression in lymphomas: a source of false diagnosis of neuroendocrine tumor at (68)Ga-DOTANOC PET/CT imaging. *Acta Oncol.* 2018;57(2):283-289. PMID: 28686510

Lenders JWM, Pacak K, Walther MM, et al. Biochemical diagnosis of pheochromocytoma: which test is best? *JAMA.* 2002;287(11):1427-1434. PMID: 11903030

91 **ANSWER: A) Dapagliflozin**

This patient has multiple indications for an SGLT-2 inhibitor, specifically dapagliflozin (Answer A), regardless of his hemoglobin A_{1c} value less than 7.0% (<53 mmol/mol). While much improvement in glycemic control would not be expected given his reduced estimated glomerular filtration rate, dapagliflozin could provide him with multiple benefits. Dapagliflozin has been shown to reduce the risk of cardiovascular death and hospitalization for heart failure in adults with heart failure with reduced ejection fraction (New York Heart Association class II-IV), as well as to reduce the risk of sustained decline in estimated glomerular filtration rate, end-stage kidney disease, and cardiovascular death and hospitalization for heart failure in adults with chronic kidney disease at risk of progression. Dapagliflozin can be initiated for the indication of chronic kidney disease as long as the estimated glomerular filtration rate is 25 mL/min per 1.73 m^2 or greater. This medication can be continued until the patient initiates dialysis. Dapagliflozin has also demonstrated benefits in patients with heart failure who have mildly reduced or preserved ejection fraction. Empagliflozin has demonstrated benefits in patients with heart failure with reduced ejection fraction and heart failure with preserved ejection fraction. The EMPA-KIDNEY outcome study with empagliflozin demonstrated a reduction in the risk of end-stage kidney disease, a sustained decrease in estimated glomerular filtration rate of 40% or more from baseline, or death of renal or cardiovascular causes with empagliflozin vs placebo. Empagliflozin can be initiated for the indication of chronic kidney disease as long as the estimated glomerular filtration rate is 20 mL/min per 1.73 m^2 or greater. In both DAPA-CKD and EMPA-KIDNEY, there was no increase in the risk of hyperkalemia observed with either of the SGLT-2 inhibitors vs placebo.

Eplerenone (Answer B), an aldosterone antagonist, as compared with placebo, has been shown to reduce morbidity and mortality among patients with acute myocardial infarction complicated by left ventricular dysfunction and heart failure. It has also been shown to reduce the risk of death and the risk of hospitalization among patients with systolic heart failure and mild symptoms. Eplerenone is not a good choice in this patient because it is contraindicated in the setting of an estimated glomerular filtration rate of 30 mL/min per 1.73 m^2 or less and because the patient has baseline hyperkalemia. While eplerenone is also indicated for the treatment of hypertension, his blood pressure is currently well controlled.

Likewise, the addition of an ACE inhibitor such as ramipril (Answer D) to lower blood pressure is not indicated nor recommended in a patient receiving an angiotensin II receptor blocker. The ONTARGET study (Ongoing Telmisartan Alone and in Combination with Ramipril Global Endpoint Trial) compared the ACE inhibitor ramipril, the angiotensin II receptor blocker telmisartan, and the combination of the 2 drugs in patients with vascular disease or diabetes who were at high risk. Telmisartan was equivalent to ramipril in effectiveness in patients with vascular disease or high-risk diabetes and was associated with less angioedema. The combination of the 2 drugs was associated with more adverse events (hypotension, syncope, kidney dysfunction, and hyperkalemia, with a trend toward an increased risk of kidney dysfunction requiring dialysis) without increased benefit. Of note, ACE inhibitors can also cause hyperkalemia and thus would not be advised in a patient with baseline hyperkalemia. Therefore, addition of an ACE inhibitor is incorrect.

While GLP-1 receptor agonists have shown promise in terms of kidney risk reduction (secondary outcome data from cardiovascular outcome trials), there are currently no data from appropriately powered prospective randomized controlled trials to determine whether there is a benefit in terms of reducing the risk of chronic kidney disease. The currently ongoing FLOW study (Effect of Semaglutide Versus Placebo on the Progression of Renal Impairment in Subjects With Type 2 Diabetes and Chronic Kidney Disease) is trying to answer this question and is estimated to be completed in August 2024 (not available at the time this vignette was authored). Although some data suggest a potential benefit in patients with heart failure, there are currently no randomized controlled trial data available that address the effect of GLP-1 receptor agonists in patients with heart failure with reduced ejection fraction. At this time, given the available data, semaglutide (Answer E) is incorrect.

Metformin (Answer C) has not been demonstrated to decreased cardiovascular risk in any appropriately powered cardiovascular outcome trials, and it is contraindicated in the setting of congestive heart failure or an estimated glomerular filtration rate less than 30 mL/min per 1.73 m^2. For these reasons, metformin is incorrect.

Educational Objective

Determine when to initiate SGLT-2 inhibitor therapy and select the drug that has demonstrated benefits in patients with heart failure with reduced ejection fraction and/or chronic kidney disease.

Reference(s)

Pitt B, Remme W, Zannad F, et al; Eplerenone Post-Acute Myocardial Infarction Heart Failure Efficacy and Survival Study Investigators. *N Engl J Med.* 2003;348:1309-1321. PMID: 12668699

ONTARGET Investigators, Yusuf S, Teo KK, et al. Telmisartan, ramipril, or both in patients at high risk for vascular events. *N Engl J Med.* 2008;358(15):1547-1559. PMID: 18378520

Zannad F, McMurray JJV, Krum H, et al; EMPHASIS-HF Study Group. Eplerenone in patients with systolic heart failure and mild symptoms. *N Engl J Med.* 2011;364(1):11-21. PMID: 21073363

Heerspink HJL, Stefansson BV, Correa-Rotter R, et al; DAPA-CKD Trial Committees and Investigators. Dapagliflozin in patients with chronic kidney disease. *N Engl J Med.* 2020;383(15):1436-1446. PMID: 32970396

McMurray JJV, Solomon SD, Inzucchi SE, et al; DAPA-HF Trial Committees and Investigators. Dapagliflozin in patients with heart failure and reduced ejection fraction. *N Engl J Med.* 2019;381(21):1995-2008. PMID: 31535829

Empa-Kidney Collaborative Group, Herrington WG, Staplin N, et al. Empagliflozin in patients with chronic kidney disease. *N Engl J Med.* 2023:388(2):117-127. PMID: 36331190

92

ANSWER: B) Combined oral contraceptive pill

Perimenopause is the time during which variations in menstrual cycle length occur, and it ends 12 months after the final menstrual period. The total duration of perimenopause varies, but it begins with early perimenopause during which time the menstrual cycle is variable in length with a 7- or more day difference in length of consecutive cycles. Early perimenopause then progresses to late perimenopause during which time the interval of amenorrhea is 60 or more days. During late perimenopause, women can also begin to experience menopause-related symptoms and declining reproductive capacity as a result of ovarian aging. However, hormonally normal and ovulatory menstrual cycles can occur up until the final menstrual period. Therefore, if pregnancy is not desired, contraception is needed if the person is engaging in sexual behavior that can lead to conception.

For this woman who is otherwise healthy and not using any form of contraception (and is thus at risk of pregnancy), a combined oral contraceptive pill (Answer B) is the best option. It has the added benefit of likely relieving her vasomotor symptoms.

A levonorgestrel-releasing intrauterine system (Answer E) would also be a good option for contraception, but it would not help to alleviate any of the hormonal fluctuations or perimenopausal symptoms.

The β-estradiol patch and oral micronized progesterone (Answer A) and conjugated estrogens and medroxyprogesterone acetate in oral formulation (Answer C) are options for menopausal hormone therapy, but neither would provide her with adequate estrogen and progestin to serve as a contraceptive method.

The estradiol acetate vaginal ring (Answer D) is approved for the treatment of moderate to severe symptoms of vulvar and vaginal atrophy due to menopause. This would not provide contraception distinct from the etonogestrel/ethinyl estradiol vaginal ring.

Educational Objective

Assess the need for and determine the appropriate type of perimenopausal contraception.

Reference(s)

Harlow SD, Gass M, Hall JE, et al; STRAW+10 Collaborative Group. Executive summary of the Stages of Reproductive Aging Workshop + 10: addressing the unfinished agenda of staging reproductive aging. *J Clin Endocrinol Metab.* 2012;97(4):1159-1168. PMID: 22344196

The 2022 hormone therapy position statement of The North American Menopause Society Advisory Panel. The 2022 hormone therapy position statement of The North American Menopause Society. *Menopause.* 2022;29(7):767-794. PMID: 35797481

Voedisch AJ, Ariel D. Perimenopausal contraception. *Curr Opin Obstet Gynecol.* 2020;32(6):399-407. PMID: 33002952

93

ANSWER: D) Refer to an otolaryngologist

Salivary glands (parotid, submandibular, and sublingual) contain the sodium-iodide symporter and are able to concentrate iodine. Thus, salivary glands can receive a significant radiation dose following radioactive iodine therapy for thyroid cancer, leading to salivary gland dysfunction. The parotid gland is more susceptible to injury than the submandibular gland due to the predominant presence of serous cells in the parotid gland. Compared with mucous cells, serous cells more readily concentrate iodine and this can explain the preferential sialadenitis of the parotid gland. Common symptoms related to sialadenitis are xerostomia and pain and swelling of the salivary glands. Submandibular gland hypofunction is believed to be a more important cause of the symptoms of xerostomia than parotid hypofunction because the submandibular gland produces 70% of saliva. Xerostomia can lead to increased incidence in dental caries. Risk factors for sialadenitis following radioactive iodine include higher dose of administered radioiodine, female sex, history of sialadenitis, and Sjogren syndrome.

The Society of Nuclear Medicine and Medical Imaging guidelines recommend preventive measures that include increased oral fluid intake, sucking candy, and chewing gum to increase salivary flow and secretion to prevent the stasis of radioactive iodine in the salivary glands and to lower the chance of radiation-induced inflammation following radioactive iodine treatment. However, the benefit of sialagogue intake remains controversial. Traditional conservative treatments consist of external massage, nonsteroidal anti-inflammatory medications, and cholinergic medications. Steroids can be used if the pain and swelling remain unchanged after use of nonsteroidal anti-inflammatory agents. Amifostine as a free radical scavenger has been shown to prevent salivary gland damage after the administration of high-dosage radioiodine treatment (not routinely prescribed). Sialendoscopy can be offered in the management of chronic sialadenitis to open the salivary duct or remove mucous plugs.

This patient is experiencing sialadenitis that is related to the high-dose radioactive iodine treatment with symptoms of dry mouth and swelling with mild pain under her right jaw and several dental amalgams. She has tried conservative measures, including massage, warm compresses, oral hydration, and nonsteroidal anti-inflammatory agents with very little relief. Therefore, the use of warm compresses twice daily (Answer A) would be unlikely to further improve her symptoms. In the setting of severe pain or swelling, oral glucocorticoid therapy could be considered.

Initiation of amoxicillin-clavulanate twice daily (Answer B) is not indicated, as there are no obvious signs of infection such as fever, chills, face swelling and pain, redness over the same side of the face, pus drainage, or foul taste.

Sialagogic agents (eg, sour candies and drops) (Answer E) are not proven to be beneficial in chronic sialadenitis and their use following radioactive iodine treatment remains controversial. Lymph node metastasis to level 1 in the neck is exceedingly uncommon in thyroid cancer, and undetectable thyroglobulin and thyroglobulin antibodies are indicative of an excellent therapeutic response. Thus, performing FNA biopsy (Answer C) would be inappropriate.

Sialendoscopic intervention is an effective treatment for the management of radioactive iodine-associated sialadenitis that is refractory to conservative management. Success rates vary from 50% to 87%. Therefore, she should be referred to an otolaryngologist (Answer D).

Educational Objective

Identify sialadenitis as an adverse effect of radioiodine treatment in a patient with thyroid cancer.

Reference(s)

Mandel SJ, Mandel L. Radioactive iodine and the salivary glands. *Thyroid.* 2003;13(3):265-271. PMID: 12729475

Bhayani MK, Acharya V, Kongkiatkamon S, et al. Sialendoscopy for patients with radioiodine-induced sialadenitis and xerostomia. *Thyroid.* 2015;25(7):834-838. PMID: 25860842

Hollingsworth B, Senter L, Zhang X, et al. Risk factors of ^{131}I-induced salivary gland damage in thyroid cancer patients. *J Clin Endocrinol Metab.* 2016;101(11):4085-4093. PMID: 27533304

Silberstein EB, Alavi A, Balon HR, et al, The SNMMI practice guideline for therapy of thyroid disease with ^{131}I 3.0. *J Nucl Med.* 2012;53(10):1633-1651. PMID: 22787108

94 ANSWER: B) CT of the abdomen/pelvis

This patient had recent worsening of glucose control in the setting of longstanding, well-controlled diabetes, which is unusual. While change in lifestyle factors and disease progression may explain such a scenario, in these circumstances, it is important to consider other potential causes. Her weight loss raises the possibility of an occult malignancy. Certainly, she should have routinely advised screening procedures such as colonoscopy and mammography. In addition, it is important to consider cancers associated with worsening diabetes or incident diabetes.

Pancreatic cancer has been associated with diabetes. Evidence suggests that the risk of pancreatic cancer in persons with type 2 diabetes is 1.8- to 2.0-fold higher than in those without diabetes. One meta-analysis suggests that among individuals with longer history of diabetes, the excess risk is reduced by 50%, supporting the hypothesis that diabetes may be an early manifestation of the cancer and suggests a causal relationship between pancreatic cancer and the development of diabetes mellitus. The latter is supported by studies suggesting that sera from patients with pancreatic cancer contain diabetogenic peptides and that insulin sensitivity improves substantially 3 months after surgery. There is evidence that this risk is 2-way; that is, diabetes may also be a risk factor for the development of pancreatic cancer. One study from a multiethnic cohort suggests that diabetes is associated with a 2-fold increase in the risk of incident pancreatic cancer. Based on this information, screening for pancreatic cancer with abdominal cross-sectional imaging (Answer B) is the best next step. The decision to investigate for pancreatic cancer in a person recently diagnosed with diabetes mellitus is challenging given that diabetes is so common. Guidelines from the American Gastroenterological Society suggest that new-onset diabetes in persons who are at high risk for developing pancreatic cancer should prompt additional investigations and/or change in screening interval. This vignette emphasizes the association between pancreatic cancer and diabetes and encourages suspicion in the appropriate clinical context to help guide the evaluation.

In this case, the clinician was astute to recognize that ongoing weight loss despite improvements in glycemic control after starting sulfonylurea therapy makes continuation of the current regimen (Answer A) without additional investigations unadvisable. The patient was found to have an ill-defined hypodensity in the pancreatic neck. Neoadjuvant chemotherapy was pursued, and 6 months later the Whipple procedure demonstrated a 1.1-cm invasive ductal adenocarcinoma of the pancreas. Other considerations would be somatostatinoma and glucagonoma, both of which are rare neuroendocrine tumors. Eighty percent of patients with glucagonoma present with a rash, classically necrolytic erythema migrans, which this patient does not have. Since glucagonomas are very rare, measuring glucagon (Answer D) is not necessary now. Somatostatinomas can present with diabetes of varying severity, biliary colic, and steatorrhea, but also with hypoglycemia and other nonspecific abdominal symptoms.

Although it was reasonable to screen for latent autoimmune diabetes because of this patient's history of Graves disease, given that glutamic acid decarboxylase 65 and islet antigen 2 antibodies were undetectable and that she had at least a partial response to sulfonylurea, additional antibody testing (Answer E) to investigate the possibility of an autoimmune cause is unlikely to be helpful.

C-peptide measurement (Answer C) in a person whose glycemic control has improved would not be helpful.

Educational Objective

Explain that persons with diabetes mellitus are at increased risk for pancreatic cancer.

Reference(s)

Huxley R, Ansary-Moghaddam A, Berrington de Gonzalez, Barzi F, Woodward M. Type-II diabetes and pancreatic cancer: a meta-analysis of 36 studies. *Br J Cancer.* 2005;92(11):2076-2083. PMID: 15886696

Aslanian HR, Lee JH, Canto MI. AGA clinical practice update on pancreas cancer screening in high-risk individuals: expert review. *Gastroenterology.* 2020;159(1):358-362. PMID: 32416142

95 ANSWER: D) Refer for overnight polysomnography

Anterior hypopituitarism can develop over time in more than one-third of patients who receive radiation. This patient takes cortisol, thyroid, and testosterone replacement and has a low IGF-1 concentration. Per Endocrine Society recommendations, a trial of GH replacement (rather than a stimulation test) can be undertaken if clinical benefit is anticipated, the IGF-1 concentration is lower than 75 ng/mL (<9.8 nmol/L), and 3 other pituitary hormone deficiencies are present. The American Association of Clinical Endocrinologists' guidelines suggest an IGF-1 Z-score of −2.0 as the cutoff for the same clinical scenario. GH replacement should be initiated after optimization of other hormones, which is supported in this case by normal free T_4 and testosterone concentrations. Energy and exercise endurance may improve with GH replacement. In addition, bone mineral density usually improves in patients taking GH injections, although fracture reduction data are not available. The patient should be counseled about the possible risks of GH replacement, including fluid retention, joint and muscle pain, paresthesias, sleep apnea, and worsened hyperglycemia. He has prediabetes and elevated LDL cholesterol and should be counseled about lifestyle modifications.

Before initiation of GH replacement (Answer E), he should be evaluated for sleep apnea (Answer D), which could be responsible for his clinical manifestations. Large neck circumference and elevated BMI are anthropometric parameters associated with obstructive sleep apnea. GH replacement can be considered after evaluation and treatment of this condition.

GH deficiency may contribute to increased cardiovascular morbidity and mortality in patients with hypopituitarism. Although cardiovascular markers improve with GH replacement, its effect on cardiovascular events and mortality has not been demonstrated. Regarding glucose metabolism, a recent meta-analysis demonstrated that GH replacement for 6 to 12 months increases fasting glucose, hemoglobin A_{1c}, and HOMA-IR (homeostatic model assessment of insulin resistance) in adults with GH deficiency. With longer duration of GH replacement therapy, only fasting plasma glucose remains elevated. A recent systematic review and meta-analysis demonstrated the overall safety of GH therapeutic use in adults without increased risk of pituitary tumor recurrence, malignancy, or stroke.

GH-stimulation testing (Answer C) is not necessary in this patient given multiple hormone deficiencies, history of brain radiation, and an IGF-1 concentration less than 75 ng/mL (<9.8 nmol/L).

A sample for serum cortisol measurement was drawn an hour after hydrocortisone administration. The patient takes a total daily hydrocortisone dose of 20 mg and does not have clinical signs of overreplacement with glucocorticoids. Therefore, decreasing the hydrocortisone dosage to 10 mg in the morning (Answer A) is incorrect.

His testosterone concentration measured 10 days after testosterone injection is adequate. Increasing the dosage (Answer B) might cause polycythemia, especially if he has untreated obstructive sleep apnea. In addition, increasing the testosterone dosage could increase his LDL-cholesterol concentration.

Educational Objective

Manage long-term hypopituitarism and identify caveats of growth hormone replacement.

Reference(s)

Fleseriu M, Hashim IA, Karavitaki N, et al. Hormonal replacement in hypopituitarism in adults: an Endocrine Society clinical practice guideline. *J Clin Endocrinol Metab.* 2016;101(11):3888-3921. PMID: 27736313

Jasim S, Alahdab F, Ahmed AT, et al. The effect of growth hormone replacement in patients with hypopituitarism on tumor recurrence, secondary cancer, and stroke. *Endocrine.* 2017;56(2):267-278. PMID: 27815769

Zhou H, Sun L, Zhang S, Wang Y, Wang G. Effect of long-term growth hormone replacement on glucose metabolism in adults with growth hormone deficiency: a systematic review and meta-analysis. *Pituitary.* 2021;24(1):130-142. PMID: 32888174

Yuen KCJ, Biller BMK, Radovick S, et al. American Association of Clinical Endocrinologists and American College of Endocrinology guidelines for management of growth hormone deficiency in adults and patients transitioning from pediatric to adult care. *Endocr Pract.* 2019;25(11):1191-1232. PMID: 31760824

Yuen KCJ, Birkegard AC, Blevins LS, et al. Development of a novel algorithm to identify people with high likelihood of adult growth hormone deficiency in a US healthcare claims database. *Int J Endocrinol.* 2022;7853786. PMID: 35761982

96 ANSWER: B) Follow-up CT in 12 months

Detection of incidental adrenal masses has increased in parallel with the broadened use of cross-sectional imaging. The prevalence of adrenal masses is higher in older individuals. The approach to such incidental adrenal masses is driven by the answers to 2 questions: (1) Is the nodule benign or malignant? and (2) Is there hormonal excess?

Malignant adrenal nodules, either primary or metastatic, are uncommon. Adrenal cortical carcinoma has an estimated population incidence of 1 to 2 per million per year. Malignant nodules are often large, with an unenhanced attenuation of greater than 20 Hounsfield units on CT. Malignant adrenal masses might have irregular margins, intratumoral heterogeneity, necrosis, and/or calcifications. Conversely, benign cortical nodules are most often lipid rich, with an unenhanced CT attenuation less than 10 Hounsfield units.

Myelolipomas are benign adrenal tumors composed of macroscopic adipose tissue and hematopoietic elements. On CT, myelolipomas are well-circumscribed, hypodense masses, with an attenuation of −90 to −120 Hounsfield units, giving them the characteristic dark appearance on both noncontrast and contrast-enhanced images, as seen in this patient. Myelolipomas are typically nonsecretory, although rare cases of mild ACTH-independent hypercortisolism have been described. Most myelolipomas are solitary and are usually asymptomatic. A minority of myelolipomas cause compressive symptoms, usually when they exceed 6 to 7 cm. Large bilateral adrenal myelolipomas can be seen in patients with congenital adrenal hyperplasia and prolonged poor disease control. Because of their benign nature, the management for most adrenal myelolipomas is observation, unless they cause mass-effect symptoms. Follow-up imaging at 1 year (Answer B) to assess for growth of the myelolipoma is appropriate in this patient because of its relatively large dimensions. Although adrenal myelolipomas might enlarge, the growth rate is typically slow. Follow-up imaging can be omitted in patients with small myelolipomas (<4 cm).

Adrenalectomy (Answer C) presents more risk than benefit in this 81-year-old patient with numerous comorbidities, and there are no concerns for mass effect or hormonal excess.

Lipid-poor, benign cortical nodules are usually homogeneous and display rapid contrast medium washout (>50% at 10 minutes). When tumors have heterogeneous attenuation, Hounsfield unit measurements and contrast washout are unreliable. In such cases, after hormonal exclusion of a pheochromocytoma, FDG-PET-CT (Answer A) is useful to distinguish between malignant (high standardized uptake value [SUV]) and benign nodules (low SUV).

Screening for pheochromocytoma with plasma metanephrines (Answer D) or 24-hour urinary metanephrines is not necessary in patients with lipid-rich adrenal tumors, which are always of cortical origin. Pheochromocytomas arise from chromaffin cells of the adrenal medulla, and all such tumors have a noncontrast attenuation greater than 10 Hounsfield units on CT.

Serum DHEA-S measurement (Answer E) can be auxiliary in the diagnosis of autonomous hypercortisolism. DHEA-S has a long half-life (7 to 22 hours), and it reflects integrated ACTH function. DHEA-S is often low in patients with autonomous hypercortisolism, but it cannot be used as the sole diagnostic tool. DHEA-S peaks in young adults and declines with aging. DHEA-S is lower in women than in men, and it is commonly very low in octogenarians. Conversely, DHEA-S might be elevated in persons with adrenal cortical carcinomas, often in conjunction with cortisol hypersecretion.

Educational Objective

Guide the evaluation and management of large adrenal incidentalomas.

Reference(s)

Calissendorff J, Juhlin CC, Sundin A, Bancos I, Falhammar H. Adrenal myelolipomas. *Lancet Diabetes Endocrinol.* 2021;9(11):767-775. PMID: 34450092

Dennedy MC, Annamalai AK, Prankerd-Smith O, et al. Low DHEAS: a sensitive and specific test for the detection of subclinical hypercortisolism in adrenal incidentalomas. *J Clin Endocrinol Metab.* 2017;102(3):786-792. PMID: 27797672

Sherlock M, Scarsbrook A, Abbas A, et al. Adrenal incidentaloma. *Endocr Rev.* 2020;41(6):775-820. PMID: 32266384

97 ANSWER: A) CT of the chest, abdomen, and pelvis

In this competitive weightlifter, routine drug testing revealed an unexpected hCG elevation. Screening for banned substances in elite athletes is an accepted routine, and the exact methodology is constantly evolving. Urine samples are commonly used because they are easy to obtain and typically contain drug and metabolite levels that are higher than in blood. Urine collection commences with the chaperoned provision by the athlete. This sample is then divided into 2 bottles labeled A and B. All testing is carried out on the A sample, typically by means of gas chromatography. A positive result requires the analysis of the second sample (B), and if this result concurs with the first, then a potential doping offense is investigated. This patient had a high level of hCG in his B sample and was referred for further evaluation. The clinical history and additional evaluation do not suggest anabolic steroid abuse (no truncal acne, no atrophic testes [although the latter could be masked by concomitant hCG use]) and he repeatedly denied use of exogenous hCG. His mild gynecomastia is consistent with hCG exposure but does not distinguish an endogenous source from an exogenous one. Hence, the possibility of endogenous hCG production must be excluded.

In young men, the most common source of endogenous hCG production is germ-cell tumors. Among extragonadal germ-cell tumors, hCG is elevated in 85% of cases of nonseminomatous germ-cell tumors and in 50% of seminomas. Given that less than 5% of germ-cell tumors are extragonadal, testicular assessment was performed first, which failed to detect a tumor. In adults, the most common sites of extragonadal germ-cell tumors are the anterior mediastinum and retroperitoneum. Therefore, cross-sectional imaging (Answer A) is the best investigation to perform next. In this patient, CT of the chest, abdomen, and pelvis demonstrated a 33-mm anterior mediastinal mass (*see image B*). Fluorodeoxyglucose avidity was observed on PET (*see image A*). There were no extrathoracic foci. He underwent video-assisted thoracoscopic excision of the lesion. The histopathologic findings were consistent with a seminoma, and hCG, gonadotropins, and serum testosterone all normalized within weeks after the operation. He was referred for adjuvant therapy but declined due to concerns about adverse effects. His gynecomastia regressed over months. When last seen 10 years after his operation, hCG, gonadotropins, and serum testosterone all remained in the normal range, with no evidence of recurrence on imaging.

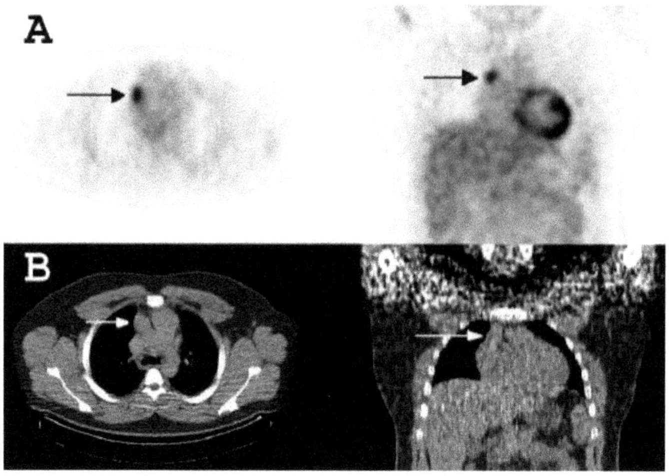

Figure 1 (A&B) from Newcomb AE, Clarke CP, Chiang CY, Jerums G. *J Thorac Cardiovasc Surg*, 2006; 132(3): 722-723. © The American Association for Thoracic Surgery.

Primary mediastinal seminomas are typically slow growing and can be very bulky by the time they cause discomfort. Most (75%) are symptomatic at the time of diagnosis (eg, cough, weight loss, chest pain, dyspnea, and/or superior vena cava syndrome). For this patient, regular screening for banned substances fortuitously led to an early diagnosis at an asymptomatic stage.

Serum α-fetoprotein (Answer C), like hCG, is a tumor marker for germ-cell tumors and is elevated in up to 85% of persons with nonseminomatous germ-cell tumors, but not in those with pure seminomas. While α-fetoprotein may be useful in the follow-up plan, it is not the best investigation to perform next because localizing the tumor is the first priority.

hCG promotes gynecomastia by stimulating ductal development via the LH receptor, which is known to be expressed in male breast tissue, and it also stimulates estradiol production by the Leydig cells. While not measured in this man, serum estradiol preoperatively would be expected to be above the male reference range. However, estradiol measurement (Answer E) would not add to the diagnostic and management approach in this case and is not indicated.

Germ-cell tumors do not express somatostatin receptors, and ^{68}Ga DOTA-octreotate (GaTate) PET-CT (Answer B) is not indicated. All pituitary glycoprotein hormones (ie, hCG, TSH, LH, and FSH) are dimers composed of a common α-subunit and a distinct β-subunit, the latter confers receptor specificity. In some pituitary tumors, isolated α-subunit secretion occurs, and in patients with incongruent thyroid function studies (ie, elevated free T_4 and free T_3 with nonsuppressed TSH not due to assay interference), a relatively elevated α-subunit is one parameter (although not 100% discriminatory) to distinguish a TSH-producing tumor from resistance to thyroid hormone (due to a dominant-negative thyroid receptor β variant). However, in this case there is no indication to measure α-subunit (Answer D).

Educational Objective

Guide the evaluation of elevated hCG in a man.

Reference(s)

Anawalt BD. Detection of anabolic androgenic steroid use by elite athletes and by members of the general public. *Mol Cell Endocrinol.* 2018;15(3);464:21-27. PMID: 28943276

Newcomb AE, Clarke CP, Chiang CY, Jerums G. Urine drug testing in an athlete leads to the diagnosis of unsuspected mediastinal germ cell tumor. *J Thorac Cardiovasc Surg.* 2006;132(3):722-723. PMID: 16935150

98 ANSWER: E) Switch to a basal-correction regimen and initiate prandial insulin when full diet is ordered

More than 25% of noncritically ill hospitalized patients have diabetes mellitus. Uncontrolled hyperglycemia in the inpatient setting is associated with increased incidence of hospital complications, among which are prolonged length of stay and increased risk of infections. Reducing hyperglycemia is, therefore, important; however, this can increase the risk of hypoglycemia.

Premixed insulin NPH 70/30 regimens are used in the outpatient setting in some patients with diabetes mellitus. Most premixed insulins contain an intermediate-acting insulin (NPH) and a short-acting prandial insulin. The main limitations of these regimens are that they have a fixed percentage of intermediate short-acting insulin and they allow limited flexibility in adjusting doses with meals. As a result, compared with using separate basal and prandial (bolus) insulin injections, premixed insulin regimens may have a higher risk of hypoglycemia, especially in situations where a patient decides to delay or skip a meal.

The hospital setting is a dynamic environment, and nutrition needs or goals can change. Hospitalized patients can have decreased appetite or nausea and vomiting. They can be placed on a clear-liquid diet and transition to full diet as tolerated. Moreover, hospitalized patients may undergo procedures, imaging studies, or surgeries. In such cases, patients are commonly placed on nothing-by-mouth status past midnight. Therefore, these inpatients do not need prandial insulin because there is no prescribed diet. They can be managed with basal and correctional insulin as needed to correct any hyperglycemia that occurs (Answer E). Once a full diet is ordered, starting prandial insulin would be appropriate.

Continuing NPH 70/30 at the current dosage (Answer A) or even at a decreased dosage (Answer B) can lead to significant hypoglycemia, as these premixed insulin regimens also provide prandial coverage. This has been shown in a large randomized clinical trial that included hospitalized patients with diabetes mellitus managed either with a basal-bolus or premixed insulin regimen. In this clinical trial, participants who received premixed insulin had higher rates of hypoglycemia and the study was terminated early due to safety concerns at the first prespecified interim analysis.

Discontinuing NPH 70/30 and initiating correctional insulin either alone or with metformin does not represent the appropriate management for this patient with type 2 diabetes. She has uncontrolled diabetes, as documented by her recent hemoglobin A_{1c} measurement, even after receiving NPH 70/30, 30 units in the morning and 20 units before dinner. It is, therefore, unlikely that using only correctional insulin (Answer C) or correctional insulin and metformin (Answer D) will optimize her glycemic control during the current hospitalization.

Educational Objective

Mitigate the risk of hypoglycemia in the hospital and recommend appropriate management in hospitalized patients with diabetes mellitus who use NPH 70/30 insulin regimens in the ambulatory setting.

Reference(s)

Garber AJ, Handelsman Y, Grunberger G, et al. Consensus statement by the American Association of Clinical Endocrinologists and American College of Endocrinology on the comprehensive type 2 diabetes management algorithm - 2020 executive summary. *Endocr Pract.* 2020;26(1):107-139. PMID: 32022600

Korytkowski MT, Muniyappa R, Antinori-Lent K, et al. Management of hyperglycemia in hospitalized adult patients in non-critical care settings: an Endocrine Society clinical practice guideline. *J Clin Endocrinol Metab.* 2022;107(8):2101-2128. PMID: 3569058

Bellido V, Suarez L, Rodriguez MG, et al. Comparison of basal-bolus and premixed insulin regimens in hospitalized patients with type 2 diabetes. *Diabetes Care.* 2015;38(12):2211-2216. PMID: 26459273

99 ANSWER: E) Discontinue liothyronine, increase levothyroxine dosage

In women with hypothyroidism on thyroid hormone replacement, it is important to reassess serum TSH approximately 6 weeks following the discontinuation of estrogen-containing oral contraceptive pills to ensure that the serum TSH concentration is maintained within the goal range, as was done for this patient. Estrogen-containing oral contraceptives may be associated with an increase in the hepatic production of thyroid-binding proteins and therefore lead to higher medication requirements in patients with hypothyroidism on thyroid hormone replacement. The converse is also true, such that the discontinuation of these medications may lead to decreased thyroid hormone requirements in some patients. Thus, thyroid function should be tested after estrogen-containing oral contraceptive pills are initiated or discontinued.

Pregnancy necessitates an approximately 50% increase in thyroid hormone production by the maternal thyroid gland. Increased thyroid hormone production is mediated by the thyrotrophic effects of hCG and an estrogen-induced increase in hepatic thyroxine-binding globulin production, which leads to a reduction in bioavailable free T_4, further promoting thyroid hormone synthesis. The fetal thyroid gland develops and begins functioning by 10 to 12 weeks' gestation; however, because fetal hypothalamic-pituitary axis maturation and TSH production do not stabilize until late midgestation, the fetus remains highly reliant on the transfer of maternal thyroid hormone.

Unlike euthyroid women, those with hypothyroidism are unable to increase thyroidal T_4 and T_3 production to meet gestational demands. Therefore, a higher dosage of exogenous thyroid hormone is usually required to maintain euthyroidism. Women are generally advised to increase their levothyroxine dosage by approximately 30% after a positive pregnancy test, and subsequent close monitoring of serum TSH concentrations is required to maintain the TSH concentration in the lower half of the trimester-specific reference range. In women who are planning pregnancy, medical treatment of hypothyroidism should be optimized before conceiving. A TSH concentration between the lower limit of the reference range and 2.5 mIU/L is recommended for women with hypothyroidism who are planning pregnancy.

Overt hypothyroidism in pregnancy has been associated with adverse pregnancy and fetal outcomes, including preeclampsia, gestational diabetes, placental abruption, postpartum hemorrhage, preterm delivery, fetal loss, low birthweight, and negative neurodevelopmental outcomes in the child (ie, reduced intelligence quotient). Although evidence is conflicting, subclinical hypothyroidism may also be associated with adverse pregnancy complications, especially for TPO antibody–positive women. Thyroid hormone is essential for normal fetal CNS development, including neuronal migration, synaptogenesis, glial-cell differentiation, and myelination. Free T_4 concentrations present in embryonal and fetal fluids are directly dependent on the maternal T_4 supply. The fetal CNS is relatively impermeable to T_3, and most T_3 in the fetal brain is derived from maternally delivered T_4.

Women receiving T_3-containing preparations are at risk for having insufficient transfer of maternal T_4 to the fetal brain. Therefore, in women who are pregnant or are planning pregnancy, treatment with levothyroxine alone is recommended and the administration of exogenous T_3 (liothyronine; desiccated thyroid) is not advised. T_3-containing preparations should be discontinued in women who are planning pregnancy (thus, Answers A, B, and C are incorrect). However, discontinuation of liothyronine necessitates an increase in the levothyroxine dosage to maintain euthyroidism (thus, Answer E is correct and Answer D is incorrect).

Educational Objective

Manage hypothyroidism in women planning pregnancy.

Reference(s)

Alexander EK, Pearce EN, Brent GA, et al. 2017 guidelines of the American Thyroid Association for the diagnosis and management of thyroid disease during pregnancy and the postpartum. *Thyroid.* 2017;27(3):315-389. PMID: 28056690

Lee SY, Pearce EN. Assessment and treatment of thyroid disorders in pregnancy and the postpartum period. *Nat Rev Endocrinol.* 2022;18(3):158-171. PMID: 34983968

100 ANSWER: A) Continue current therapy

This patient demonstrates hypocalcemia and high-normal phosphate with inappropriately low PTH and a family history indicating autosomal dominant inheritance. Several conditions can cause inherited hypoparathyroidism, including the following syndromes:

- Haploinsufficiency of GATA3 causes autosomal dominant hypoparathyroidism in association with sensorineural hearing loss and kidney anomalies.
- DiGeorge syndrome (due to 22q11.2 deletion and characterized by facial dysmorphism, low-set ears, hooded eyelids, short palpebral fissures, absent or hypoplastic thymus, cardiac abnormalities, parathyroid hypoplasia, and other abnormalities)
- CHARGE syndrome (due to pathogenic variants in the *CHD7* gene and characterized by coloboma, heart defects, choanal atresia, delayed growth, genital anomalies, hypogonadism, and ear anomalies)
- Kenny-Caffey syndrome type 2 (due to pathogenic variants in the *FAM111A* gene and characterized by short stature, skeletal dysplasia, eye abnormalities, and hypoparathyroidism)
- Various mitochondrial disorders can also cause hypoparathyroidism, but this patient's family history is inconsistent with maternal inheritance
- Autosomal dominant hypocalcemia due to activating pathogenic variants affecting either the calcium-sensing receptor gene (*CASR*) or genes involved in postreceptor signaling (such as *GNA11*)

In the absence of other clinical or syndromic features, autosomal dominant hypocalcemia is most likely caused by pathogenic variants in *CASR* or *GNA11*. In the parathyroid glands, activating pathogenic variants in *CASR* or *GNA11* result in PTH secretion being suppressed by calcium concentrations that are lower than appropriate, resulting in persistent hypocalcemia that can be difficult to manage. Both the PTH receptor and the calcium-sensing receptor are expressed in the distal renal tubule, and thus the combination of low PTH levels and the activated calcium-sensing receptor exacerbate renal calcium losses, as evidenced by this patient's elevated urinary calcium-to-creatinine ratio during treatment, despite hypocalcemia. Patients with *CASR* pathogenic variants also often have hypomagnesemia.

Compared with patients with hypoparathyroidism, those with autosomal dominant hypocalcemia appear to be even more prone to nephrocalcinosis during treatment. Consequently, to minimize hypercalciuria, recommendations have been to use the smallest treatment dosages of active vitamin D and calcium necessary to minimize symptoms. This patient has had hypocalcemic seizures in the past and does have hypocalcemic symptoms, so treatment is indicated. However, a lower serum calcium concentration should be targeted. Because he is minimally symptomatic, maintaining the current dosages (Answer A) is the best choice, but emphasizing treatment adherence may help to avoid his periodic hypocalcemic symptoms.

Increasing his calcium or calcitriol dosage (Answers C and D) would increase his serum calcium and might further decrease symptoms. However, increasing these dosages would further exacerbate his hypercalciuria and nephrocalcinosis, which is the major complication of the treatment and can lead to chronic kidney disease.

Decreasing the hydrochlorothiazide dosage (Answer B) would tend to worsen hypercalciuria and lower serum calcium. Increasing hydrochlorothiazide could be considered, acknowledging that this may increase his need for potassium supplementation to avoid hypokalemia.

Patients with this disorder are also generally hyperphosphatemic because of the low PTH. Starting sevelamer (Answer E) is an option for phosphate binding, but it is usually not necessary because administering his calcium with meals doubles as a phosphate binder and can be adjusted to keep the phosphate in the high-normal to slightly high range, although it can be difficult to normalize serum phosphate. Some small studies and case reports have described use of PTH receptor agonist injections to manage hypocalcemia in patients with autosomal dominant hypocalcemia due to *CASR* pathogenic variants, but this may not eliminate the risk of hypercalciuria as the activating calcium-sensing receptor still contributes directly to urinary calcium loss. Recent early-phase studies have used a calcilytic agent to alter the signaling at the calcium-sensing receptor in autosomal dominant hypocalcemia to raise PTH and calcium, with the goal of improving serum calcium without causing hypercalciuria. However, this treatment is not yet available.

Educational Objective

Recommend appropriate management of autosomal dominant hypocalcemia.

Reference(s)

Roszko KL, Bi RD, Mannstadt M. Autosomal dominant hypocalcemia (hypoparathyroidism) types 1 and 2. *Front Physiol.* 2016;7:458. PMID: 27803672

Winer KK, Kelly A, Johns A, et al. Long-term parathyroid hormone 1-34 replacement therapy in children with hypoparathyroidism. *J Pediatr.* 2018;203:391-399.e391. PMID: 30470382

Roberts MS, Gafni RI, Brillante B, et al. Treatment of autosomal dominant hypocalcemia type 1 with the calcilytic NPSP795 (SHP635). *J Bone Miner Res.* 2019;34(9):1609-1618. PMID: 31063613

101

ANSWER: B) Canagliflozin

This patient experienced rapid onset of painless vision loss that resulted from retinal vein occlusion. Patients with diabetes, hypertension, and hyperlipidemia are at high risk of developing this complication. The symptoms can be insidious, progressing from blurry vision to vision loss over hours to days, or abrupt, sometimes presenting with immediate complete vision loss. This invariably occurs in just 1 eye. Recently, SGLT-2 inhibitors (Answer B) have been reported to be associated with retinal vein occlusion, although the mechanism is unclear. When retinal vein occlusion occurs in a patient on SGLT-2 inhibitor therapy, this medication must be considered as a potential etiology.

In the SUSTAIN-6 trial, semaglutide (Answer E) was observed to be associated with an increased incidence of diabetic retinopathy (3.0%) vs placebo (1.8%). Vision disturbances related to retinopathy usually develop slowly, rather than progress rapidly over hours to days, as was the case in this patient. A subsequent meta-analysis reported that semaglutide was not associated with an increased risk of diabetic retinopathy. However, when semaglutide is prescribed to older patients or those with long duration of diabetes, caution should be exercised regarding risk of diabetic retinopathy.

Retinal vein occlusion has not been linked to insulin glargine (Answer C), metformin (Answer D), or atorvastatin (Answer A).

Educational Objective

Identify SGLT-2 inhibitor use as a potential etiology of retinal vein occlusion.

Reference(s)

Lee MK, Kim B, Han K, et al. Sodium-glucose cotransporter 2 inhibitors and risk of retinal vein occlusion among patients with type 2 diabetes: a propensity score-matched cohort study. *Diabetes Care.* 2021;44(10):2419-2426. PMID: 34301735

Marso SP, Bain SC, Consoli A, et al; SUSTAIN-6 Investigators. Semaglutide and cardiovascular outcomes in patients with type 2 diabetes. *N Engl J Med.* 2016;375(19):1834-1844. PMID: 27633186

Wang F, Mao Y, Wang H, Liu Y, Huang P. Semaglutide and diabetic retinopathy risk in patients with type 2 diabetes mellitus: a meta-analysis of randomized controlled trials. *Clin Drug Investig.* 2022;42(1):17-28. PMID: 34894326

102 ANSWER: C) See a dietician to discuss how to incorporate foods with lower simple carbohydrates and less salt

The patient in this vignette has several abnormal metabolic parameters: elevated hemoglobin A_{1c}, elevated triglycerides, hypertension, and elevated BMI. Lifestyle modification is the cornerstone of therapy in patients with metabolic disorders. Implementing an effective lifestyle intervention program requires a partnership between the patient and their physician that acknowledges complexities such as dietary preferences, financial considerations, cultural preferences, and the built environment in which the patient lives. A person's socioeconomic position across the course of life is inversely associated with C-reactive protein, a marker of basal inflammation and atherosclerosis. In other words, people who are socioeconomically disadvantaged are more likely than those who are not to have chronic diseases associated with high inflammatory markers. Similarly, patients who are socioeconomically disadvantaged may find it more difficult to implement standard lifestyle modification recommendations that often require resources (personal, financial, etc), which can be scarce.

A recent systematic review showed that dietary patterns of the highest quality are associated with a significant reduction in the risk of all-cause mortality, cardiovascular disease, cancer, type 2 diabetes, and neurodegenerative disorders. Dietary patterns of the highest quality have common features that include a high intake of fruits, vegetables, whole grains, nuts, and legumes and lower intake of saturated fat of animal origin and sugar-sweetened and ultra-processed foods. High dietary quality can be achieved with any cultural or ethnic dietary style.

Prior to escalating medication for impaired glucose tolerance (Answer D), the patient should be provided advice on lifestyle changes, in particular dietary modification. The most effective dietary pattern for any individual patient is one to which they will adhere. The patient in this case has stated her dietary preferences and is most likely to adhere to advice that aligns with her own values and preferences (Answer C). The Mediterranean-style dietary pattern (Answer A) has clear benefits for both the treatment and prevention of cardiometabolic disease, but it is not the best choice for this particular patient. Emphasizing common components of high-quality dietary patterns as listed above can still help this patient achieve metabolic goals while respecting cultural preferences.

Increasing physical activity (Answer B) can improve overall metabolic health, but it is less likely to be effectively implemented by this patient who has expressed time constraints as a barrier.

Stopping the oral contraceptive pill (Answer E) may improve hypertriglyceridemia and blood pressure, but it is not expected to improve glycemic control or affect her weight as much as improvements in dietary quality should.

Educational Objective

Provide care for a patient whose metabolic health is significantly influenced by social determinants of health.

Reference(s)

Berger E, Castagné R, Chadeau-Hyam M, et al. Multi-cohort study identifies social determinants of systemic inflammation over the life course. *Nat Commun.* 2019;10(1):773. PMID: 30770820

Schwingshackl L, Bogensberger B, Hoffmann G. Diet quality as assessed by the Healthy Eating Index, Alternate Healthy Eating Index, Dietary Approaches to Stop Hypertension Score, and health outcomes: an updated systematic review and meta-analysis of cohort studies. *J Acad Nutr Diet.* 2018;118(1):74-100. PMID: 29111090

103 ANSWER: A) Biopsy of the ear canal lesion

Infiltrative lesions of the hypothalamus, infundibulum, and pituitary gland are rare and require a thorough diagnostic workup. Main causes include hypophysitis (lymphocytic, granulomatous, xanthomatous, immunotherapy-induced), multisystemic disorders (eg, neurosarcoidosis, Langerhans-cell histiocytosis, Erdheim-Chester disease, IgG4-related disease), infections (eg, tuberculosis, syphilis), and lymphoproliferative malignancies (lymphoma, plasmacytoma, or metastases). Investigations should start with a complete blood cell count, inflammatory markers (eg, erythrocyte sedimentation rate, C-reactive protein), and serum calcium and creatinine measurement. This should be followed by specific testing for systemic granulomatous, infectious, or neoplastic conditions and CT or PET-CT body imaging, depending on the clinical scenario. Cerebral spinal fluid analysis is also helpful to detect infection, neurosarcoidosis, germinomas, or lymphoproliferative disorders. An empiric trial of high-dosage glucocorticoids can be undertaken if hypophysitis is suspected and the patient has mass effect symptoms, vision loss, and/or an enlarging pituitary mass. Transsphenoidal biopsy is indicated for lesions causing mass effect or for those that enlarge after short-term imaging or do not respond to glucocorticoids.

In this case, blood tests were nonrevealing and pituitary MRI identified a hypothalamic lesion and an enhancing lesion of the right parietal calvarium, which was hypermetabolic on PET-CT. Biopsy of the right ear canal lesion (Answer A) documented an infiltrative lesion composed of eosinophils, small lymphocytes, and histocytes. Most neoplastic cells stained positive for CD45, S100, CD1a, and vimentin, occasional neoplastic cells stained for CD68, which confirmed the diagnosis of Langerhans-cell histiocytosis. Treatment with monthly cytarabine was initiated with subsequent shrinkage of the hypothalamic lesion and bone lesion after 3 months. In addition, he received desmopressin, levothyroxine, and testosterone replacement.

Langerhans-cell histiocytosis is a rare granulomatous disease characterized by abnormal expansion of histiocyte-like dendritic cells with onset often during childhood, although cases have been reported in adults. The most common involved sites are the bones (especially skull, pelvis, and femur), lungs, skin, and hypothalamic-pituitary axis. Vasopressin deficiency is the most common presenting feature of hypothalamic-pituitary Langerhans-cell histiocytosis. The diagnosis is established with immunohistochemistry stains of lesion biopsies. A standardized treatment has not been established. However, chemotherapy, surgery, radiation, or a combination of these modalities has been effective in reported cases.

Cerebral spinal fluid analysis (Answer B) and transsphenoidal biopsy (Answer E) are incorrect because histopathologic evaluation of the right ear canal lesion would be able to provide the histologic diagnosis. These procedures may, however, be required if the biopsy does not reveal the diagnosis of Langerhans-cell histiocytosis.

A therapeutic trial of glucocorticoids (Answer C) is only recommended after etiological workup has been completed.

Reducing fluid intake (Answer D) in this patient with vasopressin deficiency would cause hypernatremia.

Educational Objective

Guide the diagnostic workup in a patient with an infundibular lesion and vasopressin deficiency.

Reference(s)

Oda Y, Amano K, Seki Y, et al. Clinical features and difficulty in diagnosis of Langerhans cell histiocytosis in the hypothalamic-pituitary region. *Endocr J.* 2022;69(4):441-449. PMID: 34776469

Langlois F, Varlamov EV, Fleseriu M. Hypophysitis, the growing spectrum of a rare pituitary disease. *J Clin Endocrinol Metab.* 2022;107(1):10-28. PMID: 34528683

Kadowaki Y, Nishiyama M, Nakamura M, et al. Adult-onset Langerhans cell histiocytosis changing CNS lesion from pituitary to suprasellar extension. *Endocrinol Diabetes Metab Case Rep.* 2022;2022:22-0232. PMID: 35642690

Aubart FC, Idbaih A, Emile JF, et al. Histiocytosis and the nervous system: from diagnosis to targeted therapies. *Neuro Oncol.* 2021;23(9):1433-1446. PMID: 33993305

Sagna Y, Courtillot C, Drabo JY, et al. Endocrine manifestations in a cohort of 63 adulthood and childhood onset patients with Langerhans cell histiocytosis. *Eur J Endocrinol.* 2019;181(3):275-285. PMID: 31269469

104 ANSWER: B) Continue insulin pump therapy but switch to manual mode, increase nocturnal basal rate, and change the insulin-to-carbohydrate ratio to increase prandial insulin coverage

Significant changes in diabetes management may be needed in patients who enter pregnancy and have preexisting diabetes mellitus. This young pregnant patient with type 1 diabetes had uncontrolled diabetes before pregnancy as documented by her high hemoglobin A_{1c} value, which correlates with the average glucose concentrations and the below-target time-in-range (70-180 mg/dL [3.9-10.0 mmol/L]).

Insulin changes are, therefore, needed. Glycemic targets are different in pregnant patients than in the general population, as tighter glycemic control among pregnant patients with diabetes is associated with better maternal and fetal outcomes. Glycemic targets in this population are as follows:

- Fasting preprandial and nocturnal glucose values: 70-90 mg/dL (SI: 3.9-5.0 mmol/L)
- 1-Hour postprandial glucose: 110-140 mg/dL (SI: 6.1-7.8 mmol/L)
- 2-Hour postprandial glucose: 100-120 mg/dL (SI: 5.6-6.7 mmol/L)

Reviewing patterns of glucose values from the continuous glucose monitoring report, this patient has fasting and nocturnal hyperglycemia along with 2-hour postprandial hyperglycemia. Therefore, she requires changes in basal rates overnight or early morning and changes in the insulin-to-carbohydrate ratio. Because pregnancy is associated with progressively increasing insulin requirements, patients must be evaluated frequently for insulin titration.

Insulin pump use is not contraindicated during pregnancy. Although initiation of insulin pump therapy during pregnancy may be challenging due to the learning curve for a patient who has not used this system before, continuation of insulin pump therapy during pregnancy for someone already well-versed in this insulin delivery system can be an appropriate and effective approach. Most patients who have been adequately trained using insulin pump therapy prefer to continue rather than transition to multiple daily injection therapy (Answer E).

Various hybrid closed-loop insulin systems are available in the United States and have received FDA clearance for patients with diabetes. These systems use different algorithms with a goal of achieving normoglycemia without increasing hypoglycemia. However, the role of hybrid closed-loop insulin pumps during the pregnancy is still unclear, and the FDA (at the time this vignette was written) does not recommend using these systems in pregnancy. A hybrid closed-loop system is available and is cleared for use during pregnancy in the United Kingdom and European Union but not in the United States. Limited data support the use of this technology in pregnant patients. Additionally, the glycemic targets during pregnancy are much lower than the glycemic targets that the hybrid-closed systems are trying to achieve. Although target values vary among systems (refer to manufacturers' manuals), the lowest glucose values that these systems target are between 110 and 120 mg/dL (6.1-6.7 mmol/L). During pregnancy, as described above, the fasting, preprandial, and nocturnal glycemic targets that need to be achieved are much lower.

The continued use of an insulin pump would be the best approach for this patient, but on manual mode, not auto mode (thus, Answers C and D are incorrect). However, only increasing the basal rates will not improve the hyperglycemia that occurs with meals. Increasing basal rates to counteract prandial hyperglycemia can be problematic. Although the approach of using higher basal rates (Answer A) may not lead to issues while the patient is eating frequent meals, it can cause hypoglycemia if the patient has decreased food intake (eg, secondary to illness).

In this case, the best answer is to continue insulin pump therapy but switch the settings to manual mode and titrate basal rates and the insulin-to-carbohydrate ratio. Because she has nocturnal fasting and postprandial hyperglycemia, the nocturnal basal rate needs to be increased and the insulin-to-carbohydrate ratio should be more aggressive to provide more prandial-bolus insulin coverage (Answer B).

Educational Objective

Recommend appropriate management of pregnant patients with diabetes mellitus who use hybrid closed-loop insulin delivery systems.

Reference(s)

Skajaa GO, Fuglsang J, Kampmann U, Ovesen PG. Parity increases insulin requirements in pregnant women with type 1 diabetes. *J Clin Endocrinol Metab.* 2018;103(6):2302-2308. PMID: 29584894

Alexopoulos AS, Blair R, Peters AL. Management of preexisting diabetes in pregnancy: a review. *JAMA.* 2019;321(18):1811-1819. PMID: 31087027

105 **ANSWER: A) After consultation with breast oncology, start low-dosage vaginal estrogen in the form of a 17β-estradiol vaginal ring**

About 6000 US women reach menopause every day, which is more than 2 million women per year. Given that the mean age of menopause onset is 51 years and that 80 years is the mean life expectancy of women today, on average, women are menopausal more than one-third of their lives.

Natural menopause is defined as the final menstrual period confirmed after 1 year of no menstrual bleeding. It represents the permanent cessation of menses resulting from loss of ovarian follicular function, which leads to a decrease of estradiol. This woman experienced surgical-induced menopause. Given estrogen's expansive effects on target tissues throughout the body, menopausal symptoms are wide ranging and can include vasomotor symptoms (hot flashes and night sweats), vulvovaginal symptoms such as vaginal dryness and dyspareunia, urinary stress incontinence, sleep disturbances, cognitive symptoms, psychological symptoms, and reduced libido. In determining treatment options for menopausal symptoms, both the risks and benefits must be considered, as well as relative and absolute contraindications. This requires a detailed history from the patient.

Given that this woman has a history of estrogen- and progesterone-dependent cancer, systemic menopausal hormone therapy (Answers D and E) is an absolute contraindication. In addition, there is no indication for progestogen therapy given that she does not have a uterus.

Because of her vaginal dryness and urinary stress incontinence, she would be a good candidate for local vaginal estrogen therapy (Answer A). Vaginal estrogen therapy is FDA approved for vulvovaginal atrophy and dyspareunia. Vaginal atrophy is associated with higher rates of urinary incontinence, and some data have demonstrated that local estrogen improves urinary stress incontinence, a condition this patient has. Discussion and collaboration should take place with the treating oncology team because of her history of breast cancer.

Given the accepted benefit of vaginal estrogen therapy, increasing the frequency of vaginal moisturizers (Answer B) would not be appropriate.

Because some of her symptoms can be effectively treated, even with her medical history, one should not simply recommend only behavior modifications and avoidance of triggers (Answer C). Nonhormonal management of vasomotor symptoms should also be considered in this patient with severe vasomotor symptoms. Therapies with established effectiveness include selective serotonin reuptake inhibitors (paroxetine, 7.5 mg [FDA-approved for vasomotor symptoms], as well as fluoxetine and escitalopram), serotonin and norepinephrine reuptake inhibitors, gabapentin, clonidine, clinical hypnosis, and cognitive behavioral therapy.

Educational Objective

Evaluate contraindications to and potential options for menopausal hormone therapy.

Reference(s)

Harlow SD, Gass M, Hall JE, et al; STRAW+10 Collaborative Group. Executive summary of the Stages of Reproductive Aging Workshop + 10: addressing the unfinished agenda of staging reproductive aging. *J Clin Endocrinol Metab.* 2012;97(4):1159-1168. PMID: 22344196

The North American Menopause Society. *Menopause Practice: A Clinician's Guide.* 6th ed. The North American Menopause Society, 2017.

Nonhormonal management of menopause-associated vasomotor symptoms: 2015 position statement of The North American Menopause Society. *Menopause.* 2015;22(11):1155-1172. PMID: 26382310

The 2022 hormone therapy position statement of The North American Menopause Society Advisory Panel. The 2022 hormone therapy position statement of The North American Menopause Society. *Menopause.* 2022;29(7):767-794. PMID: 35797481

Struenkel CA, Davis SA, et al. Treatment of symptoms of the menopause: an Endocrine Society clinical practice guideline. *J Clin Endocrinol Metab.* 2015;100(11):3975-4011. PMID: 26444994

106 ANSWER: C) Pathogenic variant in the gene encoding menin

Persistent or recurrent hypercalcemia after parathyroidectomy should prompt consideration of causes other than parathyroid adenomas, such as multigland hyperplasia, genetic syndromes, medications, or other etiologies of hypercalcemia. This patient had rapid recurrence of hypercalcemia after 2 parathyroidectomies. Additional clinical features or family history, if present, may provide clues to the underlying diagnosis. This patient has a congenital heart malformation (aortic stenosis), but this is not generally associated with hyperparathyroidism. He does, however, have gastrointestinal symptoms (reflux) and a lipoma. Although both findings are common in the general population, they are also features seen in multiple endocrine neoplasia type 1 due to pathogenic variants in the gene encoding menin (*MEN1*) (Answer C). These findings should prompt consideration of multiple endocrine neoplasia type 1 in patients with hyperparathyroidism, especially if hypercalcemia persists or recurs after surgery. On further testing, this patient had an elevated gastrin concentration (ideally gastrin should be measured when fasting and without taking H2 blockers or proton-pump inhibitors). Abdominal CT revealed pancreatic neuroendocrine tumors, and genetic testing confirmed the presence of an *MEN1* pathogenic variant.

Hyperparathyroidism is also associated with pathogenic variants in other genes such as *RET* (multiple endocrine neoplasia type 2) and *CDC73* (hyperparathyroidism–jaw tumor syndrome, which is associated with fibro-osseus lesions in the jaw, increased risk for parathyroid cancer, kidney cysts, and kidney tumors). Each of these conditions should be considered depending on the presence of relevant clinical features.

Persistent hypercalcemia is also expected to occur if a patient with familial hypocalciuric hypercalcemia (FHH) due to pathogenic inactivating variants in the calcium-sensing receptor gene (*CASR*) (Answer D) undergoes parathyroidectomy. When available, historical laboratory values are important in guiding the differential diagnosis. Patients with FHH generally have lifelong hypercalcemia, so a history of prior normal calcium levels would argue against FHH. Because of this patient's lifelong cardiac issues, extensive laboratory values were available, which demonstrated that hypercalcemia did not develop until after he was an adult, making FHH unlikely. Additionally, he has hypercalciuria, although interpretation of urinary calcium excretion is complicated by use of loop and thiazide diuretics. Of note, FHH can also be caused by pathogenic variants in the *GNA11* and *AP2S1* genes, both involved in postreceptor signaling at the calcium-sensing receptor. FHH is not generally symptomatic and is not associated with nephrolithiasis.

Hydrochlorothiazide (Answer B) modestly decreases urinary calcium excretion and can increase serum calcium, although not usually to this degree. However, one would expect suppression of PTH if this were the cause of the hypercalcemia, and his PTH concentration and urinary calcium excretion are both elevated.

Amiodarone can induce hyperthyroidism (Answer C), and hyperthyroidism can be a cause of hypercalcemia due to increased bone turnover. However, hyperthyroidism must be severe to cause significant hypercalcemia, and this patient's TSH is just mildly suppressed. The elevated PTH also argues against this etiology.

He has hypophosphatemia combined with hypercalciuria, which can occur in the setting of pathogenic variants in the sodium-phosphate cotransporter gene (Answer E). Variants affecting NPT2c impair kidney phosphate reabsorption, and because this is not FGF-23 mediated, the 1,25-dihydroxyvitamin D production rises, which increases both intestinal phosphate and calcium absorption. Due to hyperabsorption of calcium, these patients are hypercalciuric and prone to nephrolithiasis and nephrocalcinosis. While the full phenotype is generally inherited in an autosomal recessive manner and presents in childhood with rickets, there is evidence that heterozygous patients with pathogenic variants affecting NPT2c also have some phenotypic manifestations that may present in adulthood. Variants affecting NPT2a may also cause hypercalcemia for similar reasons. However, patients with variants affecting NPT2a or NPT2c do not typically have elevated PTH. In this patient with hyperparathyroidism, the hypophosphatemia occurs due to PTH's effect of downregulating the expression of sodium-phosphate transporters in the kidney.

Educational Objective

Diagnose and manage recurrent or persistent primary hyperparathyroidism in the setting of multiple endocrine neoplasia.

Reference(s)

Minisola S, Arnold A, Belaya Z, et al. Epidemiology, pathophysiology, and genetics of primary hyperparathyroidism. *J Bone Miner Res.* 2022;37(11):2315-2329. PMID: 36245271

Thakker RV, Newey PJ, Walls GV, et al; Endocrine Society. Clinical practice guidelines for multiple endocrine neoplasia type 1 (MEN1). *J Clin Endocrinol Metab.* 2012;97(9):2990-3011. PMID: 22723327

107 ANSWER: C) Polysomnography

Increased hematocrit (ie, erythrocytosis or polycythemia, defined as hematocrit >54% [>0.54]) is the most common adverse effect reported in randomized controlled trials of testosterone treatment in cisgender men. A meta-analysis of 4 trials including 1779 patients reported a relative risk for erythrocytosis of 8.14 (95% CI, 1.87-35.40) compared with placebo. Endocrine Society guidelines recommend measuring hematocrit at baseline, 3 to 6 months after starting treatment, and annually thereafter. Risk factors for erythrocytosis include older age, intramuscular testosterone rather than transdermal therapy (due to higher peak serum testosterone on-treatment concentrations in the former), and supraphysiologic serum testosterone concentrations. In this 58-year-old man, transdermal testosterone achieved a low-normal serum testosterone concentration, yet he developed erythrocytosis. Therefore, an underlying cause is likely. If hematocrit is greater than 54% (>0.54), Endocrine Society guidelines recommend that testosterone therapy be stopped until hematocrit decreases to a safe level. This patient should be evaluated for an underlying cause, and therapy should be reinitiated at a reduced dosage. In some cases, if no underlying treatable cause of the erythrocytosis can be identified and/or the patient's hypogonadal symptoms recur at a lower dosage, regular venesection (phlebotomy) may be needed.

This patient has several risk factors of obstructive sleep apnea, including obesity, male sex, cigarette smoking, hypertension, and older age. Obstructive sleep apnea is common, with an estimated prevalence of 15% to 30% in North American men, and up to 60% in those with obesity (BMI >30 kg/m^2). In this patient, while libido improved with testosterone treatment as expected, his fatigue, and consequently his energy levels, did not. On further inquiry, his fatigue was mostly related to daytime sleepiness. Collateral history from a bed partner was not available (to document snoring, choking, gasping during sleep), as he was single. Most sleep experts do not routinely use evaluation tools (eg, STOP-Bang questionnaire or the Epworth Sleepiness Scale) to select those at risk for obstructive sleep apnea who need a sleep study because none of these tools has been shown to be superior to a history and physical examination and their poor accuracy makes them imperfect diagnostic tools. Low testosterone is associated with obstructive sleep apnea, but current evidence suggests that this association is mediated largely, if not exclusively, by obesity (which in itself is a strong risk factor for both obstructive sleep apnea and low serum testosterone). Given the high pretest probability, this patient was referred for attended, in-laboratory, full-night polysomnography (Answer C) and severe obstructive sleep apnea was diagnosed.

After successful cessation of cigarette smoking and implemented and optimized continuous positive airway pressure therapy, his fatigue and energy improved markedly. With continuous positive airway pressure and withholding topical testosterone for 6 weeks, his hematocrit improved to 48% (0.48). Topical testosterone was reinitiated at a full replacement dosage, maintaining a serum testosterone concentration around 450 ng/dL (15.6 nmol/L) with resolution of hypogonadal symptoms. His hematocrit remained stable (48% [0.48]) over subsequent months.

Testosterone-mediated increase in hematocrit in patients with risk factors should prompt consideration of undiagnosed obstructive sleep apnea. In a retrospective study of 474 testosterone-treated men, 62 (13.1%) developed erythrocytosis, and there was a strong correlation between erythrocytosis and a concomitant diagnosis of obstructive sleep apnea, which persisted even after adjusting for age, BMI, and peak on-treatment serum testosterone concentrations with an adjusted odds ratio of 2.09 (95% CI, 1.17-3.76). BMI was the only risk factor for obstructive sleep apnea in this study. Although Endocrine Society guidelines list untreated severe obstructive sleep apnea as a contraindication to testosterone treatment, whether testosterone treatment worsens obstructive sleep apnea is not clear, with the only 12-week randomized controlled trial reporting that testosterone therapy in men with obesity and severe obstructive sleep apnea mildly worsens sleep-disordered breathing in a time-limited manner (at 7 weeks but not at 12 weeks). However, it is prudent that at-risk men be evaluated for obstructive sleep apnea in an individualized manner (depending on clinical suspicion) before testosterone treatment is started.

While it is reasonable to consider other underlying causes of erythrocytosis that could be unmasked by testosterone treatment (eg, hypoxia diagnosed on a 6-minute walk test [Answer E], a *JAK2* pathogenic variant [Answer B], or, very rarely, an erythropoietin-producing tumor, most commonly in the kidneys or liver, located by CT of the abdomen and pelvis [Answer A]), these alternative diagnoses are, given the clinical presentation, much less likely.

Because the clinical history does not suggest relative erythrocytosis (eg, due to hypovolemia), and given the known erythropoietic actions of testosterone, red blood cell mass is probably increased in this patient. Therefore, measurement of red blood cell mass (Answer D) is unlikely to be helpful. He is on SGLT-2 inhibitor therapy, and anecdotal evidence suggests that concomitant SGLT-2 inhibitor treatment could increase the risk of testosterone treatment–associated erythrocytosis. Postulated mechanisms include their diuretic effect and potentially stimulation of erythropoietin secretion. However, in the 2 reported cases to date, this occurred within months of SGLT-2 inhibitor initiation, whereas this patient had been on SGLT-2 inhibitor treatment for about 2 years.

Educational Objective

Suspect undiagnosed sleep apnea as a common cause of increased hematocrit and persistent fatigue in a hypogonadal man on testosterone replacement.

Reference(s)

Ponce OJ, Spencer-Bonilla G, Alvarez-Villalobos N, et al. The efficacy and adverse events of testosterone replacement therapy in hypogonadal men: a systematic review and meta-analysis of randomized, placebo-controlled trials. *J Clin Endocrinol Metab.* 2018 [Online ahead of print] PMID: 29562341

Bhasin S, Brito JP, Cunningham GR, et al. Testosterone therapy in men with hypogonadism: an Endocrine Society clinical practice guideline. *J Clin Endocrinol Metab.* 2018;103(5):1715-1744. PMID: 29562364

Lundy SD, Parekh NV, Shoskes DA. Obstructive sleep apnea is associated with polycythemia in hypogonadal men on testosterone replacement therapy. *J Sex Med.* 2020;17(7):1297-1303. PMID: 32307242

Clarke BM, Vincent AD, Martin S, et al. Obstructive sleep apnea is not an independent determinant of testosterone in men. *Eur J Endocrinol.* 2020;183(1):31-39. PMID: 32348955

Hoyos CM, Killick R, Yee BL, Grunstein RR, Liu PY. Effects of testosterone therapy on sleep and breathing in obese men with severe obstructive sleep apnoea: a randomized placebo-controlled trial. *Clin Endocrinol (Oxf).* 2012;77(4):599-607. PMID: 22512435

Motta G, Zavattaro M, Romeo F, Lanfranco F, Broglio F. Risk of erythrocytosis during concomitant testosterone and SGLT2-inhibitor treatment: a warning from two clinical cases. *J Clin Endocrinol Metab.* 2019;104(3):819-822. PMID: 30395251

108 ANSWER: E) Start moderate-intensity statin therapy

Unlike LDL-cholesterol levels, the relationship between HDL-cholesterol levels and atherosclerotic cardiovascular disease (ASCVD) events is not linear and is sometimes difficult to predict. While low HDL-cholesterol levels are known to be associated with increased ASCVD risk, there is no clear evidence that high HDL-cholesterol levels decrease the risk. In a recent large prospective study of participants enrolled in the United Kingdom Biobank, men with very high HDL cholesterol (>80 mg/dL [>2.07 mmol/L]) had an almost 2-fold increased risk of cardiovascular and all-cause mortality compared with risk of men with HDL-cholesterol values in the normal range (40-60 mg/dL [1.04-1.55 mmol/L]). Men with HDL-cholesterol values between 60 and 80 mg/dL (1.55-2.07 mmol/L) did not have either higher or lower risk. While a similar increased risk was not observed in women, there was no protective effect of high HDL cholesterol either. Even though current guidelines do not suggest considering high HDL cholesterol to be a risk factor, it would be prudent to be aggressive with risk factor modification in patients with high HDL cholesterol rather than consider it to be a protective factor. This patient has other risk factors, including impaired fasting glucose, and has a 10-year estimated ASCVD risk of 8.2%. Starting a moderate-intensity statin (Answer E) is therefore the appropriate choice. Withholding statin therapy because of presumed protective effect of high HDL cholesterol is not correct.

Patients with extreme elevations of HDL cholesterol often have an underlying genetic basis such as pathogenic variants in the genes encoding cholesteryl ester transfer protein (*CETP*), hepatic lipase (*LIPC*), or scavenger receptor class B type I (*SCARB1*). While there are some reports of decreased ASCVD risk in patients with *CETP* pathogenic variants, it has not been a consistent observation. Genetic testing (Answer B) is unlikely to help guide therapeutic choices in patients with high HDL cholesterol and is currently not recommended. Testing should be considered only in patients with suspected familial hypercholesterolemia, familial chylomicronemia syndrome, or other rare monogenic disorders such as sitosterolemia, cerebrotendinous xanthomatosis, and lysosomal acid lipase deficiency.

Metformin therapy (Answer D) in patients with impaired fasting glucose has not been shown to reduce ASCVD risk.

While there is some evidence that fibrates (Answer C) may reduce ASCVD risk in patients with hypertriglyceridemia and low HDL cholesterol, it would not be appropriate in this patient who does not have these features.

Abstinence from alcohol (Answer A) should be recommended for patients with severe hypertriglyceridemia.

Educational Objective

Identify LDL cholesterol as the primary risk factor for ASCVD and explain that a very high HDL-cholesterol concentration may not be protective and may even increase ASCVD risk.

Reference(s)

Liu C, Dhindsa D, Almuwaqqat Z, Sun YV, Quyyumi AA. Very high high-density lipoprotein cholesterol levels and cardiovascular mortality. *Am J Cardiol.* 2022;167:43-53. PMID: 35039162

Berberich AJ, Hegele RA. A modern approach to dyslipidemia. *Endocr Rev.* 2022;43(4):611-653. PMID: 34676866

Brown EE, Sturm AC, Cuchel M, et al. Genetic testing in dyslipidemia: a scientific statement from the National Lipid Association. *J Clin Lipidol.* 2020;14(4):398-413. PMID: 32507592

109 ANSWER: C) Ultrasound-guided FNA of left thyroid nodule

This patient has subclinical hyperthyroidism with a serum TSH value less than 0.1 mIU/L in the context of a multinodular thyroid gland. Correlation of thyroid ultrasonography and thyroid scintigraphy images can be used to determine the etiology of thyroid hormone excess and identify hyperfunctioning and nonfunctioning thyroid nodules, which are managed differently.

On review of the radionuclide thyroid scan images, the nodule in the right thyroid lobe is hyperfunctioning ("hot"), while that in the left nodule demonstrates lower-than-normal uptake that is similar to that of the surrounding normal thyroid tissue (isofunctioning or "warm"). Since hyperfunctioning nodules rarely harbor malignancy, no cytologic evaluation of the right thyroid nodule (Answers D and E) is warranted. The left thyroid nodule is hypoechoic and solid without high-suspicion features on the corresponding ultrasound images. It is consistent with the intermediate-suspicion pattern per the 2015 American Thyroid Association guidelines for thyroid nodules and cancer, or TR-4 according to the American College of Radiology TI-RADS system. Based on the nodule's sonographic appearance, ultrasound-guided FNA would be indicated for this nodule at a size threshold greater than 1 cm per the American Thyroid Association and greater than 1.5 cm per the American College of Radiology. The best next step in this patient's management would thus be to perform ultrasound-guided FNA of the left thyroid nodule (Answer C). Although right thyroid lobectomy (Answer A) or radioactive iodine therapy (not a listed answer option) would be possible definitive treatment strategies for this patient's subclinical hyperthyroidism, neither would be the best next step in her management, as the presence of thyroid malignancy in the contralateral lobe must first be excluded.

Measurement of TRAb (Answer B) would not aid in the diagnosis or management of this patient who has a right toxic adenoma as an established cause of her hyperthyroidism.

Educational Objective

Correlate thyroid ultrasound imaging and thyroid scintigraphy in the context of hyperthyroidism and multinodular goiter.

Reference(s)

Haugen BR, Alexander EK, Bible KC, et al. 2015 American Thyroid Association management guidelines for adult patients with thyroid nodules and differentiated thyroid cancer: the American Thyroid Association Guidelines Task Force on Thyroid Nodules and Differentiated Thyroid Cancer. *Thyroid.* 2016;26(1):1-133. PMID: 26462967

Tessler FN, Middleton WD, Grant EG, et al. ACR Thyroid Imaging, Reporting and Data System (TI-RADS): white paper of the ACR TI-RADS Committee. *J Am Coll Radiol.* 2017;14(5):587-595. PMID: 28372962

110 ANSWER: E) Start sitagliptin and low-dose insulin aspart correction

This patient is at high risk for inpatient hypoglycemia and is currently experiencing hyperglycemia due to recent surgery (increased stress state). While correctional doses of insulin (or insulin sliding scale) can be used on day 1 to 2 to estimate insulin requirements, proceeding with only correctional/sliding scale insulin (Answer A) throughout the hospital stay is not ideal, as the overall goal would be to prevent and not react to hyperglycemia.

Most studies support the use of basal-bolus therapy while hospitalized. However, this patient has already experienced hypoglycemia, is at high risk to continue to develop hypoglycemia given his age and prior minimal outpatient requirements, and most likely will have reduced insulin requirements as he continues to heal. The addition of a DPP-4 inhibitor (Answer E) reduces prandial insulin requirements and frequency of hypoglycemia with no difference in time-in-range as compared with basal-bolus therapy, and this is the best option for this patient. DPP-4 inhibitors can therefore be used in patients with mild hyperglycemia who have adequate glycemic control with noninsulin therapies preadmission.

Starting insulin glargine, 10 units at bedtime, and scheduling 3 units of insulin aspart before each meal (Answer C) or starting insulin glargine, 14 units at bedtime, and low-dose insulin aspart correction (Answer D) will result in a higher dose of insulin administered compared with the prior day's requirements and therefore will result in hypoglycemia.

Sulfonylureas (Answer B) are associated with hypoglycemia, more so when caloric intake is variable and in older adults. Starting glipizide would increase this patient's risk of hypoglycemia and should not be used in the acute hospital setting.

Educational Objective

Recommend use of DPP-4 inhibitors for inpatient glucose management in the setting of mild hyperglycemia.

Reference(s)

Korytkowski MT, Muniyappa R, Antinori-Lent K, et al. Management of hyperglycemia in hospitalized adult patients in non-critical care settings: an Endocrine Society clinical practice guideline. *J Clin Endocrinol Metab.* 2022;107(8):2101-2128. PMID: 35690958

Vellanki P, Rasouli N, Baldwin D, et al; Linagliptin Inpatient Research Group. Glycaemic efficacy and safety of linagliptin compared to a basal-bolus insulin regimen in patients with type 2 diabetes undergoing non-cardiac surgery: a multicentre randomized clinical trial. *Diabetes Obes Metab.* 2019;21(4):837-843. PMID: 30456796

Lorenzo-González C, Atienza-Sánchez E, Reyes-Umpierrez D, et al. Safety and efficacy of DDP4-inhibitors for management of hospitalized general medicine and surgery patients with type 2 diabetes. *Endocr Pract.* 2020;26(7):722-728. PMID: 33471640

111 ANSWER: E) Review diet and over-the-counter supplements

This patient has low-renin hypertension and hypokalemia, requiring potassium supplementation despite taking lisinopril and having a mild elevation of creatinine. This phenotype is suggestive of mineralocorticoid receptor overactivation. Apart from a high-salt diet, the most common form of low-renin hypertension is primary aldosteronism, followed by Cushing syndrome (*see box*). Cortisol is a mineralocorticoid receptor agonist with affinity and potency similar to those of aldosterone. Physiologic cortisol concentrations far exceed those of aldosterone. However, tissues expressing mineralocorticoid receptors, including the kidney, inactivate cortisol to cortisone via 11β-dehydrogenase type 2 (HSD11B2). This enzyme is saturated in patients with supraphysiologic concentrations of cortisol, such as in the setting of Cushing syndrome or glucocorticoid resistance syndrome. Glucocorticoid resistance syndrome is due to autosomal recessive pathogenic variants in the *NR3C1* gene, which encodes the glucocorticoid receptor. Glucocorticoid-receptor insensitivity leads to ACTH elevation and subsequently cortisol elevation.

The syndrome of apparent mineralocorticoid excess is an autosomal recessive disorder caused by pathogenic variants in the *HSD11B2* gene. This results in higher local concentrations of cortisol, which can readily activate the mineralocorticoid receptors, leading to sodium retention, intravascular volume expansion, and sometimes hypokalemia. Patients with apparent mineralocorticoid excess have a high 24-hour urinary cortisol-to-cortisone ratio (Answer B) and an elevated ratio of cortisol to cortisone metabolites (tetrahydrocortisol plus allotetrahydrocortisol to tetrahydrocortisone ([THF+aTHF])/THE). More commonly, HSD11B2 is inhibited by exogenous substances, allowing physiologic cortisol concentrations to activate the mineralocorticoid receptor. A well-known HSD11B2 inhibitor is glycyrrhizic acid, found in black licorice. Thus, reviewing dietary preferences and over-the-counter supplements (Answer E) is important in patients with hypertension and hypokalemia who have low renin, low aldosterone, and no clinical evidence of cortisol excess.

Rare forms of low-renin hypertension mediated by the mineralocorticoid 11-deoxycorticosterone include congenital adrenal hyperplasia due to 17-hydroxylase (CYP17A1) deficiency or 11β-hydroxylase (CYP11B1) deficiency and 11-deoxycorticosterone–secreting tumors.

Additional mechanisms of low-renin hypertension include activating pathogenic variants in the gene encoding the mineralocorticoid receptor (described in a single family) and gain-of-function variants in the gene encoding the epithelial sodium channel, leading to sodium reabsorption in the distal nephron, hypokalemia, and hypertension (Liddle syndrome).

A 1-mg dexamethasone-suppression test (Answer C) is the most sensitive way to detect mild autonomous cortisol excess. This patient does not have any clinical stigmata of hypercortisolism.

Salt-loading tests (Answer D), either oral or intravenous, are used in patients with positive screening results for primary aldosteronism. This patient had a low plasma aldosterone concentration.

Spironolactone is 1 of 2 steroidal mineralocorticoid receptor antagonists available in the United States. Mineralocorticoid receptor antagonists are highly effective not only in primary aldosteronism, but in other forms of low-renin hypertension and as add-on therapy in patients with drug-resistant hypertension. Spironolactone (Answer A) would be effective for treating both hypertension and hypokalemia in this patient. Eliciting a careful history revealed that she was consuming copious amounts of black licorice while working from home (a stress-coping mechanism). Once she stopped eating licorice, her hypertension control improved dramatically and hypokalemia resolved.

Box. Forms of Low-Renin Hypertension

Genetic causes
Familial forms of primary aldosteronism
Liddle syndrome
Apparent mineralocorticoid excess
CYP11B1 deficiency
CYP17A1 deficiency
Glucocorticoid receptor resistance
Mineralocorticoid receptor–activating pathogenic variant
Acquired causes
Sporadic primary aldosteronism
Cushing syndrome
11-Deoxycorticosterone–secreting tumors
Excess consumption of black licorice
Low-renin primary hypertension
High-salt diet

Educational Objective

Construct the differential diagnosis of low-renin hypertension.

Reference(s)

Monticone S, Losano I, Tetti M, Buffolo F, Veglio F, Mulatero P. Diagnostic approach to low-renin hypertension. *Clin Endocrinol (Oxf).* 2018;89(4):385-396. PMID: 29758100

112 ANSWER: A) Heterophilic antibody interference with the TSH assay

In the setting of mild elevated TSH and normal free T_4, the differential diagnosis is broad. The most common diagnosis is subclinical hypothyroidism, and many physicians often initiate levothyroxine when this is suspected. In general, interference should be considered when there is any discrepancy between the clinical presentation and the laboratory results. Not considering this possibility can lead to misdiagnosis and unnecessary treatment. In this vignette, levothyroxine was started but the patient's serum TSH levels remained elevated/unchanged with a progressively increasing free T_4 concentration despite adjusting the levothyroxine dosage. These laboratory findings are a clue to the presence of heterophile antibodies (Answer A). Human antimouse monoclonal antibodies (HAMA) are a type of heterophile antibody. HAMA occurs in up to 10% of the general population. This heterophilic antibody interference with the TSH assay happens when patients have antibodies that recognize the mouse monoclonal antibody in the sandwich assay for TSH. Preincubation of the patient's serum with nonimmune mouse antibodies is an easy step in the assay method to eliminate the effect of HAMA. In addition, nonlinearity of TSH measurements with serial dilution of the patient's serum also strongly suggests assay interference. Commercial assays exist for detecting HAMA.

This patient does not have malabsorption (Answer C), as her serum free T_4 levels have increased from baseline with a higher levothyroxine dosage.

In a patient with resistance to thyroid hormone (Answer D), the free T_4 concentration would be elevated along with a normal or high serum TSH concentration, which is not the case here.

In addition to normal or high TSH with elevated free T_4, a patient with a TSH-secreting pituitary adenoma (Answer E) would be clinically hyperthyroid, while the patient in this vignette is euthyroid.

Macro TSH (Answer B) is less common than HAMA with a prevalence ranging from 0.6% to 1.6%. Macro TSH is a large circulating form of TSH composed of monomeric TSH complexed with immunoglobulin G (IgG). It can be detected either by gel filtration chromatography or by polyethylene glycol precipitation. Patients with macro TSH typically have markedly elevated TSH with normal free T_4 and free T_3 concentrations.

Educational Objective

Identify the presence of heterophilic antibodies as a cause of elevated serum TSH.

Reference(s)

Favresse J, Burlacu MC, Maiter D, Gruson D. Interferences with thyroid function immunoassays: clinical implications and detection algorithm. *Endocr Rev.* 2018;39(5):830-850. PMID: 29982406

Santhana Krishnan SG, Pathalapati R, Kaplan L, Cobbs RK. Falsely raised TSH levels due to human anti-mouse antibody interfering with thyrotropin assay. *Postgrad Med J.* 2006;82(973):e27. PMID: 17099084

113 ANSWER: B) Evaluate for adrenal insufficiency

Pituitary gland dysfunction after traumatic brain injury (TBI) is associated with abnormal pituitary function in up to one-third of patients, with higher prevalence after severe TBI. The abnormalities predominantly affect anterior pituitary hormone secretion The mechanism of hypopituitarism entails a primary phase of mechanical disruption of the blood vessels and neurons, followed by a secondary phase of inflammatory, metabolic, and neurodegenerative processes. Genetic and/or autoimmune factors also have a role. Ischemic changes after TBI predominantly affect the somatotroph and gonadotroph cells situated in the lateral parts of the gland with supply from the hypothalamic-pituitary portal vessels. However, corticotroph and thyrotroph cells are less affected because they are situated in the medial part and receive dual blood supply from the portal vessels and anterior pituitary artery.

Clinical manifestations of hypopituitarism overlap with those caused by TBI and are often nonspecific. In the acute phase, it is important to diagnose cortisol deficiency in patients with suggestive manifestations. Also, water metabolism perturbations can occur, including the syndrome of inappropriate antidiuretic hormone secretion or vasopressin deficiency, both of which are usually transient. In the secondary phase, patients may experience fatigue, decreased well-being and exercise endurance, social isolation, anxiety and/or depression, decreased focus and concentration, weight gain, decreased muscle mass, and increased adipose tissue. In the second phase of TBI, endocrinology evaluation is usually done after stagnation of physical and/or psychological recovery despite adequate rehabilitation. Confounders in some patients are chronic pain and use of opioids, which can interfere with cortisol and testosterone regulation. The 2022 Lancet Neurology Commission on TBI recommended screening for GH and gonadotroph deficiency after 3 to 6 months for symptomatic patients who were admitted for more than 48 hours as a result of TBI. Previous recommendations from other professional societies are in broad agreement, recommending GH testing 6 to 12 months after TBI for patients experiencing suggestive manifestations. Postponing dynamic testing is adequate given the spontaneous recovery of pituitary function after TBI in most patients. This is attributed to the regeneration of portal system vessels and pituitary stem-cell activation. The choice of which stimulation test to use in the TBI patient population has not been established. GHRH-arginine, glucagon, and insulin tolerance tests have been used in different studies. The latter is contraindicated in patients with TBI who have a history of seizures.

Similar to the treatment approach to patients with other etiologies of hypopituitarism, GH replacement in patients with TBI should be considered if there is an expected clinical benefit and started only after the other pituitary axes are evaluated and hormone replacement is optimized. Benefits demonstrated in studies of patients with TBI include improved quality of life (especially in the domains of socialization, self-confidence, and tenseness), cognitive function, body composition, LDL cholesterol, and diastolic blood pressure. Further studies are needed to confirm aerobic capacity and physical endurance improvements in the setting of GH deficiency after TBI. Dosing should follow the same principles as for GH deficiency replacement in general; start with smaller dosages and titrate based on clinical benefit, tolerance, and age-appropriate IGF-1 levels. Dosages up to 0.6 mg daily were used in clinical studies of patients with TBI.

Testing for ACTH deficiency (Answer B) is reasonable because of the patient's history of TBI and opioid use. Serum cortisol should be measured in the early morning due to diurnal variation of this hormone; depending on results, cosyntropin-stimulation testing could be indicated.

Starting hydrocortisone replacement (Answer D) is incorrect because the diagnosis of hypocortisolism has not been proven.

Starting testosterone replacement (Answer E) is incorrect because his testosterone value is not low. While hypogonadotropic hypogonadism is the second most common deficiency after GH (in a recent meta-analysis, 22% patients had GH deficiency, 10% had hypogonadotropic hypogonadism, 9.9% had central hypocortisolism, and 6% had hypothyroidism), this patient had a borderline-low testosterone concentration on a blood sample drawn in the afternoon. Measuring testosterone in the early morning is indicated.

Performing a 6-month trial of GH replacement (Answer C) is incorrect because testing for GH deficiency has not been performed.

While his IGF-1 concentration is normal, advising against GH injections based on this fact (Answer A) is incorrect because most patients with GH deficiency as a result of TBI have low-normal IGF-1 values. The diagnosis is made with GH-stimulation testing after the other pituitary hormone axes have been tested and optimized and after at least 12 months have elapsed since TBI. The IGF-1 concentration is used for dosage titration after GH replacement is started.

Educational Objective

Evaluate for hormone abnormalities after traumatic brain injury.

Reference(s)

Maas AIR, Menon DK, Manley GT, et al; InTBIR Participants and Investigators. Traumatic brain injury: progress and challenges in prevention, clinical care, and research. *Lancet Neurol.* 2022;21(11):1004-1060. PMID: 36183712

Yuen KCJ, Masel B, Jaffe MS, et al. A consensus on optimization of care in patients with growth hormone deficiency and mild traumatic brain injury. *Growth Horm IGF Res.* 2022;66:101495. PMID: 35933894

Emelifeonwu JA, Flower H, Loan JJ, McGivern K, Andrews PJD. Prevalence of anterior pituitary dysfunction twelve months or more following traumatic brain injury in adults: a systematic review and meta-analysis. *J Neurotrauma.* 2020;37(2):217-226. PMID: 31111791

Yuen KCJ, Biller BMK, Radovick S, et al. American Association of Clinical Endocrinologists and American College of Endocrinology guidelines for management of growth hormone deficiency in adults and patients transitioning from pediatric to adult care. *Endocr Pract.* 2019;25(11):1191-1232. PMID: 31760824

Gasco V, Cambria V, Bioletto F, Ghigo E, Grottoli S. Traumatic brain injury as frequent cause of hypopituitarism and growth hormone deficiency: epidemiology, diagnosis, and treatment. *Front Endocrinol (Lausanne).* 2021;12:634415. PMID: 33790864

114 ANSWER: B) Perform fetal ultrasonography starting week 26 of pregnancy and treat with insulin if macrosomia is observed

Persons with *GCK*-related maturity-onset diabetes of the young (MODY) are not at increased risk for complications from hyperglycemia and are typically not treated with glucose-lowering medication in the nonpregnant state. However, pregnant women with *GCK*-related MODY have an increased risk of miscarriage and fetal macrosomia. These outcomes are dependent on fetal *GCK* variant status. If the fetus has inherited the pathogenic variant, there is no increased risk for macrosomia. However, unaffected offspring can have increased insulin release and macrosomia. In addition, if the *GCK* variant is paternally inherited, and the mother is unaffected, the fetus has an increased risk of being small-for-gestational-age. Current guidelines do not recommend invasive testing such as amniocentesis (Answer A) to assess fetal *GCK* status. Instead, the recommendation is to perform fetal ultrasonography in the second trimester, starting at week 16, with repeated imaging every 2 weeks until delivery. If there is accelerated growth (defined as fetal abdominal circumference greater than the 75th percentile), insulin should be initiated (Answer B). When accelerated growth is observed, delivery should be induced at 38 weeks' gestation.

Insufficient data are available to confirm any benefit of insulin administration before conception or early in pregnancy (Answers D and E). Insulin treatment can cause hypoglycemia in women with *GCK*-related MODY. A dosage of 1 unit/kg per day may be required to adequately suppress hyperglycemia to avoid macrosomia. This insulin dosage may not be well-tolerated, and therefore management should account for maternal and fetal needs.

Information is sparse on sulfonylurea use (Answer C) in the management of hyperglycemia during pregnancy in patients with *GCK*-related MODY.

Notably, about 1% of patients with gestational diabetes mellitus have *GCK*-related MODY.

Educational Objective

Guide peripartum glucose management of women with GCK-related maturity-onset diabetes of the young.

Reference(s)

Colom C, Corcoy R. Maturity onset diabetes of the young and pregnancy. *Best Pract Res Clin Endocrinol Metab.* 2010;24(4):605-615. PMID: 20832739

Dickens L, Naylor R. Clinical management of women with monogenic diabetes during pregnancy. *Curr Diab Rep.* 2018;(3):12. PMID: 29450745

115 **ANSWER: A) Being operated on by a low-volume thyroid surgeon**

Significant disparities exist in thyroid cancer care and thyroid cancer–related outcomes. Thyroid cancer is the second most common malignancy in Hispanic and Asian/Pacific Islander women, and these groups have the highest rates of thyroid cancer mortality. Compared with White patients, racial and ethnic minorities are more likely to present with larger thyroid tumors and more advanced disease (thus, Answer C is incorrect).

One of the most important determinants of thyroid cancer–related outcomes is the initial thyroid cancer operation. Thyroid operations performed by low-volume surgeons are associated with a higher risk of postoperative complications compared with risk when thyroid operations are performed by higher-volume surgeons/hospitals. Black and Hispanic patients are more likely than White patients to be operated on by low-volume thyroid surgeons (Answer A) and at low-volume hospitals throughout the United States. A population-based study found that Black patients had reduced access to high-volume surgeons, a higher likelihood of receiving a total thyroidectomy vs lobectomy for thyroid cancer treatment, a higher rate of postoperative complications, longer mean hospital stays, and a higher overall cost of care. Consistent with these findings, Black patients are also less likely to receive care at an academic medical center (thus, Answer D is incorrect), and to be treated with radioactive iodine (thus, Answer E is incorrect). Adherence to the American Thyroid Association guidelines for radioactive iodine administration has been demonstrated to be the lowest for patients older than 65 years and for those who are Black.

Worry about thyroid cancer–related outcomes (Answer B), including risk of recurrence and death, is common among thyroid cancer survivors with a good prognosis. Worry is more prevalent among patients with lower education, women, and patients of Hispanic ethnicity or Asian race, but it has not been demonstrated to occur at a higher rate in Black patients.

Educational Objective

Identify disparities in access to high-volume thyroid surgical care.

Reference(s)

Asamoah EO, Caraballo G, Castro MR. Identifying and addressing health disparities in thyroid cancer care. *J Clin Endocrinol Metab.* 2022;107(5):e2190-e2191. PMID: 34871424

Chen DW, Yeh MW. Disparities in thyroid care. *Endocrinol Metab Clin North Am.* 2022;51(2):229-241. PMID: 35662439

Papaleontiou M, Reyes-Gastelum D, Gay BL, et al. Worry in thyroid cancer survivors with a favorable prognosis. *Thyroid.* 2019;29(8):1080-1088. PMID: 31232194

Shah SA, Adam MA, Thomas SM, et al. Racial disparities in differentiated thyroid cancer: have we bridged the gap? *Thyroid.* 2017;27(6):762-772. PMID: 28294040

116 **ANSWER: A) Add finerenone**

The best next step in this patient's management is to add finerenone (Answer A), which will address residual chronic kidney disease and cardiovascular disease risk. This drug is a nonsteroidal mineralocorticoid receptor antagonist indicated to reduce the risk of declining estimated glomerular filtration rate, end-stage kidney disease, cardiovascular death, nonfatal myocardial infarction, and hospitalization for heart failure in adult patients with chronic kidney disease associated with type 2 diabetes.

Finerenone was studied in the FIDELIO-DKD and FIGARO-DKD randomized placebo controlled trials. The FIDELIO-DKD trial was conducted to evaluate the effect of finerenone on chronic kidney disease outcomes in patients with type 2 diabetes. It included 5734 patients with chronic kidney disease and type 2 diabetes. Patients were required to have a urinary albumin-to-creatinine ratio ≥30 and <300 mg/g and estimated glomerular filtration rate ≥25 and <75 mL/min per 1.73 m^2 and diabetic retinopathy, or urinary albumin-to-creatinine ratio ≥300 and ≤5000 mg/g and estimated glomerular filtration rate ≥25 and <75 mL/min per 1.73 m^2. All patients were treated with RAS blockade. The primary composite outcome, assessed in a time-to-event analysis, was kidney failure, a sustained decrease of at least 40% in the estimated glomerular filtration rate from baseline, or death of renal causes. During a median follow-up of 2.6 years, finerenone reduced the risk of the primary composite outcome (hazard ratio, 0.82; 95% CI, 0.73-0.93; $P < .001$). The FIGARO-DKD trial was conducted to evaluate the effect of finerenone on cardiovascular outcomes. It included 7437 patients with chronic kidney disease and type 2 diabetes. Patients were required to have a urinary albumin-to-creatinine ratio ≥30 and <300 mg/g and an estimated glomerular filtration rate ≥25 and <75 mL/min per 1.73 m^2, or a urinary albumin-to-creatinine ratio ≥300 and ≤5000 mg/g and estimated glomerular filtration rate ≥60 mL/min per 1.73 m^2. All patients were treated with RAS blockade. The primary outcome, assessed in a time-to-event analysis, was a composite of death of cardiovascular causes, nonfatal myocardial infarction, nonfatal stroke, or hospitalization for heart failure. During a median follow-up of 3.4 years, finerenone reduced the risk of the primary composite outcome (hazard ratio, 0.87; 95% CI, 0.76-0.98; $P = .03$).

Compared with placebo, finerenone was associated with a higher overall risk of hyperkalemia in both trials. However, discontinuation of the trial regimen due to hyperkalemia was infrequent in patients who received finerenone (2.3% vs 0.9% with placebo in FIDELIO-DKD and 1.2% vs 0.4% with placebo in FIGARO-DKD) and markedly lower than what was observed in trials of dual RAS blockade (4.8% with combination therapy with a direct renin inhibitor and an ACE inhibitor or angiotensin receptor blocker and 9.2% with dual ACE inhibitor and angiotensin receptor blocker).

The patient is not fluid overloaded, so there is no reason to change the diuretic or the diuretic dosage (Answers B and D).

He is already taking high-intensity statin therapy and has an LDL-cholesterol value at goal (<55 mg/dL [<1.42 mmol/L]). Thus, there is no indication to switch to rosuvastatin (Answer E).

His blood pressure is controlled, so the lisinopril dosage does not need to be increased (Answer C). While a further increase in the lisinopril dosage might be tolerated and could provide additional kidney benefits (eg, reducing albuminuria), adding finerenone is the best choice because of the patient's reduced glomerular filtration rate and established cardiovascular disease.

Although not provided as an answer choice, steroidal mineralocorticoid receptor antagonists (spironolactone and eplerenone) may also be considered as therapeutic options in this patient. These agents are often used to reduce the risk of chronic kidney disease progression. However, unlike finerenone, spironolactone and eplerenone do not have any appropriately powered kidney outcome studies. Compared with finerenone, these medications are also associated with a higher risk of hyperkalemia and this often prevents their use. The benefits of these steroidal mineralocorticoid receptor antagonists have largely been demonstrated in patients with heart failure. Spironolactone has been demonstrated to substantially reduce the risk of both morbidity and death among patients with severe heart failure, and eplerenone has been shown to reduce morbidity and mortality among patients with acute myocardial infarction complicated by left ventricular dysfunction and heart failure.

Educational Objective

Determine when it is appropriate to add the nonsteroidal mineralocorticoid antagonist finerenone to the regimen of a patient with type 2 diabetes mellitus and chronic kidney disease.

Reference(s)

Jellinger PS, Handelsman Y, Rosenblit PD, et al. American Association of Clinical Endocrinologists and American College of Endocrinology Guidelines for Management of Dyslipidemia and Prevention of Cardiovascular Disease. *Endocr Pract.* 2017;23(Suppl 2):1-87. PMID: 28437620

Bakris GL, Agarwal R, Anker SD, et al; FIDELIO-DKD Investigators. Effect of finerenone on chronic kidney disease outcomes in type 2 diabetes. *N Engl J Med.* 2020;383(23):2219-2229. PMID: 33264825

Pitt B, Filippatos G, Agarwal R, et al; FIGARO-DKD Investigators. Cardiovascular events with finerenone in kidney disease and type 2 diabetes. *N Engl J Med.* 2021;385(24):2252-2263.

Pitt B, Remme W, Zannad F, et al; Eplerenone Post-Acute Myocardial Infarction Heart Failure Efficacy and Survival Study Investigators. Eplerenone, a selective aldosterone blocker, in patients with left ventricular dysfunction after myocardial infarction. *N Engl J Med.* 2003;348(14):1309-1321. PMID: 12668699

Pitt B, Zannad, F, Remme WJ, et al. The effect of spironolactone on morbidity and mortality in patients with severe heart failure. Randomized Aldactone Evaluation Study Investigators. *N Engl J Med.* 1999;341(10):709-717. PMID: 10471456

117 ANSWER: E) Type 1 diabetes mellitus

While advancing age is certainly a risk, other important factors also increase the risk for fragility fractures. Alcohol consumption (Answer A) is a known risk factor for fractures, especially when 3 more servings are consumed daily. The mechanisms of how alcohol consumption affects bone cells and microarchitecture are unclear. With higher consumption, the risk of falls and subsequent fractures increases. In one meta-analysis by Berg et al, the relative risk ratio for any type of fracture was 1.23 (CI, 1.06-1.43) with intake of more than 3 servings daily.

The effects of proton-pump inhibitors (Answer B) to increase fracture risk were first reported in 2005. Since then, there have been numerous reports of such an association. In a meta-analysis by Yu et al, the relative risk for hip fractures was 1.30 (CI, 1.19-1.43). Other published meta-analyses have reported similar modest increases in the risk of fractures with proton-pump inhibitor use. The mechanism is thought to be due in part to decreased gastrointestinal absorption of calcium when gastric pH is higher, although data to date have not been conclusive. Importantly, a recent randomized controlled clinical trial did not show an increased risk for fractures with proton-pump inhibitor use.

An increased fracture risk has also been observed with selective serotonin reuptake inhibitor use (Answer C). However, the mechanisms behind this association remain unclear. In the meta-analysis of Wu et al, the relative risk for any fracture was 1.72 (CI, 1.51-1.95), with other similar studies reporting modest increases.

Thiazide diuretics (Answer D) affect calcium homeostasis by increasing renal calcium reabsorption and thus reducing renal calcium wasting. In fact, thiazide diuretics increase bone density and reduce fracture risk. A Cochrane Group meta-analysis reported a reduced risk of hip fractures with a relative risk of 0.76 (CI, 0.64-0.89).

Type 1 diabetes (Answer E) is associated with a significantly higher risk of fractures, especially of the hip, compared with the risks discussed above. In several meta-analyses, the risk for fractures is 3 to 8 times greater in persons with type 1 diabetes than in those without. A similar increase in fracture risk exists for persons with type 2 diabetes, but the absolute risk is not as high. Proposed mechanisms for increased bone fragility include accumulation of advanced-glycation end products of the bone matrix leading to architectural deterioration, changes in bone marrow adiposity, and a decline in osteocyte function and viability. As with any organ with high metabolic demands, a reduction in oxygen and nutrient supply from diabetes-related microvascular damage also impairs normal bone modeling and repair and may also contribute to the observed increase in fracture risk.

Educational Objective

Identify type 1 diabetes mellitus as a factor associated with a 6-fold increased risk of fragility fractures.

Reference(s)

Moayyedi P, Eikelboom JW, Bosch J, et al; COMPASS Investigators. Safety of proton pump inhibitors based on a large, multi-year, randomized trial of patients receiving rivaroxaban or aspirin. *Gastroenterology.* 2019;157(3):682-691. PMID: 31152740

Wu Q, Bencaz AF, Hentz JG, Crowell MD. Selective serotonin reuptake inhibitor treatment and risk of fractures: a meta-analysis of cohort and case-control studies. *Osteoporos Int.* 2012;23(1):365-375. PMID: 21904950

Shah VN, Shah CS, Snell-Bergeon JK. Type 1 diabetes and risk of fracture: meta-analysis and review of the literature. *Diabet Med.* 2015;32(9):1134-1142. PMID: 26096918

Vestergaard P. Discrepancies in bone mineral density and fracture risk in patients with type 1 and type 2 diabetes--a meta-analysis. *Osteoporos Int.* 2007;18(4):427-444. PMID: 17068657

Thong EP, Herath M, Weber DR, et al. Fracture risk in young and middle-aged adults with type 1 diabetes mellitus: a systematic review and meta-analysis. *Clin Endocrinol (Oxf).* 2018;89(3):314-323. PMID: 29876960

118 ANSWER: B) Refer to an eating disorder clinic

This man presents with the anorectic classic triad of disordered eating with low BMI, most likely low bone mass (tibial stress fracture), and hypogonadotropic hypogonadism. The history suggests that restrictive eating (the probable cause of his constipation) is also the primary cause of his energy deficit, with excessive exercise a possible contributor. The effects of energy deficit on reproductive function, while well recognized in women, have received relatively scant attention in men. Up to 30% of patients diagnosed with the *Diagnostic and Statistical Manual of Mental Disorders, Fifth Edition* condition "avoidant and restrictive food intake disorders" are male. This condition is probably underrecognized, and there are limited epidemiologic data to raise public awareness of the issue. This is particularly important given significant societal pressure to attain what is perceived to be the "ideal" male body image. Of note, a recent retrospective cohort study of 683 boys presenting with delayed puberty to a tertiary referral center estimated that 3.7% of cases were caused by relative energy deficit (disordered eating and/or excessive exercise).

Preclinical and experimental studies in men suggest that both acute and chronic caloric restriction suppress the hypothalamic-pituitary-gonadal (HPG) axis at the central level, and that the severity of HPG-axis suppression correlates with the severity of the caloric deficit. Implicated mechanisms include low leptin (reducing kisspeptin-induced activation of the HPG axis) and suppression of GnRH secretion due to hypothalamic-pituitary axis activation and increased proinflammatory cytokines. Men with energy deficit caused primarily by restrictive eating typically have a low BMI. Unlike in women, where loss of menstrual function is obvious and prompts action, dysregulation of the HPG axis under these circumstances may go unnoticed in men.

A 2019 review described clinical features in 23 men with HPG-axis dysregulation due to energy deficit (mainly caused by anorexia) who were identified mostly from single case reports. Common clinical features included low libido, fatigue, bradycardia and, in some cases, reduced exercise performance and stress fractures. Median age was 20 years (range, 16-33 years), median BMI was 15.9 kg/m^2 (range, 12.5-20.5 kg/m^2), and median total testosterone concentration was 86.5 ng/dL (range, 17.3-613.8 ng/dL) (SI: 3.0 nmol/L [range, 0.6-21.3 mmol/L]). Such men sometimes display multiple endocrine abnormalities, as illustrated in this case with hypercortisolemia and evidence of euthyroid sick syndrome. SHBG, a sensitive marker of energy deficit, is typically elevated, as in this case. Mild anemia due hypogonadism and/or nutritional deficits is not uncommon. If tested, there can be evidence of hepatic GH resistance with elevated GH and low IGF-1. There is a high prevalence of comorbid depression, anxiety, and/or body image disorders. Obsessive attention to exercise, combined with some degree of restrictive eating, may not result in a low BMI, although there may be history of weight loss. If significant resistance exercise is being undertaken, there may be a toned and muscular appearance; however, the percentage of body fat is reduced. Over a 20-year period, a retrospective study at a large academic center identified 10 men with hypogonadotropic hypogonadism due to excessive exercise. Affected men were young, aged 18 to 33 years old, with decreased training performance and low libido being the most common presenting symptoms. Mean BMI was 20.3 ± 2.1 kg/m^2, mean serum total testosterone was 123.9 ng/dL (SI: 4.3 nmol/L), and body fat ranged from 4.1% to 13%.

Similar to what is observed in women, HPG-axis suppression due to energy deficit in men is functional and reversible with correction of the energy deficit (ie, increasing caloric intake and, if appropriate, reducing excessive exercise). During weight regain in men with anorexia nervosa, increases in circulating leptin closely correlate with HPG-axis recovery. Thus, restoring the energy deficit is key to recovery of the HPG axis. In men in whom HPG-axis dysfunction persists despite restoration of the energy deficit, other causes should be excluded (eg, organic HPG-axis pathology, covert exogenous androgen use, or other substance abuse). In men with body dysmorphic disorders, associated depression, or exogenous androgen dependence, psychiatric input may be required. Therefore, referral to an eating disorder clinic (Answer B) with the aim of achieving a healthy body weight is the best step to address this patient's hypogonadism.

There is no evidence that testosterone treatment in men with HPG-axis dysregulation due to energy deficit improves clinically important outcomes. Indeed, given that malnutrition-associated HPG-axis dysregulation is functional and reversible, testosterone treatment (Answer E) inhibits endogenous HPG-axis recovery and is not recommended.

Likewise, there is no evidence to suggest that selective estrogen-receptor modulators (Answer D) or aromatase inhibitors (the latter carry a risk of further reducing bone density) are beneficial for the treatment of HPG-axis dysregulation due to energy deficit.

MRI shows an incidental pituitary microadenoma. Given that this patient's serum prolactin concentration is normal, his hypogonadotropic hypogonadism is not due to a prolactinoma, and dopamine agonist therapy (Answer C) is not indicated.

Macroprolactin is a nonbioactive prolactin isoform usually composed of prolactin monomers and immunoglobulin G molecules. It prolongs prolactin clearance rates similar to the effect of immunoglobulins. Macroprolactin measurement (Answer A) is indicated when serum prolactin is elevated but the clinical picture is not consistent with prolactin excess, and his serum prolactin concentration was normal.

Educational Objective

Diagnose anorexia in men and recognize that it can be associated with functional hypogonadism.

Reference(s)

Jonsdottir-Lewis E, Feld A, Ciarlo R, Denhoff E, Feldman HA, Chan Y-M. Timing of pubertal onset in girls and boys with constitutional delay. *J Clin Endocrinol Metab.* 2021;106(9):e3693-e3703. PMID: 33890108

Wong HK, Hoermann R, Grossmann M. Reversible male hypogonadotropic hypogonadism due to energy deficit. *Clin Endocrinol (Oxf).* 2019;91(1):3-9. PMID: 30903626

Dwyer AA, Chavan NR, Lewkowitz-Shpuntoff H, et al. Functional hypogonadotropic hypogonadism in men: Underlying neuroendocrine mechanisms and natural history. *J Clin Endocrinol Metab.* 2019;104(8):3403-3414. PMID: 31220265

Grossmann M, Wittert GA. Dysregulation of the hypothalamic-pituitary-testicular axis due to energy deficit. *J Clin Endocrinol Metab.* 2021;106(12):e4861-e4871. PMID: 34264314

119 **ANSWER: D) Lifestyle counseling**

When approaching patients with severe hypertriglyceridemia, the initial step should be to address lifestyle factors (Answer D) that can exacerbate hypertriglyceridemia and then to consider pharmacotherapy depending on whether they are at high risk for developing atherosclerotic cardiovascular disease (ASCVD) or pancreatitis. While a fasting serum triglyceride concentration greater than 500 mg/dL (>5.65 mmol/L) is often considered to place a person at high risk for development of pancreatitis and is a threshold for initiating primary triglyceride-lowering therapies, most patients with hypertriglyceridemic pancreatitis have triglyceride concentrations greater than 2000 mg/dL (>22.60 mmol/L). It would be reasonable to consider starting fenofibrate (Answer C) or omega-3 fatty acids (Answer E) if triglycerides remain consistently elevated above 500 mg/dL (>5.65 mmol/L) even after adequate lifestyle intervention, as these patients can experience rapid increase in triglycerides due to brief exposure to secondary exacerbating factors (alcohol, high saturated fat intake). However, the initial step should be lifestyle modification to achieve ideal body weight, reduction of refined carbohydrate and saturated fat intake, alcohol abstinence, and regular physical exercise. The lipid panel can be repeated in 4 to 6 weeks after initiation of lifestyle changes to see if serum triglycerides remain higher than 500 mg/dL, which would require initiation of pharmacotherapy.

Patients with moderate hypertriglyceridemia are at increased risk for ASCVD and benefit from statin therapy. When considering this patient's risk for ASCVD, it is important to understand the cause of his dyslipidemia. The 2 common causes of elevated triglyceride levels in multiple family members are familial combined hyperlipidemia and familial hypertriglyceridemia. These are not monogenic disorders, and unfortunately genetic testing would not be helpful in distinguishing between them. Familial combined hyperlipidemia, which is strongly associated with ASCVD, can generally be distinguished from the more benign familial hypertriglyceridemia by elevated apolipoprotein B levels and often a family history of premature coronary artery disease. This patient has a relatively low apolipoprotein B concentration, making familial combined hyperlipidemia an unlikely diagnosis. Therefore, initiating statin monotherapy (Answer A) or a combination of statin and omega-3 fatty acids (Answer B) for primary prevention of ASCVD is not necessary now.

While non–HDL cholesterol can be a simple and satisfactory measure of overall atherogenic lipid content in patients with hypertriglyceridemia, measurement of apolipoprotein B is of greater value in distinguishing between these 2 types of genetic hypertriglyceridemia. Apolipoprotein B measurement has also been recommended by some guidelines to help decide whether to initiate lipid-lowering therapy, as well as whether to intensify lipid-lowering therapy. The American College of Cardiology/American Heart Association recommends statin initiation if the apolipoprotein B value is greater than 130 mg/dL and identifies a concentration less than 90 mg/dL as being desirable. The European Society of Cardiology recommends escalation of lipid-lowering therapy if apolipoprotein B levels are greater than 100 mg/dL in patients at moderate risk, greater than 80 mg/dL in those at high risk, and greater than 65 mg/dL in those at very high risk.

Educational Objective

Explain the importance of measuring apolipoprotein B in patients with familial hypertriglyceridemia.

Reference(s)

Simha V. Management of hypertriglyceridemia. *BMJ.* 2020;371:m3109. PMID: 33046451

Sniderman AD, Thanassoulis G, Glavinovic T, et al. Apolipoprotein B particles and cardiovascular disease: a narrative review. *JAMA Cardiol.* 2019;4(12):1287-1295. PMID: 31642874

Berberich AJ, Hegele RA. A modern approach to dyslipidemia. *Endocr Rev.* 2022;43(4):611-653. PMID: 34676866

Mach F, Baigent C, Catapano AL, et al; ESC Scientific Document Group. 2019 ESC/EAS guidelines for the management of dyslipidaemias: lipid modification to reduce cardiovascular risk. *Eur Heart J.* 2020;41(1):111-188. PMID: 31504418

120 **ANSWER: B) Check complete blood cell count and calculate Fibrosis-4 score**

Patients with type 2 diabetes mellitus have important comorbidities to manage. In this patient, management of cardiovascular risk is important, and it appears that he has been appropriately placed on a moderate-intensity statin as primary prevention. Guidelines suggest that in persons aged 40 to 75 years who are at higher cardiovascular risk, use of a higher-intensity statin is recommended. Therefore, given his hypertension, increasing intensity of statin treatment and targeting an LDL-cholesterol concentration to less than 70 mg/dL (<1.81 mmol/L) would be reasonable. Serum lipoprotein(a) concentrations (Answer D) greater than 30 mg/dL (>1.07 µmol/L) are associated with increased coronary risk in prospective studies, but there are no guidelines regarding which populations should be screened. In persons with diabetes, a coronary calcium score (Answer C) of 0 is associated with a low coronary heart disease event rate over 10 years. As this patient is already taking a statin, these tools to assess coronary heart disease risk would not help make further management decisions.

Another important comorbidity is metabolic dysfunction-associated steatotic liver disease (MASLD) (formerly termed nonalcoholic fatty liver disease [NAFLD]), a term that encompasses metabolic dysfunction-associated steatosis and metabolic dysfunction-associated steatohepatitis (MASH) (formerly termed nonalcoholic steatohepatitis [NASH]). MASH is defined histologically as having 5% or more hepatic steatosis that is associated with inflammation and hepatocyte injury (hepatocyte ballooning), with or without evidence of liver fibrosis. Steatohepatitis is present in 50% of persons with diabetes and is thought to drive the development of fibrosis and is a major risk factor for hepatocellular carcinoma. Despite this association, studies suggest that MASH is underdiagnosed. Recent guidelines endorse the use of the Fibrosis-4 score (Answer B), which estimates the risk for fibrosis based on AST, ALT, and platelet count as the most cost-effective primary screening tool to identify persons at risk for developing fibrosis and cirrhosis. MASH may be present even in those with AST and ALT concentrations less than 40 U/L (<0.67 µkat/L), so it is important to calculate the Fibrosis-4 score. Patients at intermediate or high risk based on the Fibrosis-4 score are advised to undergo further confirmatory testing with liver stiffness measurement using transient elastography or, if this test is not available, with commercial blood fibrosis markers. Other tests such as magnetic resonance elastography or liver biopsy (which is the gold standard) should be ordered or performed by specialists. Abdominal ultrasonography (Answer E) is not considered to be adequately sensitive or specific to screen for MASLD. Older persons with diabetes are at increased risk for cognitive decline and institutionalization. There is increased risk for Alzheimer disease, vascular dementia, and all-cause dementia when compared with persons with normal glucose tolerance. Yet symptoms can be quite subtle, at least initially. Therefore, assessment of cognitive function using a validated tool such as the Montreal Cognitive Assessment (Answer A) is recommended to be done in all persons aged 65 years or older or in whom there is clinical suspicion. Assessment of cognitive function is not indicated for this patient.

If MASLD is identified, patients should be counseled to abstain from alcohol and should receive appropriate vaccinations for hepatitis A and B. Priority should be placed on weight loss, and in those persons with type 2 diabetes, added consideration should be given to medications that have been shown to improve aspects of MASLD. In patients with biopsy-proven MASH, pioglitazone reduces inflammation and fibrosis. The other potentially beneficial class of agents is GLP-1 receptor agonists. Liraglutide has been shown to reduce progression to fibrosis. Compared with placebo, semaglutide has shown higher rates of histologic resolution of MASH but not improvement in liver fibrosis stage.

Educational Objective

Assess for comorbidities in persons with type 2 diabetes mellitus and explain the importance of screening for nonalcoholic steatohepatitis.

Reference(s)

ElSayed NA, Aleppo G, Aroda VR, et al; American Diabetes Association. 4. Comprehensive medical evaluation and assessment of comorbidities: *standards of care in diabetes-2023. Diabetes Care.* 2023;46(Suppl 1):S49-S67. PMID: 36507651

Kanwal F, Shubrook JH, Younossi Z, et al. Preparing for the NASH epidemic: a call to action. *Diabetes Care.* 2021;44(9):2162-2172. PMID: 34312182

Question-Mapping Index

ENDOCRINE SELF-ASSESSMENT PROGRAM 2024

Part III

This question-mapping index groups question topics according to the 8 umbrella sections of ESAP (Adrenal, Bone-Calcium, Diabetes, Lipids-Obesity, Pituitary, Reproduction [Female], Reproduction [Male], and Thyroid). Relevant ***question numbers*** *follow each topic.*

REPRODUCTION, FEMALE

REPRODUCTION, MALE

THYROID

www.ingramcontent.com/pod-product-compliance
Ingram Content Group UK Ltd.
Pitfield, Milton Keynes, MK11 3LW, UK
UKHW051040091026
15624UKWH00011B/615

9 781936 704385